LIFE
IN THE
MIDDLE

LIFE

IN THE

MIDDLE

PSYCHOLOGICAL AND SOCIAL
DEVELOPMENT IN MIDDLE AGE

EDITED BY

SHERRY L. WILLIS

Department of Human Development and Family Studies
College of Health and Human Development
Pennsylvania State University
University Park, Pennsylvania

JAMES D. REID

Department of Psychology
Washington University
St. Louis, Missouri

ACADEMIC PRESS

SAN DIEGO   LONDON   BOSTON   NEW YORK   SYDNEY   TOKYO   TORONTO

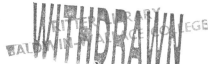

Academic Press
a division of Harcourt Brace & Company
525 B Street, Suite 1900, San Diego, California 92101-4495, USA
http://www.apnet.com

Academic Press
24-28 Oval Road, London NW1 7DX, UK
http://www.hbuk.co.uk/ap/

Library of Congress Catalog Card Number: 98-87563

International Standard Book Number: 0-12-757230-9

PRINTED IN THE UNITED STATES OF AMERICA
98 99 00 01 02 03 BB 9 8 7 6 5 4 3 2 1

Contents

PART I

Theoretical Perspectives on Midlife

1 Midlife Development in a Life Course Context
Phyllis Moen and Elaine Wethington

2   *The Developing Self in Midlife*

Susan Krauss Whitbourne and Loren Angiullo Connolly

3   *The Midlife Crisis Revisited*

Stanley D. Rosenberg, Harriet J. Rosenberg, and Michael P. Farrell

PART II

Biological Functioning and Physical Health at Midlife

6   *Cardiovascular Health: A Challenge for Midlife*
**Ilene C. Siegler, Berton H. Kaplan, Dean D. Von Dras,
and Daniel B. Mark**

PART III

Psychosocial Functioning at Midlife

7   *Psychological Well-Being in Midlife*
Corey Lee M. Keyes and Carol D. Ryff

8   *The Sense of Control in Midlife*
Margaret Clark-Plaskie and Margie E. Lachman

9   *Gender Roles and Gender Identity in Midlife*

Margaret Hellie Huyck

10   *Intellectual Functioning in Midlife*

Sherry L. Willis and K. Warner Schaie

11 *A Life-Span Framework for Assessing the Impact of Work on White-Collar Workers*

Bruce J. Avolio and John J. Sosik

12 *Middle Age: New Thoughts, New Directions*

James D. Reid and Sherry L. Willis

Contributors

Numbers in parentheses indicate the pages on which the authors' contributions begin.

Nancy E. Avis (105)
Institute for Women's Research
New England Research Institutes
Watertown, Massachusetts 02472

Bruce J. Avolio (249)
Center for Leadership Studies and School of
    Management
Binghamton University
Binghamton, New York 13902-6015

Margaret Clark-Plaskie (181)
Empire State College–The State University
    of New York
Corning, New York 14830

Loren Angiullo Connolly (25)
Philadelphia Geriatric Center
Philadelphia, Pennsylvania 19141-2996

Michael P. Farrell (47)
State University of New York
    at Buffalo
Buffalo, New York 14623

Margaret Hellie Huyck (209)
Institute of Psychology
Illinois Institute of Technology
Chicago, Illinois 60616

Berton H. Kaplan (147)
Department of Epidemiology
School of Public Health
University of North Carolina
Durham, North Carolina

Corey Lee M. Keyes (161)
Department of Sociology
Emory University
Atlanta, Georgia 30322; and
Department of Behavioral Sciences and
    Health Education
The Rollins School of Public Health
Atlanta, Georgia

Margie E. Lachman (181)
Department of Psychology
Brandeis University
Waltham, Massachusetts 02254-9110

Daniel B. Mark (147)
Department of Medicine
Duke University Medical Center
Durham, North Carolina 27710

Susan S. Merrill (77)
California Medical Review Incorporated
    (CMRI)
San Francisco, California 94105

Phyllis Moen (3)
Bronfenbrenner Life Course Center
Cornell University
Ithaca, New York 14853-4401

James D. Reid (175)
Department of Psychology
Washington University
St. Louis, Missouri 63103-4899

Harriet J. Rosenberg (47)
Dartmouth Medical School
Lebanon, New Hampshire 03756

Stanley D. Rosenberg (47)
Dartmouth Medical School
Lebanon, New Hampshire 03756

Carol D. Ryff (161)
Department of Psychology
The Institute on Aging and
    Adult Life
University of Wisconsin
Madison, Wisconsin 53706

K. Warner Schaie (233)
The Pennsylvania State University
University Park, Pennsylvania 16802

Ilene C. Siegler (147)
Department of Psychiatry and Behavioral
    Sciences

Duke University Medical Center; and
    School of Public Health,
University of North Carolina
Durham, North Carolina

John J. Sosik (249)
School of Management
Penn State Great Valley

Lois M. Verbrugge (77)
Institute of Gerontology
University of Michigan
Ann Arbor, Michigan 48109-2007

Dean D. Von Dras (147)
Department of Psychology
Washington University
St. Louis, Missouri 63103-4899

Elaine Wethington (3)
Brofenbrenner Life Course Center
Cornell University
Ithaca, New York 14853-4401

Susan Krauss Whitbourne (25)
Department of Psychology
University of Massachusetts at Amherst
Amherst, Massachusetts 01002

Sherry L. Willis (233,275)
The Pennsylvania State University
University Park, Pennsylvania 16802

Preface

Of all the periods in the life-span, middle age has received the least attention in terms of scholarly writing. Midlife has largely been the domain of pop psychology since the late 1960s when the term "midlife crisis" was introduced into the national psyche. Of the sixty or so books published in the past two decades, less than ten represent a scholarly approach to the topic of middle age. By all accounts, Neugarten's 1968 *Middle Age and Aging* (Chicago: University of Chicago Press) remains a classic.

This previously ignored age period will become the focus of increasing scholarly attention in the next two decades, as the largest cohorts in United States history move through the middle years. From 1960 to 1985, those aged 45–64 increased to 45 million, a 24% increase. From 1990 to 2015, middle-agers will increase from 47 to 80 million, a 72% increase. Given the size of these cohorts, the median age of the United States population will increase from 33 years in 1990 to 42 years in 2050, reflecting the movement of the "baby boomers" through middle age. The baby boomers are of interest not only because of their size, but also because they represent the best educated and most affluent cohorts to pass through middle age. Some attention has been given to the societal and health care demands that will arise when these cohorts reach *old age,* but optimal physical and psychological development in late life will depend largely on the experiences of baby boomers during *middle age.*

Given these demographic trends, there is increasing demand for academic texts and courses on this age period. There is a growing body of scientific knowledge regarding development during the middle years and the societal and historical context in which development occurs. However, the information is not readily accessible to the reader who searches under terms such as midlife or middle age. Often such information is part of larger longitudinal data sets, which do not specifically mention midlife in the title. Similarly, research that focuses on major concerns of midlife is often published in journals and texts that are discipline specific.

This textbook represents an attempt to bring together in one volume scholarly writings that focus on individual growth and development during midlife. We begin with the assumption that adult development is characterized by increasing inter-individual variability. We reject the old-fashioned notion of middle age as a period of relative stability followed by inevitable decrement and decline of old age. There is no one developmental course or trajectory that can succinctly describe and explain the midlife years for each individual. Rather, individual development encompasses the dynamic interaction of biological, psychological, and social (including cultural and historical) forces.

Influenced by the significant and pioneering theoretical postulates of Daniel Levinson in 1986 (A concept of adult development, *American Psychologist, 41,* 3–13), we believe that psychological development in middle age is a process of alternating periods of stability followed by periods of change. These alternating patterns can be observed in biological, psychological, and social functioning. Individual differences in middle age may be conceptualized within a framework of variability in patterns of biopsychosocial functioning. Indeed, it is the dynamic interaction among these major aspects of functioning that makes midlife such a unique and challenging area of theory, research, and clinical applications.

Our goal for this book is to stimulate further interest in adult development. Indeed, the knowledge base is small. We are, however, encouraged by the growing body of research in this area. Both basic and applied research are needed in all areas of biopsychosocial functioning during midlife. Particularly in the area of physical health and psychological well-being, research is needed to identify lifestyle factors, personality styles, and cognitive perspectives that lead to optimal functioning in midlife. The research agenda for the future might benefit by shifting the focus in the literature away from normal or usual functioning. Rather, our goal should be to focus on pathways to optimal biopsychosocial functioning during midlife.

As indicated by the title, *Life in the Middle,* a life cycle perspective is incorporated. Focusing on middle age draws the reader's attention to the broad process of development from birth to death. Hence, this volume attempts to place midlife development within the context of an entire life cycle.

We were fortunate to have assembled a remarkable group of contributors to this volume. The chapters are organized into three major parts. The first part of the book focuses on important theoretical perspectives and issues that relate to the psychology of midlife. Within this part, the context of development is explored from the perspective of a historical/cultural period and within the context of dynamic social change. In addition, this part of the book takes a fresh look at theories of identity and personality functioning in middle age. The second part of the book investigates more closely specific issues that relate to biological functioning and physical health during midlife. These chapters include important issues of physical health and disease, including cardiovascular and women's health. Psychosocial issues during middle age are reviewed in the third part of the text. Chapters are presented that focus on psychological and social functioning including subjective well-being, issues of autonomy and control, gender, cognitive development, and occupational functioning. The overall goal of the volume is to present our readers with a holistic and integrative approach to life in the middle.

We are greatly appreciative of the stellar group of authors who worked with us so patiently on this project. As the field of adult development continues its own development, we are pleased to be both observers and contributors to the process of human growth and development during middle age.

Sherry L. Willis and James D. Reid

Theoretical Perspectives on Midlife

We begin this volume with a fresh look at important conceptual and theoretical issues that relate to midlife development. In their chapter, "Midlife Development in a Life Course Context," Phyllis Moen and Elaine Wethington articulate a sociological perspective that provides a larger picture of midlife development. From this starting point, Susan Krauss Whitbourne and Loren Angiullo Connolly go on to provide a unique review and important extension of the theoretical works of Erikson and Piaget as they relate to identity development in their chapter, "The Developing Self in Midlife." Finally, Stanley D. Rosenberg, Harriet J. Rosenberg, and Michael P. Farrell provide the reader with an important opportunity to look at the literature on midlife crisis in their chapter, "The Midlife Crisis Revisited."

CHAPTER 1

Midlife Development in a Life Course Context

Phyllis Moen and Elaine Wethington

Bronfenbrenner Life Course Center, Cornell University, Ithaca, New York

INTRODUCTION

Midlife as a Life Stage

The belief that "midlife" comprises a separate and distinct stage of life is a recent cultural construction, originating only in the twentieth century (Skolnick, 1991). The emergence of midlife as a life stage is linked to two related demographic trends: the increase in human longevity and the decline in fertility. As the average length of life has increased and the time spent rearing children has decreased, people have come to perceive the life course as divided into more distinct stages of youth, early adulthood, midlife, and old age. These two demographic changes are particularly relevant in defining midlife for women, given the gender gap in longevity and the greater salience of family roles for women. But these demographic trends have also worked in tandem with the transformations in the economy and in career paths to produce the constellation of social roles that characterize an adult life course in transition. While distinct stages of parenthood, marriage, and career have previously defined midlife as a separate period in the life course, over the latter half of the twentieth century, we are now witnessing a reconfiguring of the middle years of adulthood.

Given individual, gender, and social class variations in the type and timing of role transitions, it is difficult to set precise ages when midlife begins or ends (Farrell & Rosenberg, 1981); the boundaries of midlife are "fluid." However, it is popularly thought to begin at age 35, and to encompass the middle stages of parenting, the period during which children move into school age, adolescence, and early adulthood (Brooks-Gunn & Kirsh, 1984). Still other markers of midlife boundaries are career "peaking" (Brim, 1992), transitions in employment as mothers return to the labor force or shift to full-time work schedules in tandem with declining parental obligations (Long & Porter, 1984; Moen, Downey, & Bolger 1990; Smith & Moen, 1988), and, for some, early retirement (Moen, 1994). Consistent with a social role and life course perspective on midlife, one could also view midlife as the time when people are enacting a full set of social and personal responsibilities, with the later stages of midlife being a time of relinquishing, or contemplating relinquishing, their employment role and the parenting of (preadult) children.

The middle years, moreover, have been until recently a phase of adulthood neglected by research, often depicted as little more than a "staging area on the way to old age" (Baruch & Brooks-Gunn, 1984, p. 1). The entrance of the large "Baby Boom" generation into midlife, however, has created a demand for information about midlife as a social and developmental stage (Wethington, Cooper, & Holmes, 1997). It is perhaps ironic that new interest in examining what is distinctive about midlife as a stage of life has arisen in a period when both the social consensus and psychological expectations about social roles and age-appropriate behavior have fragmented, led by the baby boom generation itself (Jones, 1980; Moen, 1998).

A Life Course Perspective

In the light of emerging shifts in the nature and perceptions of midlife, we believe a *life course* approach, with a focus on both objective and subjective aspects of role pathways, offers the freshest and most flexible means of viewing the middle years of adulthood. From this theoretical approach, transitions in the middle years of adulthood cannot be specified without some reference to the multiple meanings of age: as a biological aging process, a social life stage, and a historical and generational context (Elder, 1975, 1985; Hagestad & Neugarten, 1984; Riley, 1982, 1987; Settersten & Mayer, 1997). Midlife represents physical changes, exemplified, for women, in the menopause transition. But it also incorporates social norms and expectations about appropriate roles and behavior for those in their middle years. And it locates individuals historically; individuals entering midlife at the beginning of the twenty-first century are vastly different in their resources, expectations, and experiences from those entering midlife in the 1950s or at the beginning of the twentieth century.

Studies of the life course have recently become prominent as social researchers focus on process and change in life experience and life chances, consider the links between individual lives and broad social changes, and draw on panel data and innovative methodological techniques to study transitions and trajectories, rather than cross-sectional links at any one point in time (Elder, 1994, 1998; Riley, Foner, & Waring, 1988). An enduring theme of life course analysis is one of *social change,* that is, recognition of the interplay between macro-level social change and individual life chances and experiences at the micro-level. Thus, the middle years of adulthood for the baby boom cohort are vastly different than this same period for those born in the Great Depression. A second theme is a focus on *life pathways,* emphasizing continuities and discontinuities in roles and relationships over time. The life course depicts the interweave of age-graded trajectories, such as work and family careers, that change in conjunction with age as well as with changing circumstances and options that each generation encounters (Elder, 1998). A third distinctive theme in the life course approach is its *subjective* side, the way individuals define themselves and their lives, and the active role they take in designing and redesigning their life biographies. A final life course theme is the importance of *context;* individuals located in different social ecologies experience their middle years in vastly disparate ways.

A life course perspective challenges traditional ways of investigating midlife. Instead of considering snapshots of individual lives at one point in time, a life course approach focuses on life *pathways,* considering role and developmental transitions, trajectories, and turning points in lives over time. In fact, one useful way of depicting the life course is as a series of movements in and out of various roles and relationships. As individuals move through their life course they also take on or relinquish various components of their *identity,* defining and redefining themselves as husbands, wives, divorcées, widows, grandparents, caregivers, workers, volunteers, retirees. The life course approach attends to the social and psychological connections between transitions and trajectories in various roles, relationships, and identities across time, the dynamics of multiple, interlocking pathways. For example, becoming divorced or widowed in midlife can affect the duration of time women continue to work, while taking on the caregiving role does not appear to facilitate leaving one's job (Moen, Robison, & Fields, 1994). And women who (re)enter the workforce in midlife on a permanent basis are apt to retire from their career jobs earlier than those who have a history of intermittent participation (Han & Moen, 1998). Individual lives can thus be characterized as a series of interrelated trajectories through schooling, occupation, marriage, parenthood, and caregiving, as well as volunteer and community participation. An important theoretical and practical implication of this approach is that occupying particular roles at any one point in time may matter less in terms of psychological adjustment than the duration of role occupation, the number and predictability of role entries and exits over the middle years, and their timing in relation to age as well as other roles occupied. Role continuities and changes, in turn, are tied to developmental trajectories: shifts in physical health, emotional well-being, and subjective orientations throughout midlife.

An understanding of how past experiences affect midlife, as well as how experiences in midlife shape subsequent aging, is critical to a life course approach to individual lives. Numerous studies of people in midlife focus exclusively on their middle years, without considering how their life history of role involvements and relationships throughout adulthood might shape the quality of their present lives. The tacit assumption of the typical approach is that past experiences matter little. But recent theoretical advances view the developmental course of adulthood within a life course and continuity theoretical framework, recognizing that individuals are products of a life history of events, relationships, and behavior (e.g., Atchley, 1989; Donahue, Robins, Roberts, & John, 1993; Elder, 1998; Morgan, 1986; O'Rand, Henretta, & Krecker, 1992; Rosow, 1985; Sorensen, Weinert, & Sherrod, 1986). Increasingly, empirical studies of adjustment at midlife consider past experiences in terms of the pattern and type of roles and role transitions throughout adulthood (e.g., Donahue et al., 1993; Moen & Fields, 1998). Situational demands, opportunities, and barriers, including current and anticipated health problems, may also shape the course of midlife (Whitbourne, 1986). As these studies show, the life course story is frequently one of the cumulation of advantage or disadvantage, with educated, healthy, active individuals who are socially integrated through marriage and/or challenging jobs or volunteer work being the best able to cope with the biological, social, and psychological changes associated with the middle years. But there are other stories as well, involving important turning points in midlife—such as divorce, remarriage, returning to school, a career change—that can shape the direction of middle and late adulthood.

This chapter is organized around the four themes that characterize a life course approach to the middle years: locating lives in structural *context,* an emphasis on interlocking *transitions and trajectories,* attention to *subjective definitions,* and acknowledgment of the interplay between *social change and individual lives.*

LIVES IN CONTEXT

The role choices and life paths of those in midlife are embedded in existing social structures and situational imperatives that delimit both opportunities and constraints (Bronfenbrenner, 1979; Elder, 1998; Riley, Kahn, & Foner, 1994). We consider five contextual factors that figure prominently in shaping the middle life course: social class, education, gender, race, and health. These attributes affect midlife opportunities and expectations, as well as individual motivations, generally, to seek out new roles or to remain in existing ones (Brim, 1992).

Social Class and Education

In order to understand alternative life course pathways it is important to locate individuals in the broader social structure. Individuals in midlife with the prestige, security, and challenges associated with high socioeconomic status clearly benefit from these resources financially, psychologically, and cognitively (Kohn & Schooler, 1985), both contemporaneously as well as long-term. Early educational attainment and occupational success have a profound effect on men's role acquisitions, such as marriage and parenthood (see Wilson, 1987) and their psychological identity (Weiss, 1990). As Brim (1992) has noted, moreover, successful management of a number of major life roles such as marriage, occupation, and parenthood is associated with more successful psychological adjustment in midlife.

A life course paradigm as well suggests that the effects of socioeconomic resources on role choices may well change over the individual life course. For example, Clausen and Gilens (1990), using follow-up data from the Berkeley Guidance and Oakland Growth Studies, found that the husband's occupational status becomes less important than the woman's own educational attainment in estimating the labor force involvement of women in their late 40s and 50s. And Esterberg, Moen, and Dempster-McClain (1994) have found that women's returning to school in midlife increases their likelihood of subsequent divorce. The fact that divorce also promotes returning to school (Bradburn, Moen, & Dempster-McClain, 1995) points to the complexity of and interdependence of life course choices and transitions. Socioeconomic status in midlife may well change with divorce or remarriage, with unemployment, downsizing, or promotion, or with a return to school or to the work force.

Gender

Historically, gender relations have had a profound influence on the role options of men and women (Fennell & Walker, 1986). The fact that women have been allocated the major responsibility for child care, homemaking, and kin relations has traditionally restricted their participation in nonfamilial activities (Gove & Tudor, 1973), and increased the likelihood of their becoming caregivers of impaired relatives in midlife (Moen et al., 1994). Men have traditionally benefited psychologically from their closer and more continuous attachment to the labor force (Moen & Fields, 1998; Thoits, 1986), and some research has demonstrated the positive impact of more continuous labor force attachment for women (Wethington & Kessler, 1989). But the fact that women typically focus on family roles in earlier adulthood has broad implications for their employment and financial well-being in midlife and beyond (e.g., O'Rand & Landerman, 1984). Both men and women typically experience a decline in family and nonfamily roles in the later years of midlife, as their children leave home, their marriages frequently dissolve, and they move out of the labor force (Moen, Dempster-McClain, & Williams, 1992; Smith & Moen, 1986).

Fundamental changes in social attitudes and dispositions regarding fertility, labor force participation, families, and gender roles have effectively begun to broaden the opportunities available to women, in midlife as well as at other life stages (Moen,

1994; 1995a). Although the significance of these changes is enormous for society at large, their effects have been the most far-reaching for the baby boom cohort now entering midlife. Most tellingly, the employment patterns across the life course of women now in their middle years is coming to more closely resemble those of men now in midlife (Contemporary Research Press, 1993).

Race

The experience of members of racial and ethnic minorities at midlife is almost completely unexplored (Ramseur, 1989). The life course perspective, however, would suggest that racial group differences in role acquisitions and experiences across the life course, particularly those involving occupation, marriage, parenting, and community involvement, would profoundly affect experiences at midlife. Cross-sectional research also demonstrates that role involvement is associated with well-being (Gove & Tudor, 1973) and perception of the self (Thoits, 1983), regardless of race.

Racial and ethnic differences in role acquisitions are very closely related to differences in economic opportunity. Garfinkel and McLanahan's (1986) study of the impact of single motherhood on subsequent role acquisition demonstrates that early life deprivation and lack of occupational opportunity can restrict alternatives and opportunities in midlife. Wilson's (1987) research on the lack of occupational opportunities for African-American males in inner cities shows clearly the interdependency of role acquisition and midlife "success," including the addition of marriage and involved parenthood to role repertoires. Some suggest that the discontinuous work history of black males makes the retirement transition a different experience for black as opposed to white men (Fillenbaum, George, & Palmore, 1985; Gibson, 1991).

It is essential, however, to avoid the inference that midlife is a less satisfactory experience for members of minority groups, even for those most afflicted by racial discrimination and lack of economic opportunity. Racial groups may be more similar than different, challenging the notion of the inevitability of a cumulation of disadvantage accompanying discrimination. For example, Danigelis and McIntosh (1993), comparing involvement in productive activities among those aged 60 and older, found differences in productive activity between men and women but not between whites and blacks. Similarly, psychological research on adults who are members of minority groups (e.g., Ramseur, 1989) refutes the view that more negative views of the self and psychopathology are the norm.

Health

An individual's history of physical and mental health has an important impact on role transitions and trajectories in midlife. Physical illness and disability, as well as chronic mental health problems, have been shown to impede role acquisition or prevent the management of multiple simultaneous roles (Moen et al., 1992; Verbrugge, 1989). In addition, a particularly demanding role at midlife (e.g., being a single mother of several children) might not only prevent a woman from acquiring more roles outside the household, but also lead to more emotional and physical distress (Angel & Angel, 1993). Moreover, health (and attendant behavioral) problems in childhood and youth are known to have an impact on the acquisition of the occupational role in early adulthood (e.g., Kandel, Davies, & Raveis, 1985). Unfortunately, study of the interplay of role trajectories and health in midlife is still relatively uncommon, although cross-sectional studies of role incumbency and health are numerous (e.g., Verbrugge, 1983). As Verbrugge points out, the issue is one of social causation versus social selection. Social *causation* assumes that social integration (occupying multiple roles) influences health. By contrast, social *selection* assumes that healthy people are the ones most likely to take on and maintain multiple social roles. But the social causation versus social selection argument is less crucial than an understanding of the pathways to health and social integration in middle and later adulthood. What is required is a dynamic approach to health and social integration, examining the extent to which experiences throughout the life course shape physical abilities and involvement in multiple roles in midlife and beyond (e.g., Moen et al., 1992; Moen & Fields, 1998).

ALTERNATIVE PATHWAYS: TRANSITIONS AND TRAJECTORIES

We submit that the pattern and types of roles throughout adulthood are critical to an understanding of the lives and choices of those in their middle years. However, situational demands, opportunities, and barriers, including current and anticipated health problems and the life experiences of significant others, also shape midlife choices and trajectories. Given the age stratification system, social positions are allocated on the basis of age, producing widespread social conceptions about appropriate and expected roles at various life stages (Riley, 1987; Riley et al., 1994). The two most central roles in contemporary adulthood relate to paid work and family; however, other roles such as volunteering are also salient for significant numbers of individuals. We consider continuities and changes in three interlocking pathways: family, employment, and volunteering.

Family Roles and Relationships

A life course formulation points to the *interdependency of lives,* with continuities and changes in family roles shaping midlife relationships and resources. Women's midlife experiences, compared to men's, are more closely linked to the choices and contingencies of other family members (Moen, 1992). Women's responsibilities and options shift as children leave (or return) home; husbands change jobs, become down-sized, retire, become impaired, leave, or die; parents become frail or die. Men's midlife experiences are typically more linked to their working conditions and their roles as family providers (e.g., Farrell & Rosenberg, 1981; Weiss, 1990).

In addition to a focus on the impact of role changes and transitions, the *timing* of family role transitions may be important in understanding midlife development. Timing has to do with when a role transition occurs in an individual's life course. For example, becoming widowed or divorced in one's 40s or 50s may be a vastly different experience than losing a spouse in one's 70s, because individuals in early midlife are likely to have other role identities and sources of support beyond mar-riage, including an attachment to job or career. On the other hand, older individuals may be better prepared psychologically for marital dissolution, especially widow-hood, which is normatively "on time" for the aged, but not for those in midlife (Wortman & Silver, 1990). Similarly, becoming a grandparent in one's 30s may be less welcome than in one's 50s.

Also critical to an understanding of the middle years is the *degree of predictability* of transitions, that is, whether or not a transition is expected. For example, having the last child leave home can be long anticipated and planned for, whereas divorce or the death of one's spouse more typically is not (Wheaton, 1990; White & Ed-wards, 1990). Grandparenthood is frequently an expected, and welcome, role ac-quisition in the middle life course (Cherlin & Furstenberg, 1987),

Providing care for family members and other relatives (ailing husbands, frail parents, or developmentally disabled children), on the other hand, is often an un-anticipated obligation confronted in the middle years of adulthood. Caregiving for ailing or infirm family members is an increasingly likely role for midlife women (Moen et al., 1994; Robison, Moen, & Dempster-McClain, 1995). Being a care-giver appears to have a negative effect on well-being, because the role obligations may well outweigh any integrative effects (Brody, 1985; Cantor, 1983; George & Gwyther, 1986). From a larger perspective on gender roles, Gove and Hughes (1979) and Veroff, Douvan, and Kulka (1981) suggest that women's responsibility for the welfare of children, husbands, and ailing relatives may have deleterious consequences for their own well-being (see also Kessler & McLeod, 1984). Despite these potential deleterious effects, women living alone are likely to be more vulnerable than are those who share life with a child or a spouse (e.g., Pearlin & Johnson, 1977).

Employment

For many adults, paid work is a major, if not the principal, source of purposive activity, social relations, independence, identity, and self-respect (Jahoda, 1982). It is the way that we become integrated and acknowledged as members of the larger community. An increasingly significant late midlife transition is retirement from employment, as growing numbers of workers move into early retirement in their fifties, both by choice and as a consequence of corporate restructuring (Han & Moen, 1998). Social researchers are coming to regard retirement not as an "either–or" proposition but as a process, possibly extending over several years, involving a number of transitions between paid and unpaid work (Lowenthal & Robinson, 1976; Moen, 1998; Reimers & Honig, 1989). In describing the phases of retirement, Atchley (1993) suggests that many experience a postretirement period of low activity of several years, followed by a resumption of active engagement. This underscores the importance of conducting longitudinal studies of the retirement transition, focusing on retirement expectations and planning of workers in midlife as well as trajectories and transitions during the postretirement period.

Current trends in retirement reflect decisions made by men and women about their career jobs in light of social security rules, employer pension plans, and corporate restructuring. Although they have documented trends in early exits, social scientists have not sufficiently modeled the process by which these timing decisions are made, as well as decisions regarding subsequent productive activity in paid and volunteer work (but see Han & Moen, 1998; Moen & Fields, 1998). Given the centrality of paid employment in American society, what can be said about the social value, as well as the lives, lifestyles, and prospects, of individuals in midlife who, whether by choice or circumstance, retire early from their full-time career jobs?

One possible option is to embark on a second or third career—whether an entirely different type of job or a continuance of one's previous work but at a reduced level. A second possibility is unpaid work—as a volunteer or as an active participant in a voluntary association. The first, post-retirement employment, is an extension of the productive activity typically representative of adulthood in our society. The second, volunteer participation, may be either a continuation of activities begun in earlier and middle adulthood or a qualitative shift in relative emphasis from paid work to unpaid volunteer labor. Both options afford opportunities for productive activity, social interaction, and identity-defining status within society. But neither has been institutionalized as a means of drawing on the talents of and integrating those who find themselves retired in later midlife into the larger society in a meaningful way. Although an expanded definition of "productive activity" can incorporate housework, child care, and help to family and friends as well as community participation (Fischer, Mueller, & Cooper, 1991; Herzog, Kahn, Morgan, Jackson, & Antonucci, 1989; Moen, 1998), paid work remains the principal mechanism for activities promoting sustained social integration in our society.

The evidence has shown that significant numbers of retirees undergo "partial" retirement, moving to part-time employment by either reducing working hours on their career jobs or taking on new (and frequently lower paying) jobs (Honig & Hanoch, 1985; Han & Moen, 1998; Reimers & Honig, 1989). Self-employed men are especially apt to continue paid employment, either on the same job or on a new job, and nearly a third of the men who take on a part-time job do not do so until 2 years after their retirement (Burkhauser & Quinn, 1989).

Volunteer Work

Volunteering can be defined as unpaid work, as "the giving freely of an individual's time, talents, and energy" (Anderson, 1991, p. 74). Volunteer activity represents a pervasive but typically overlooked and underrated experience in women's and men's lives. It is estimated that 89 million Americans were engaged in volunteer activities in 1985 (Anderson, 1991). Yet, despite its prevalence, we have little reliable knowledge about the enduring influence of volunteering on lives or about the pathways leading men and women into and out of unpaid work in their middle years. Neither do we understand the processes by which volunteering or participation in voluntary associations may serve to promote health and well-being.

Participation in voluntary associations is an important form of social integration, especially as those in late midlife leave their paid jobs (Moen, 1997; Moen & Fields, 1998). Postretirement community involvement may well be a function of lifelong patterns of participation (Wilensky, 1961). Herzog and colleagues (1989) point out that volunteer work in community organizations is similar to paid employment, with volunteers engaging in work with "clear market value" (p. S134). Previous volunteering in earlier adulthood should also be related to volunteering in midlife (Chambré, 1987; Cohen-Mansfield, 1989; Moen, 1997; Moen, Dempster-McClain, & Williams, 1992).

A key consideration in the productive activity (whether paid or unpaid) of those in midlife is health and illness. For example, Reimers and Honig (1989) show that men aged 58–70 are more likely to move into full retirement (no wage earnings) if they experience a health limitation. Poor health promotes the transition of those in midlife to retirement (Parnes & Nestel, 1974), and may be an important consideration, but less of an impediment, to volunteer work (Chambré, 1987; Moen & Fields, 1998).

It is not clear whether voluntary participation in the middle years is responsive to the same motivators and constraints as paid labor force participation. The fact that volunteer work apparently does not become a substitute for paid work following retirement suggests the possible lack of opportunities or perceived opportunities (Chambré, 1987; Herzog et al., 1989; Moen & Fields, 1998). What is required are longitudinal studies that capture the community activity patterns and choices of those in the middle life course.

Interlocking Roles

We have discussed family, work, and volunteer roles separately, for ease of presentation, but clearly these are interlocking, interdependent trajectories. Individual choices in one domain are always contingent on other responsibilities and relationships. Such a focus on the interplay across life domains is especially important when looking at women's lives in their middle years, since women's social integration into the larger society has been circumscribed by the primacy of their family obliga-tions. Women are also more likely than men to spend their middle adulthood alone, without the presence (and support) of a spouse. Women in late midlife are particularly susceptible to social isolation as they leave or lose employment and other roles as well as, frequently, the wife role, through divorce or widowhood (Smith & Moen, 1988).

SUBJECTIVE DEFINITIONS

Thus far we have focused on external events and objective role trajectories and transitions in describing a life course approach to the middle years. But the life course perspective also recognizes the importance of subjective and psychological changes, particularly as shaped by objective experiences (MacDermid, Franz, & De Reus, 1998; Markus & Wurf, 1987; Stryker & Statham, 1985). For example, individuals' identities and self-evaluations are to some degree molded by their ob-jective experiences (Clausen, 1990; Donahue et al., 1993). In establishing a personal identity, most adults in midlife primarily define themselves by their jobs (Jahoda, 1982), and this is increasingly true of women as well as men (Moen, 1992; Stewart, 1989; Weiss, 1990). Other role involvements, such as marriage and parenthood, are also critical to individuals' self-concepts (e.g., Antonucci & Mikus, 1988; Ryff, Schmutte, & Less, 1996; Umberson, 1987, 1992).

A number of sociological and psychological theorists (e.g., Brandstaedter & Baltes-Goetz, 1990; Labouvie-Vief, 1982; Perun & Bielby, 1980; Riegel, 1975) have adopted a dynamic (or "dialectical") view of the relationship between role transitions, life events, and psychological development in the middle years. For example, the accumulation and loss of social roles/identities have been linked to corresponding changes in psychological distress over time (Moen, 1997; Thoits, 1986); changes and acquisitions of identities linked to typical midlife roles have been associated with the development of mature coping styles and defense processes (Labouvie-Vief, Hakim-Larson, & Hobart, 1987); and lack of identity "integra-tion" at midlife has been found to be associated with a history of frequent role change over the life course to that point (Donahue et al., 1993).

Midlife is typically viewed as the stage at which adults attain "full maturity," as their responsibilities become more complex. The psychosocial view of midlife im-plies that it is a period of life characterized by personal growth (Clausen, 1986; Labouvie-Vief, 1982; Riegel, 1975; Vaillant, 1977). An idea shared by many perspectives on psychological processes in midlife (Levinson, Darrow, Klein, Levin-son, & McKee, 1977; McCrae & Costa, 1990) is that changes in identity, ways of thinking and reasoning, and self-concept may be brought on by normative life transitions and unexpected life events. The literature on the psychological impact of life transitions and events is vast (e.g., Dohrenwend & Dohrenwend, 1981); unfortunately, most of it lacks a focus on personality growth or changes in identity.

The concept of life "turning point" is one way to connect objective role transitions to changes in identity and subjective definitions in midlife (Clausen, 1990, 1993; Wethington et al., 1997). *Transitions* refer to objective changes in roles and relationships; *turning points* are salient transitions that individuals define as changing the direction of their lives.

Turning Points

Following Clausen (1990), we define a psychological turning point in midlife as a new insight into one's self, a significant other, or important life situation; this insight becomes a motive that leads to redirecting, changing, or improving one's life. The experiences of a "psychological turning point" are thus a marker of when important shifts in thinking and insights into self and other occur during the course of life. Psychosocial transitions typical of midlife—entry and exit from marriage, parenthood, employment, and shifts in commitment within these roles—may be important precursors of undergoing a psychological turning point (Clausen, 1995; Perun & Bielby, 1980; Wethington et al., 1997).

According to Clausen (1990), a psychological turning point occurs after an experience or a realization that causes someone to reinterpret past experiences in a way that changes long-held, fundamental assumptions. A turning point is a profound reinterpretation or reorientation (attitudinal or behavioral) directed at the self, a relationship with a significant other, or activities in a major life role. Clausen's empirical work (using the Berkeley Growth studies) uncovered four types of turning points: a change or reformulation of commitment to a major life role, activities in a major life role, or relationship with a close, significant other; a major change regarding perspective on life; a change in important life goals; and a major change in views regarding the self. Not all changes of these sorts qualify as turning points. To qualify, the experiences must also involve *new insights* or evidence that redirection followed (or was attempted) because of this insight.

Wethington, Kessler, and Holmes (1992) operationalized these four definitions of turning points in two qualitative studies of adults aged 25 through 70 (study 1, N = 70; study 2, N = 125). Turning points were found to fall into two general categories: self-insights regarding new understanding or awareness of one's motives, personal limitations, and talents; and insights into situational factors, such as the character of significant others and limits to control over specific situations. Participants frequently described how turning points involved a need to control their emotional reactions, expressed either through psychological endurance and compensation or behavioral change such as conscious diversion into other activities (Wethington et al., 1997).

The two qualitative studies used convenient, nonrepresentative samples. The turning point questions were then further refined by the investigators, and used in two nationally representative studies. (The first was a small telephone pilot study,

N = 132; the second was a self-administered version of the questions administered to 3032 participants in a nationally representative study of midlife adults, conducted by the John D. and Catherine T. MacArthur Foundation Research Network on Successful Midlife Development.) The two nationally representative studies made it possible to estimate the prevalence and distribution of turning points.

Overall, women were more likely than men to report psychological turning points (Wethington et al., 1997), and these reports were least frequent among those over age 55 (Wethington et al., 1997; Wethington & Pixley, 1998). The report of a psychological turning point was most frequently associated with the recent occurrence of a negative life event or life transition of a severely threatening nature (Wethington, Brown, & Kessler, 1995); psychological growth was most likely to be reported in regard to severe events which were successfully resolved (Wethington & Pixley, 1998). (See also Thoits, 1994.)

Identity

The experience of a turning point may involve a change in identity; however, the notion of identity also implies stability, as well as change, over time. Identity can be described as the self-perceptions and self-evaluations that matter to the individual (George, 1980, p. 14). Self and identity are intimately tied to one's social roles. As Turner (1978, p. 2) points out, "In the broadest sense the person consists of all the roles in an individual's repertoire." Role identities are ways individuals describe and think about themselves in terms of their statuses within society and their relationships with those around them. As Rosow (1974) suggests, self-image and identification correspond to actual group membership.

Continuity and Accentuation

A life course approach posits a process of accentuation, with past dispositions and attributes (including one's identity) both shaping and persisting in new situations (Elder, 1998). This suggests a certain cumulative process: patterns of actual role occupancy throughout the life course should figure into one's sense of self in midlife (Stryker, 1980). For example, Bielby and Bielby (1989) suggest that the greater the time invested in a role, the greater the subjective identification with it.

A life course approach, in combination with role theory, also posits that some roles may be more salient than others, having lasting impact on one's self-identification in midlife, even beyond the years of actual role occupancy (Merton, 1957; Stryker & Serpe, 1982; Turner, 1978).

Transitions and Expectations

Midlife can represent shifts in identity as much as shifts in roles. Although *role loss* appears in fact to be concomitant with aging (e.g., Moen, 1997; Moen et al., 1992), we know little about how individuals perceive themselves in terms of their salient *role identities* as they move through midlife, or what they *anticipate* to be salient role-identities in old age. How are *currently* salient role identities in midlife related to *previous* role identities, earlier in adulthood, or role identities *anticipated* to be salient in old age? How is identity in midlife affected by actual role occupancy, now and throughout adulthood? Only a few researchers (e.g. Donahue et al., 1993) have attempted to address these questions.

Expected role identities are important in that they serve to structure one's anticipations and plans for the future (Brim & Ryff, 1980). As Neugarten (1977) points out, we rehearse transitions that we anticipate to be "on time" in terms of some age-graded, and normative, calendar. These self-views may, in turn, become important frames of reference, playing a causal role in the acquisition, or letting go, of activities and roles concomitant with aging in midlife and beyond (Filipp & Klauer, 1986; Neugarten, 1977, Stryker, 1980). It has been found that the externally driven loss of social roles and, consequently, one's social identity concomitant with aging, has tremendous negative, and for the most part private, repercussions for the lives of the old (Rosow, 1974). However, self-directed role loss or change can have positive consequences if it resolves long-term difficulties (Thoits, 1994; Wheaton, 1990).

Because identity is a product of life experiences, one could assume that changes in roles, relationships, and responsibilities would produce similar changes in personal identity. But the process by which self-perceptions are modified by role changes, or themselves serve to shape role trajectories and transitions, is far from clear. Some roles and some identities are obviously more salient than others; whether this salience shifts in the middle years, and whether normative transitions trigger this shift, is a topic for future research. Current research (e.g. Donahue et al., 1993; Helson & Roberts, 1992; Wethington et al., 1997) has used samples from special groups or volunteers rather than representative samples. Wethington and Pixley (1998) are the first to report using a nationally representative sample.

SOCIAL CHANGE AND INDIVIDUAL LIVES

We have seen that a life course perspective characterizes midlife as the dynamic interplay between a biological age period, a social clustering of roles, resources, and relationships, and a subjective perception of one's self and one's possibilities. But viewing the developmental course of middle adulthood within a life course framework also recognizes that individuals are embedded in a changing social, cultural, and economic environment. As Riley (1987, p. 9) points out, "More salient for many people undergoing a transition may be the changes that occur, not *in* their personal lives, but around them in the environing social structures." This means that different cohorts of individuals, born at different historical times, have unique experiences, including the experience of midlife (Stewart, 1989; see also Helson & Wink, 1992, and, popularly, Samuelson, 1996). In these times of rapid social change in gender and other roles, individuals in different age-cohorts come to their middle years with different motivations, impediments, and opportunities. This is important because age differences may reflect cohort differences regarding normative expectations. For example, the women's movement has transformed the employment and educational possibilities of midlife women (Bradburn et al., 1994; Moen, 1995b). Thus, what it means to be in one's middle years is vastly different for the baby boomers, as opposed to those born at the turn of the twentieth century who faced midlife during the Great Depression years (Forest, Moen, & Dempster-McClain, 1995). As we enter a new millennium, growing numbers of women see their middle years as a time of opportunity; their grandmothers may have viewed them as the absence of opportunity, or even as the beginning of old age. At the same time, men in midlife may be facing uncertainties and job insecurities that their fathers did not experience at a similar age (Glassner, 1994) as corporations restructure and the lifetime career contract is being recast (Moen, 1998). Corporate downsizing and mergers are causing the early retirement and displacement of thousands of middle-aged men and women who expected to be employed at increasing rates of pay until age 65 (Newman, 1993). Their re-employment may be hampered by employers' preferences to hire younger, less expensive workers.

What characterizes contemporary midlife is a growing diversity in roles, resources, and relationships, as people who are the same age are at vastly different family or career stages. Old norms and cultural expectations are out of date, with no emerging consensus as to timetables regarding career, family, or community pathways (Gotlib & Wheaton, 1997; Settersten & Mayer, 1997). For example, a trend toward stronger work commitments even while rearing children (Moen, 1992; Waite, Haggstrom, & Kanouse, 1985) has reorganized the childrearing phase of midlife for a number of women (see also Contemporary Research Press, 1993). Similarly, the overall decline (with some recent leveling) in the average female fertility rate has produced a very large number of women and men who will remain childless (Norton & Moorman, 1987), while other men and women spend their middle years as parents of young children. The large number of women who bear children while young and unmarried may be entering the "elder" role of grandparent in their 40s, a decade long characterized as comprising the peak of midlife. The high divorce rate has produced a number of people who are unpartnered during a significant portion of midlife, as well as a large number of people who have multiple marriages or sexual relationships of relatively short duration through this period (Glick, 1990). And two trends, the increase in longevity and progressively earlier retirement, mean that retirement may no longer be defined as the upper boundary of midlife, as men and women in their 50s and 60s face an extended post-retirement phase of activity and vitality (Han & Moen, 1998; Moen, 1994).

Midlife in the early twenty-first century is in a state of flux, with economic, demographic, technological, social, and cultural changes producing unprecedented variability for those in this life stage. This brings to mind a final life course theme: that individuals help to construct their own lives and their own environments (Elder,

1998). These remarkable social changes offer challenges but also opportunities: for individuals to customize their middle years according to their own interests and inclinations and for society to create new structures that will serve to expand the life chances and choices for those in the middle life course.

ACKNOWLEDGMENTS

The first author's research on this chapter was supported by a grant from the Alfred P. Sloan Foundation (#96-6-9) and a grant from the National Institute on Aging (IT50 AG11711). The work of the second author was supported by the John D. and Catherine T. MacArthur Foundation Research Network on Successful Midlife Development.

REFERENCES

Anderson, D. (1991). Retirees: Community service resources. In *Resourceful aging: Today and tomorrow* (Conference Proceedings, Volume II, pp. 73–78). Washington, DC: American Association of Retired Persons.

Angel, R. L., & Angel, J. L. (1993). *Painful inheritance: Health and the new generation of fatherless families.* Madison, WI: University of Wisconsin Press.

Antonucci, T. C., & Mikus, K. (1988). The power of parenthood: Personality and attitudinal changes during the transition to parenthood. In G. Y. Michaels & W. A. Goldberg (Eds.), *The transition to parenthood* (pp. 62–84). Cambridge: Cambridge University Press.

Atchley, R. C. (1989). A continuity theory of normal aging. *The Gerontologist, 29,* 183–190.

Atchley, R. C. (1993). Critical perspectives on retirement. In T. R. Cole, W. A. Achenbaum, P. L. Jakobi, & R. Kastenbaum (Eds.), *Voices and visions of aging: Toward a critical gerontology* (pp. 3–19). New York: Springer Publishing Co.

Baruch, G., & Brooks-Gunn, J. (Eds.). (1984). *Women in midlife.* New York: Plenum.

Bielby, W., & Bielby, D. (1989). Family ties: Balancing commitments to work and family in dual earner households. *American Sociological Review, 54,* 776–789.

Bradburn, E. M., Moen P., & Dempster-McClain, D. (1995). An event history analysis of women's return to school. *Social Forces, 73,* 1517–1551.

Brandstaedter, J., & Baltes-Goetz, B. (1990). Personal control over development and quality of life perspectives in adulthood. In P. Baltes & M. M. Baltes (Eds.), *Successful aging: Perspectives from the behavioral sciences* (pp. 197–224). Cambridge: Cambridge University Press.

Brim, G. (1992). *Ambition: How we manage success and failure throughout our lives.* New York: Basic.

Brim, O. G., & Ryff, C. (1980). On the properties of life events. In P. B. Baltes & O. G. Brim (Eds.), *Life-span development and behavior* (Vol. 3, pp. 367–388). New York: Academic Press.

Brody, E. M. (1985). Parent care as a normative family stress. *The Gerontologist, 25,* 19–29.

Bronfenbrenner, U. (1979). *The ecology of human development.* Cambridge: Harvard University Press.

Brooks-Gunn, J., & Kirsh, B. (1984). Life events and the boundaries of midlife for women. In G. K. Baruch & J. Brooks-Gunn (Eds.), *Women in midlife* (pp. 11–30). New York: Plenum.

Burkhauser, R. V., & Quinn, J. F. (1989). American patterns of work and retirement. In W. Schmall (Ed.), *Redefining the process of retirement: An international perspective* (pp. 91–114). Berlin: Springer-Verlag.

Cantor, M. (1983). Strain among caregivers: A study of experience in the United States. *The Gerontologist, 23,* 597–604.

Chambré, S. M. (1987). *Good deeds in old age: Volunteering by the new leisure class.* Lexington, MA: Lexington Books.

Cherlin, A. J., & Furstenberg, F. F. (1987). *The new American grandparenthood: A place in the family, a life apart.* New York: Basic.

Clausen, J. A. (1986). *The life course: A sociological perspective.* Englewood Cliffs, NJ: Prentice-Hall.

Clausen, J. A. (1990, August). *Turning point as a life course concept.* Paper presented at the annual meetings of the American Sociological Association, Washington, DC.

Clausen, J. A. (1993). *American lives: Looking back at the children of the Great Depression.* New York: Free Press.

Clausen, J. A. (1995). Gender, context, and turning points in adults' lives. In P. E. Moen, G. Elder, & K. Lüscher (Eds.), *Examining lives in context: Perspectives on the ecology of human development* (pp. 365–389). Washington, DC: American Psychological Association.

Clausen, J. A., & Gilens, M. I. (1990). Personality and labor force participation across the life course: A longitudinal study of women's careers. *Sociological Forum, 5,* 595–618.

Cohen-Mansfield, J. (1989). Employment and volunteering roles for the elderly: Characteristics, attributions, and strategies. *Journal of Leisure Research, 21,* 214–227.

Contemporary Research Press. (1993). *American working women: A statistical handbook.* Dallas, TX: Author.

Danigelis, N. L., & McIntosh, B. R. (1993). Resources and the productive activity of elders: Race and gender as contexts. *Journal of Gerontology: Social Sciences, 48,* S192–S293.

Dohrenwend, B. P., & Dohrenwend, B. S. (1981). *Stressful life events and their contexts.* New Brunswick, NJ: Rutgers University Press.

Donahue, E. M., Robins, R. W., Roberts, B. W., & John, O. P. (1993). The divided self: Concurrent and longitudinal effects of psychological adjustment and social roles on self-concept differentiation. *Journal of Personality and Social Psychology, 64,* 834–846.

Elder, G. H., Jr. (1975). Age differentiation and the life course. *Annual Review of Sociology, 1,* 165–190.

Elder, G. H., Jr. (Ed.). (1985). Perspectives on the life course. In *Life course dynamics: Trajectories and transitions, 1968–1980* (pp. 23–49). Ithaca, NY: Cornell University Press.

Elder, G. H., Jr. (1994). The life course paradigm: Historical, comparative, and developmental perspectives. In P. Moen, G. H. Elder, Jr., & K. Lüscher (Eds.), *Linking lives and contexts: Perspectives on the ecology of human development.* Washington, DC: American Psychological Association.

Elder, G. H., Jr. (1998). The life course as developmental theory. *Child Development, 69,* 1–12.

Esterberg, K. G., Moen, P., & Dempster-McClain, D. (1994). Transition to divorce: A life-course approach to women's marital duration and dissolution. *The Sociological Quarterly, 35,* 289–307.

Farrell, M. P., & Rosenberg, S. D. (1981). *Men at midlife.* Boston: Auburn House.

Fennell, M., & Walker, H. (1986). Gender differences in role differentiation and organizational task performance. *Annual Review of Sociology, 12,* 255–275.

Filipp, S-H., & Klauer, T. (1986). Conceptions of self over the life span: Reflections on the dialectics of change. In M. M. Baltes & P. B. Baltes (Eds.), *The psychology of control and aging* (pp. 167–206). Hillsdale, NJ: Erlbaum.

Fillenbaum, G. G., George, L. K., & Palmore, E. B. (1985). Determinants and consequences of retirement among men of different races and economic levels. *Journal of Gerontology, 40,* 85–94.

Fischer, L. R., Mueller, D. P., & Cooper, P. W. (1991). Older volunteers: A discussion of the Minnesota Senior Study. *The Gerontologist, 31,* 183–194.

Forest, K. B., Moen, P., & Dempster-McClain, D. 1995. Cohort differences in the transition to motherhood: The variable effects of education and employment before marriage. *The Sociological Quarterly, 36,* 315–336.

Garfinkel, I., & McLanahan, S. S. (1986). *Single mothers and their children: A new American dilemma.* Washington, DC: Urban Institute Press.

George, L. K. (1980). *Role transitions in later life.* Belmont, CA: Wadsworth.

George, L. K., & Gwyther, L. P. (1986). Caregiver well-being: A multidimensional examination of family caregivers of demented adults. *The Gerontologist, 34,* 253–259.

Gibson, R. (1991). Age-by-race differences in the health and functioning of elderly persons. *Journal of Aging and Health, 3,* 335–351.

Glassner, B. (1994). *Career crash: America's new crisis—and who survives.* New York: Simon and Schuster.

Glick, P. C. (1990). American families: As they were and are. *Sociology and Social Research, 74,* 139–145.

Gotlib, I. H., & Wheaton, B. (Eds.). (1997). *Stress and adversity over the life course: Trajectories and turning points.* New York: Cambridge University Press.

Gove, W. R., & Hughes, M. (1979). Possible causes of the apparent sex differences in physical health: An empirical investigation. *American Sociological Review, 44,* 126–146.

Gove, W. R., & Tudor, J. F. (1973). Adult sex roles and mental illness. *American Journal of Sociology, 78,* 812–835.

Hagestad, G. O., & Neugarten, B. L. (1984). Age and the life course. In R. H. Binstock & E. Shanas (Eds.), *Handbook of aging and the social sciences* (2nd ed., pp. 35–61). New York: Van Nostrand Reinhold.

Han, S.-K., & Moen, P. (1998). Clocking out: Multiplex time in retirement. Bronfenbrenner Life Course Center Working Paper Series #98-03. Ithaca, NY: Cornell University.

Helson, R., & Roberts, B. (1992). The personality of young adult couples and wives' work patterns. *Journal of Personality, 60,* 575–597.

Helson, R. & Wink, P. (1992). Personality change in women from the early 40s to the early 50s. *Psychology and Aging, 7,* 46–55.

Herzog, A. R., Kahn, R. L., Morgan, J. N., Jackson, J. S., & Antonucci, T. C. (1989). Age differences in productive activities. *Journal of Gerontology: Social Sciences, 44,* S129–S138.

Honig, M., & Hanoch, G. (1985). Partial retirement as a separate mode of retirement behavior. *Journal of Human Resources, 20,* 21–46.

Jahoda, M. (1982). *Employment and unemployment: A social psychological analysis.* Cambridge: Cambridge University Press.

Jones, L. (1980). *Great expectations: America and the Baby Boom generation.* New York: Ballantine.

Kandel, D. B., Davies, M. & Raveis, V. H. (1985). The stressfulness of daily social roles for women: Marital, occupational and household roles. *Journal of Health and Social Behavior, 26,* 64–78.

Kessler, R. C., & McLeod, J. D. (1984). Sex differences in vulnerability to undesirable life events. *American Sociological Review, 49,* 620–631.

Kohn, M. L., & Schooler, C. (1985). Job conditions and personality: A longitudinal assessment of their reciprocal effects. *American Journal of Sociology, 87,* 1257–1286.

Labouvie-Vief, G. (1982). Dynamic development and mature autonomy. *Human Development, 25,* 161–191.

Labouvie-Vief, G., Hakim-Larson, J., & Hobart, C. J. (1987). Age, ego level, and the life-span development of coping and defense processes. *Psychology and Aging, 3,* 286–293.

Levinson, D., Darrow, C. N., Klein, E. B., Levinson, M. H., & McKee, B. (1977). *The seasons of a man's life.* New York: Knopf.

Long, J., & Porter, K. L. (1984). Multiple roles of midlife women: A case for new directions in theory, research, and policy. In G. Baruch & J. Brooks-Gunn, (Eds.), *Women in midlife* (pp. 109–154). New York: Plenum.

Lowenthal, M. F., & Robinson, B. (1976). Social networks and isolation. In R. H. Binstock & E. Shanas (Eds.), *Handbook of aging and the social sciences* (1st ed., pp. 432–456). New York: Van Nostrand Reinhold.

MacDermid, S. M., Franz, C. E., & De Reus, L. A. (1998). Generativity: At the crossroads of social roles and personality. In D. P. McAdams & E. de St. Aubin (Eds.), *Generativity and adult development: How and why we care for the next generation,* (pp. 181–226). New York: American Psychological Association.

Markus, H., & Wurf, E. (1987). The dynamic self-concept: A sociological perspective. *Annual Review of Psychology, 38,* 299–337.

McCrae, R., & Costa, P. (1990). *Personality in adulthood.* New York: Guilford.

Merton, R. K. (1957). *Social theory and social structure.* Glencoe, IL: Free Press.

Moen, P. (1992). *Women's two roles: A contemporary dilemma.* Westport, CT: Auburn House.

Moen, P. (1994). Women, work, and family: A sociological perspective on changing roles. In M. W. Riley, R. L. Kahn, & A. Foner (Eds.), *Age and structural lag: The mismatch between people's lives and opportunities in work, family, and leisure.* New York: Wiley, forthcoming.

Moen, P. (1995a). Gender, age, and the life course. In R. H. Binstock & L. George (Eds.), *Handbook of aging and the social sciences* (4th ed., pp. 171–187). San Diego, CA: Academic Press.

Moen, P. (1995b). A life course approach to post-retirement roles and well-being. In L. A. Bond, S. J. Cutler, & A. E. Grams (Eds.), *Promoting successful and productive aging* (pp. 239–256). Newbury Park, CA: Sage.

Moen, P. (1997). Women's Roles and Resilience: Trajectories of Advantage or Turning Points? In I. H. Gotlib & B. Wheaton (Eds.), *Stress and adversity over the life course: Trajectories and turning points* (pp. 133–156). New York: Cambridge University Press.

Moen, P. (1998). Recasting careers: Changing reference groups, risks, and realities. *Generations, 22,* 40–45.

Moen, P., Dempster-McClain, D., & Williams, R. (1992). Successful aging: A life-course perspective on women's roles and health. *American Journal of Sociology, 97,* 1612–1638.

Moen, P., Downey, G., & Bolger, N. (1990). Labor force re-entry among U.S. homemakers in midlife: A life-course perspective. *Gender and Society, 4,* 230–243.

Moen, P., & Fields, V. (1998). Retirement, social capital, and well-being: Does community participation replace paid work? Bronfenbrenner Life Course Center Working Paper Series #98-10. Ithaca, NY: Cornell University.

Moen, P., Robison, J., & Fields, V. (1994). Women's work and caregiving roles: A life-course approach. *Journal of Gerontology: Social Sciences, 49,* S176–S186.

Morgan, J. N. (1986). Unpaid productive activity over the life course. In Committee on Aging Society (Ed.), *Productive roles in an older society* (pp. 73–109). Washington, DC: National Academy Press.

Neugarten, B. L. (1977). Personality and aging. In J. E. Birren & K. W. Schaie (Eds.), *Handbook of the psychology of aging* (pp. 626–649). New York: Van Nostrand Reinhold.

Newman, K. (1993). *Declining fortunes: The withering of the American dream.* New York: Basic.

Norton, A. J., & Moorman, J. E. (1987). Current trends in marriage and divorce among American women. *Journal of Marriage and the Family, 49,* 3–14.

O'Rand, A. M., Henretta, J. C., & Krecker, M. L. (1992). Family pathways to retirement. In M. Szinovacz, D. J. Ekerdt, & B. H. Vinick (Eds.), *Families and retirement* (pp. 81–98). Newbury Park, CA: Sage.

O'Rand, A. M., & Landerman, R. (1984). Women's and men's retirement income: Early family role effects. *Research on Aging, 6,* 25–44.

Parnes, H. S., & Nestel, G. (1974). Early retirement. In H. S. Parnes, A. V. Adams, P. Andrisani, A. I. Kohen, & G. Nestel (Eds.), *The pre-retirement years* (Vol. 4, *Five years in the work lives of middle-aged men,* pp. 153–196). Columbus, OH: Center for Human Resource Research, Ohio State University.

Pearlin, L. I., & Johnson, J. S. (1977). Marital status, life-strains, and depression. *American Sociological Review, 42,* 704–715.

Perun, P. J., & Bielby, D. D. (1980). Structure and dynamics of the individual life course. In K. W. Back (Ed.), *Life course: Integrative theories and exemplary populations* (pp. 97–119). Boulder, CO: Westview.

Ramseur, H. (1989). Psychologically healthy Black adults: A review of theory and research. In R. L. Jones (Ed.), *Black adult development and aging* (pp. 215–241). Berkeley, CA: Cobb & Henry Publishers.

Reimers, C., & Honig, M. (1989). The retirement process in the United States: Mobility among full-time work, partial retirement, and full retirement. In W. Schmall (Ed.), *Redefining the process of retirement: An international perspective* (pp. 115–131). New York: Springer-Verlag.

Riegel, K. (1975). Adult life crises: Toward a dialectical theory of development. In N. Datan & L. Ginsberg (Eds.), *Life span development and psychology: Normative life crises* (pp. 99–123). New York: Academic Press.

Riley, M. W. (1982). Implications for the middle and later years. In P. W. Bermand & E. R. Ramey (Eds.), *Women: A developmental perspective* (pp. 399–405). NIH Publication No. 82-2298. Rockville, MD: Department of Health and Human Services.

Riley, M. W. (1987). On the significance of age in sociology. *American Sociological Review, 52,* 1–14.

Riley, M. W., Foner, A., & Waring, J. (1988). Sociology of age. In N. J. Smelser (Ed.), *Handbook of sociology* (pp. 243–290). Newbury Park, CA: Sage.

Riley, M. W., Kahn, R. L., & Foner, A. (1994). *Age and structural lag: The mismatch between people's lives and opportunities in work, family, and leisure.* New York: Wiley.

Robison, J., Moen, P., & Dempster-McClain, D. (1995). Women's caregiving: A life course perspective. *Journal of Gerontology: Social Sciences, 50B,* S362–S373.

Rosow, I. (1974). *Socialization to old age.* Berkeley, CA: University of California Press.

Rosow, I. (1985). Status and role change through the life cycle. In R. H. Binstock & E. Shanas (Eds.), *Handbook of aging and the social sciences* (2nd ed., pp. 62–93). New York: Van Nostrand Reinhold.

Ryff, C. D., Schmutte, P. S., & Less, Y. H. (1996). How children turn out: Implications for parental self-evaluation. In C. D. Ryff & M. M. Seltzer (Eds.), *The parental experience in midlife* (pp. 383–422). Chicago: University of Chicago Press.

Samuelson, R. (1996). *The good life and its discontents: The American dream in the age of entitlement, 1945–1995.* New York: Times Books.

Settersten, R. A., & Mayer, K. U. (1997). The measurement of age, age structuring, and the life course. *Annual Review of Sociology, 23,* 233–261.

Skolnick, A. (1991). *Embattled paradise.* New York: Basic.

Smith, K. R., & Moen, P. (1986). Women at work: Commitment and behavior over the life course. *Sociological Forum, 1,* 450–475.

Smith, K. R., & Moen, P. (1988). Passage through midlife: Women's changing family roles and economic well-being. *Sociological Quarterly, 29,* 503–524.

Sorensen, A. B., Weinert, F. E., & Sherrod, L. R. (Eds.). (1986). *Human development and the life course.* Hillsdale, NJ: Erlbaum.

Stewart, A. (1989). Linking individual development to social changes. *American Psychologist, 44,* 30–42.

Stryker, S. (1980). *Symbolic interactionism: A social structural version.* Menlo Park, CA: Benjamin/Cummings.

Stryker, S., & Serpe, R. (1982). Commitment, identity salience, and role behavior: Theory and research. In W. Ickes & E. Knowles (Eds.), *Personality, roles, and social behavior.* New York: Springer-Verlag.

Stryker, S., & Statham, A. (1985). Symbolic interaction in role theory. In G. Lindsey & E. Aronson (Eds.), *Handbook of social psychology* (3rd ed., Vol. 1, pp. 311–378). Hillsdale, NJ: Erlbaum.

Thoits, P. A. (1983). Multiple identities and psychological well-being: A reformulation and test of the social isolation hypothesis. *American Sociological Review, 48,* 174–187.

Thoits, P. A. (1986). Multiple identities: Examining gender and marital status differences in distress. *American Sociological Review, 51,* 259–272.

Thoits, P. A. (1994). Stressors and problem-solving: The individual as psychological activist. *Journal of Health and Social Behavior, 35,* 143–159.

Turner, R. (1978). The role and the person. *American Journal of Sociology, 84,* 1–23.

Umberson, D. (1987). Family status and health behaviors: Social control as a dimension of social integration. *Journal of Health and Social Behavior, 28,* 306–319.

Umberson, D. (1992). Relationships between adult children and their parents. *Journal of Marriage and the Family, 54,* 664–674.

Vaillant, G. (1977). *Adaptation to life.* Boston: Little, Brown.

Verbrugge, L. M. (1983). Multiple roles and physical health of women and men. *Journal of Health and Social Behavior, 24,* 16–30.

Verbrugge, L. M. (1989). Gender, aging, and health. In K. S. Markides (Ed.), *Aging and Health* (pp. 23–78). Newbury Park, CA: Sage.

Veroff, J. R., Douvan, E., & Kulka, R. (1981). *The inner American.* New York: Basic.

Waite, L. J., Haggstrom, G. W., & Kanouse, D. E. (1985). Changes in the employment activities of new parents. *American Sociological Review, 50,* 263–272.

Weiss, R. S. (1990). *Staying the course.* New York: Free Press.

Wethington, E., Brown, G. W., & Kessler, R. C. (1995). Interview measurement of stressful life events. In S. Cohen, R. C. Kessler, & L. U. Gordon (Eds.), *Measuring stress: A guide for health and social scientists* (pp. 59–79). New York: Oxford University Press.

Wethington, E., Cooper, H., & Holmes, C. (1997). Turning points in midlife. In I. Gotlib & B. Wheaton (Eds.), *Stress and adversity across the life course: Trajectories and turning points* (pp. 215–231). New York: Cambridge University Press.

Wethington, E., & Kessler, R. C. (1989). Employment, parenting responsibility, and psychological distress: A longitudinal study of married women. *Journal of Family Issues, 10,* 527–546.

Wethington, E., & Kessler, R. C. & Holmes, C. (1992, August). *The nature of psychological experiences at midlife: A report on exploratory studies of "turning points."* Paper presented at the annual meeting of the American Psychological Association. Washington, DC.

Wethington, E., & Pixley, J. (1998). Life transitions, life events, and generativity across the life course. In A. Rossi (Ed.), *Multiple dimensions of social responsibility.* Chicago: University of Chicago Press. Forthcoming.

Wheaton, B. (1990). Life transitions, role histories, and mental health. *American Sociological Review, 55,* 209–223.

Whitbourne, S. K. (1986). Openness to experience, identity flexibility, and life change in adults. *Journal of Personality and Social Psychology, 50,* 163–168.

White, L., & Edwards, J. N. (1990). Emptying the nest and parental well-being. *American Sociological Review, 55,* 235–242.

Wilensky, H. (1961). Life cycle, work situation, and participation in formal associations. In R. W. Kleemeier (Ed.), *Aging and leisure: A research perspective into the meaningful use of time.* New York: Oxford University Press.

Wilson, W. J. (1987). *The truly disadvantaged.* Chicago: University of Chicago Press.

Wortman, C. B., & Silver, R. C. (1990). Successful mastery of bereavement and widowhood: A life-course perspective. In P. B. Baltes & M. M. Baltes (Eds.), *Successful aging: Perspectives from the behavioral sciences* (pp. 225–264). New York: Cambridge University Press.

CHAPTER 2

The Developing Self in Midlife

Susan Krauss Whitbourne

Department of Psychology, University of Massachusetts at Amherst, Amherst, Massachusetts

Loren Angiullo Connolly

Department of Clinical Psychology, Philadelphia Geriatric Center, Philadelphia, Pennsylvania

The concept of adult development, a term once thought to be an oxymoron, has become a staple of discussion in self-help books, movies, the media, and the commercial market of games and party supplies. The messages conveyed in these popular sources, though intended to be humorous, are generally pessimistic ones revolving around the themes that after the age of 40 one is "over the hill" or in the midst of a devastating "midlife crisis." Magazine and newspaper articles increasingly devote attention to the desires of middle-aged people to remain healthy and attractive, with the assumption that these qualities can no longer be taken for granted after one has reached that certain age. Although this media attention tends to emphasize the concept of adulthood as a time of inevitable decline, there is also the more hopeful message that proper diet, exercise, and a willingness to evaluate one's priorities can help adults overcome the downward progression of life after 40.

THEORETICAL PERSPECTIVES ON PERSONALITY DEVELOPMENT IN MIDLIFE

Current fads contrast markedly with the long-held tradition within the scholarly discipline of psychology in which the middle years of adulthood are seen as a time of quiescence between the formative years of adolescence and early adulthood and the declining years of old age. This tradition has its origins partly in the writings of

Freud, who believed that personality change past the age of 50 years was virtually impossible. According to Freud, the mental processes in middle-aged individuals lack the "elasticity on which the treatment depends" (Freud, 1906/1942). Although arriving at this position from an entirely different starting point, trait theorists such as Eysenck (1967) and Cattell (1982) regard personality structure as invariant from a very early age onward, reflecting the influence of genetic and constitutional factors on enduring personal dispositions.

Since the time of Freud's work, some psychoanalysts have broken from the Freudian model and proposed that middle adulthood is a time when personality ripens and matures to newer and healthier forms than could be attained in the earlier years. Jung (1968) believed that fully mature development is not likely to occur before the middle years of adulthood (40s–50s) when the individual's psyche becomes fully individuated. More recent psychodynamic models incorporated the idea that the individual's ego defenses continue to evolve into higher levels of maturity throughout the middle years (Vaillant, 1977). Applications of psychoanalytic methods to the treatment of middle-aged and older adults provide further evidence of the possibility of significant personality change well into the later years (Nemiroff & Colarusso, 1985; Sadavoy & Leszcz, 1987).

Humanistic models of personality also propose that middle adulthood brings with it the opportunity for continued growth. According to Maslow (1962), the state of self-actualization, in which one's potential is fully being realized, cannot develop until a person is past the period of youth. Maslow's biographical and empirical analyses have received some support in the adult development literature, with growth reported in scales measuring self-actualization in midlife women (Hyman, 1988). Rogers (1961) described the fully functioning individual as one who has achieved congruence between the self and experiences, a process that is constantly evolving and changing. Although these theorists were not developmental in the traditional sense, their observations on the "mature" or "healthy" personality point to the expected movement in midlife toward an optimum of individual functioning.

In Erikson's (1963) eight-stage psychosocial model of the life cycle, it is assumed that change occurs systematically throughout the years of adulthood. Erikson proposed that after adolescence, with its often tumultuous search for identity, adults pass through three psychosocial crisis stages. The stages corresponding to the early and middle adult years focus on the establishment of close interpersonal relationships (intimacy vs. isolation), and passing on to the future one's creative products (generativity vs. stagnation). In the final stage (ego integrity vs. despair), the individual must resolve conflicted feelings about the past, adapt to the changes associated with the aging process, and come to grips with the inevitability of death. Erikson's ideas, although difficult to operationalize, have provided a major intellectual inspiration to workers in the field of adult personality development. The writings of Levinson (1978), Gould (1978), and Vaillant (1977) are based on the fundamental ideas of Erikson's theory that changing circumstances and values in work and family relationships are the major preoccupations of adults, and that resolution of feelings about aging and mortality becomes increasingly important in the later adult years. The work of these authors supports Erikson's fundamental proposal that personality continues to develop in important ways throughout life.

THE CENTRAL ROLE OF IDENTITY IN ADULT PERSONALITY DEVELOPMENT

In Erikson's model, each psychosocial crisis is theorized to offer an opportunity for the development of a new function or facet of the ego. However, the crisis involving identity has special significance, as it establishes the most important functions of the ego: self-definition and self-awareness. Following the development of identity, according to Erikson, additional functions of the ego evolve beyond those identified by Freud, including love, care, and wisdom. Although Erikson focused on the role of the ego in personality, he never departed from orthodox Freudian tradition. The ego functions theorized to be added by resolution of later psychosocial stages do not alter the dynamic features of personality involving the interaction among conscious and unconscious processes. The content of the unconscious does not change with the addition of generativity to the functions of the ego; instead, the ego is broadened and operates across a broader domain of experience.

The genuine contribution of Erikson's theory is in regarding adolescence as a time in which the ego becomes fully articulated within personality as the center of the "self." In this stage, as in the prior stages, Erikson differed from Freud in placing greater emphasis on the role of parents, peers, and society in influencing this process. Furthermore, from this point on, the ego is theorized to exert a far greater influence within the psyche than is generally recognized by Freud. However, Freud did not neglect the demands placed on personality by subsequent adult experiences. The ability to "love and work" was seen by Freud as a major accomplishment of mature genitality, the final stage of psychosexual development. Yet, these abilities did not alter the fundamental structure of id, ego, and superego set in the early childhood years. Erikson's writings, then, can be seen as not dissimilar from Freud, as both described a set of tasks that the individual (ego) must confront once the basic parameters of personality become established.

If these new demands to "love and work" do not add to the adaptive functions of the ego, what is their role in adult personality development? One possibility is that intimacy, generativity, and ego integrity, the psychosocial crises defined by Erikson, are better conceived of as developmental tasks. It has long been an assumption of life-span theories that certain demands present themselves at particular choice points in adulthood (Havighurst, 1972). Adults must find intimate partners, find a way to leave something of themselves behind for future generations, and resolve ambivalent feelings toward mortality. Other developmental tasks involve more specific challenges in the work setting, the family, and the larger community. For example, retirement is a central developmental task of later adulthood, and is only tangentially related at a conceptual level to generativity and/or ego integrity. It may be argued that Erikson has described three of a larger possible set of developmental tasks in the middle and later adult years, then, rather than a new set of components that become added to the individual's existing personality structure.

Viewing Erikson's theory of middle adulthood as a compelling (if not comprehensive) developmental task theory recasts its focus considerably. Developmental task theories are useful in providing descriptions of adult life issues, but limited in that they remain at a descriptive rather than explanatory level. Yet, such a recasting of Erikson's theory seems warranted. Consider further the epigenetic principle, the proposition that each stage unfolds in a predetermined sequence and that the resolution of one stage sets the parameters for resolution of subsequent stages. This proposition is a testable hypothesis, but again it is descriptive rather than explanatory.

Another important point regarding the epigenetic principle is that it is exclusively focused on the ego. It is this structure of personality that is presumed to develop through the stages set by the matrix of age periods and psychosocial issues. Yet, the epigenetic principle does not involve the proposal of a structure unique to the personality other than the ego. We are left, then, with the ego as the main focus of Erikson's theory throughout the adult stages. It is the ego, translated into the individual's self or identity, that forms the central theme of Erikson's developmental scenario of adulthood and old age.

By placing identity squarely at the center of adult psychosocial development, it is possible to link conceptualizations of adult development to the theoretically rich literature on the self. Adult developmental processes, rather than being seen as a breed separate from the functioning of the self or identity, can then be understood within the broader context of psychology's attempts to understand the nature and function of self-conceptualizations. The processes of assimilation and accommodation theorized to be responsible for consistency and change in the self can then be seen as central to an analysis of development over adulthood in the individual's sense of identity.

A THEORETICAL MODEL OF ADULT IDENTITY DEVELOPMENT

A starting point for examining the development of the self in adulthood is a model based on the conceptualization of identity as the source of self-definition within personality. In this model (Whitbourne, 1986b; 1996), identity is theorized to form an organizing schema through which the individual's experiences are interpreted. Identity is defined as the individual's self-appraisal of a variety of attributes along the dimensions of physical and cognitive abilities, personal traits and motives, and the multiplicity of social roles including worker, family member, and community citizen. The affective content of identity, for psychologically healthy adults, takes the positive self-referential form encapsulated in the expression "I am a competent, loving, and good person," competent at work, loving in family life, and morally righteous.

The individual's experiences, both past and present, are postulated to relate to identity through processes of assimilation and accommodation. The process of identity assimilation is defined as the interpretation of life events relevant to the self in terms of the cognitive and affective schemas that are incorporated in identity. The events and experiences to which the assimilation function applies can include major life events, cumulative interactions with the environment over time, or seemingly minor incidents that nevertheless can have a potential impact on identity. Thus, the experiences interpreted through identity assimilation can include physical changes associated with the onset of the aging process in the middle adult years or involvement in a gratifying social role, such as community volunteer. Each type of experience can have different meanings among individuals, depending on the nature of their current self-conceptualizations in identity.

The process of identity accommodation, by contrast, involves changing one's identity in response to identity-relevant experiences. Identity might change in content in response to one of these events when, for example, an illness or accident causes the individual to acknowledge new health limitations in middle age. Individuals may also take more deliberate actions to alter their identities by seeking accommodative experiences. The search for personal change through psychotherapy or counseling constitutes a self-initiated move toward identity accommodation.

There is no theoretical reason to expect that the identity processes would differ systematically with respect to age in adulthood; what may be theorized to vary from early to middle to later adulthood are the specific life events that trigger the identity processes. It is also consistent with the model to propose that individuals may change in their relative use of assimilation versus accommodation over the adult years if they are stimulated to change either through personal growth experiences or changing interpersonal interactions as in, for example, long-standing close relationships. Examples of these identity-relevant experiences in middle adulthood will be described below.

As in Piaget's (1975/1977) discussion of the equilibration process in the development of intelligence, it is assumed that the most desirable state is one in which the individual's identity is in a dynamic balance with the environment so that alternation takes place between assimilation and accommodation. In this state, the individual's identity is flexible enough to change when warranted but not unstructured to the point that every new experience causes the person to question fundamental assumptions about the self's integrity and unity. Thus, equilibrium is not a static mode, but involves movement back and forth between assimilation and accommodation. However, it is also assumed that the directionality of processes is, as in Piaget, from assimilation to accommodation, with assimilation being the preferred mode for psychologically healthy adults who like and strive to see themselves in relation to events in a positive light. Accommodation is assumed to be prompted when assimilation can no longer fit new events into the individual's existing identity.

In this regard, the so-called "midlife crisis" may be seen as an extreme accommodative reaction to a set of experiences that no longer can be processed through identity assimilation (Whitbourne, 1986a).

There are a myriad of potential sources of identity growth and change in the middle adult years any of which can stimulate the operation of identity assimilation and accommodation. The increasing recognition of physical aging on the part of the individual beginning in the decade of the 40s may be seen as constituting an important stimulus for identity development throughout the middle years. To the extent that middle-aged adults are conscious of their changing bodily shape and performance, they may be seen as faced constantly with new experiences to integrate into their existing identities. Although physical changes are typically the most readily observed and salient to many adults, changes in sensory, perceptual, and cognitive abilities can be seen as another set of important challenges to the maintenance of a stable identity over the decades of midlife. In addition to these developmental changes as sources of identity change are the consequences of life patterns and decisions that the individual makes throughout the decades from early through middle adulthood. The outcome of these behaviors may, in turn, serve as stimuli to further identity change.

The idea of applying the equilibration model to identity development in adulthood and old age emerged originally from a theoretical analysis of the literature on adult personality development and identity development in late adolescence. The conceptual starting point for this analysis was the construct of identity statuses (Marcia, 1966), which are defined as alternative modes of resolving the psychosocial stage of identity versus identity diffusion (Erikson, 1963). These modes of resolution differ in the extent to which they involve having firm commitments and a clear sense of self compared to being insecure and seeking to find one's identity through exploration.

Each of the identity statuses can be related to the identity processes of assimilation and accommodation. The identity achievement status involves the favorable resolution of the identity crisis, as individuals who are identity achieved have a clear set of commitments at which they have arrived through a process of serious exploration. These individuals may be seen as having arrived at a balance between identity assimilation and accommodation. Individuals who are in the foreclosed status have a sense of clear commitments but they have not gone through a process of exploration of alternatives. In this sense, the foreclosed status may be seen as involving a high degree of identity assimilation. The third identity status, moratorium, applies to individuals who are in the midst of the classic "identity crisis." They do not have firm commitments, and are earnestly seeking to define these for themselves. The identity-diffuse status applies to individuals who do not have a clear set of commitments, but have no strong desire to arrive at a clear identity. Persons exemplifying both the moratorium and identity-diffuse statuses may be seen as relying heavily on the process of identity accommodation, as neither have a strong identity that they impose onto their experiences. Instead, they may be swayed by their experiences to alter their self-conceptions. Persons in the moratorium status, however, may be seen as moving toward a consolidation of the self, compared to those in the diffuse status; who will remain in a chronic state of weak self-definition.

Research on identity statuses in adulthood has proven to have mixed value. As expected, midlife brings with it a movement toward greater identity achievement (Kroger & Haslett, 1991; Whitbourne & VanManen, 1996). Furthermore, identity resolutions achieved by late adolescence and adulthood can have implications for the development of intimacy in young and middle adulthood (Kahn, Zimmerman, Czikszentmihalyi, & Getzels, 1985; Tesch & Whitbourne, 1982). However, the identity status construct has limited applicability past the early years of adulthood (Kroger & Haslett, 1991; Whitbourne, 1986a). A model focusing on identity processes presents a more viable life-span framework (Grotevant, 1987), as it does not require assessment of the individual's passage through a specific "crisis" period. Instead, individuals can be evaluated according to their predominant approach at the moment to identity-related life events and experiences.

IDENTITY STYLES IN MIDDLE ADULTHOOD

Given the approximate correspondence between the identity statuses and the identity processes, a set of identity styles has been proposed to apply to a more process-oriented adult form of the identity statuses (Whitbourne, 1987). These forms represent the three possible kinds of relationships between the two identity processes: assimilation outweighing accommodation, accommodation outweighing assimilation, and assimilation and accommodation in approximate balance. Each of the identity styles has associated with it proposed approaches to life experiences in middle adulthood. Furthermore, each can lead to characteristic problematic patterns of behavior that cause the individual to seek psychotherapy or counseling.

Assimilative Identity Style

The assimilative identity style is applied to individuals who use identity assimilation as a predominant approach to their experiences. They would be expected to impose on their experiences a view of themselves as successful in their relationships, at work, and in their community involvements. In middle age, they are likely to see themselves as unchanging over the decades of the 30s, 40s, and 50s even as their physical appearance gradually becomes transformed. Underlying their desire to see themselves in as positive a light as possible is a theorized protective desire to avoid recognizing weaknesses or inadequacies in the self. These individuals, whose identities are not based on a secure conviction of their own potential for competence and mastery, fear signs that they might not be as successful, important, or physically fit as they like to believe they are. Through assimilative processes such as denial and rationalization they distort experiences that are discrepant with their identities so that they can remain untouched by knowledge of their weaknesses or limitations.

Individuals with an assimilative identity style may be likely to spend the early decades of their adulthood living out patterns dictated by their family experiences in childhood and early adolescence in an extension of a foreclosed identity status resolution in late adolescence. This life pattern may be maintained throughout the later decades of adulthood, or, if significant challenges to identity are presented by particular experiences, they may move rapidly toward an accommodative mode. For example, a man who is carrying forward the family tradition of succeeding as a business executive may experience a lack of personal fulfillment that becomes evident only after two or three decades in this career trajectory when he realizes that his personal needs are not being met. In other cases, failure to succeed in this life path may stimulate the individual to reconsider past choices. Should this executive lose his job through company reorganization, he may be faced with having to question his actual competence. The resulting period of disequilibrium that can follow from such experiences may pull the individual toward an accommodative mode until a new balance can be achieved.

Accommodative Identity Style

The accommodative identity style describes people who tend to use identity accommodation much more than identity assimilation. Individuals who adopt this style have a weak and incoherent identity and are easily influenced by whatever experiences they have to change their identities accordingly. Over the course of adulthood, these may be the individuals who remain identity diffuse in that they develop no consistent set of goals or commitments (Josselson, 1987). They react to criticism by intimate partners or co-workers by agreeing with this criticism rather than blaming the person who is on the attack. In relations with children, they are indecisive and uncertain, and may experience a certain amount of role reversal as their children grow into adulthood. Just as likely, their children may fail to develop a coherent or consistent identity because they lack a strong parental model with whom to identify.

The individual with the accommodative identity style can be seen as overreacting to the changes associated with the aging process that first become evident in the middle years of adulthood. Even the more innocuous signs of impending middle age, such as the first gray hair or shortness of breath after running, can lead these individuals to conclude that they must desperately seek ways to prevent themselves from sliding "over the hill." Conversely, they may decide to give into the inevitable decline that begins in middle age and start to act and appear "old" decades before their time.

The types of problems encountered by accommodative individuals in adulthood revolve around their lack of clear self-definition and overreactivity to their environment. They may be subject to particular forms of personality disorder involving poorly formed boundaries around the self, weakly articulated life goals, and instability in relationships. Clinicians might recognize these individuals in extreme form as having borderline personality disorder, with its characteristic lack of identity, emotional lability, and extreme need for close relationships for self-verification. A chronic sense of dissatisfaction and aimlessness may lead the accommodative individuals into seeking help through counseling or psychotherapy, particularly when those around them prove no longer willing to be helpful or supportive.

Balanced Identity Style

The individual who is able to adapt to experiences in middle adulthood by integrating them realistically into identity would be regarded as having a balanced identity style. Negative experiences with others, at home, or at work would be approached without either rejection or panic, and instead would be evaluated on the basis of their apparent truth. A balanced identity style seems closest to what most personality theorists and clinicians would regard as a "healthy," or "mature" approach, in that such an individual would have a sense of goals and inner purpose yet be flexible enough to adapt to changing circumstances through the vagaries of adult life. The adaptiveness of this identity style may be reflected in the gains shown in the ability to integrate flexibly cognitive and affective modes of thought and behavior. Individuals with this identity style may be expected to be at the height of their "executive" powers in midlife (Schaie, 1977–1978).

With regard to specific developmental changes experienced through the middle years of adulthood, the individual with the balanced identity style would recognize the need to adapt to whatever age-related changes in physical and cognitive functioning occur, but would do so in a measured, rational manner. When possible, such an individual would attempt to overcome potential deficiencies and age-related limitations through exercise and the appropriate use of health precautions, but would not become demoralized should these efforts not be entirely successful.

EMPIRICAL RESEARCH ON THE SELF IN MIDDLE ADULTHOOD

The period of middle adulthood, although occupying a significant share of the life course, is not an area that is heavily researched within psychology as a specific topic of study. This relative disregard can perhaps be traced to the Freudian and trait models in which the middle years are regarded as a time of stability. The majority of available data are connected with the notion of midlife crisis or represent attempts to verify trait models of consistency over time in basic personal dispositions. The range of available empirical work narrows even further when considering the development of the self or identity. Sequential research on psychosocial development in midlife (Whitbourne, Zuschlag, Elliot, & Waterman, 1992) indicates a pattern of growth consistent with the predictions of Erikson's theory. In line with these findings is evidence that adults become more self-confident, accepting, and decisive as they move through the middle years (Helson & Wink, 1992; Ryff, 1991). These data are suggestive but limited in enlightening theoretical models of the self in midlife.

In recent years, however, a social-cognitive model of the self in adulthood has emerged from several alternative sources. Whitbourne (1985) has described a model of the "life-span construct," an organizing schema that represents the individual's conceptualizations of future scenarios and past life stories. The life-span construct is theorized to influence the way that individuals interpret events in the present, recollect experiences from the past, and anticipate events in the future. The life-span construct is assessed through a "life drawing," a projective measure of the life-span construct that relates to the individual's sense of time perspective and well-being over the middle and later adult years (Whitbourne & Dannefer, 1985–1986; Whitbourne & Powers, 1994).

In terms of identity styles, there is suggestive evidence to support this construct from related research on personality traits in the middle adult years. Individuals who are high on the personality trait of openness to experience may be more likely to use identity accommodation. In a study of middle-aged adults, Whitbourne (1986c) found that those adults who were open to considering alternatives to their present life situations had higher openness to experience scores. Identity flexibility, as it was referred to in this study, was also predictive of actual life changes within 12 months of initial assessment. It may be inferred, then, that adults who are low on the trait of openness to experience are also more likely to use identity assimilation when approaching new events in adulthood. In general, to the extent that personality traits remain stable over the adult years (Conley, 1985; McCrae & Costa, 1990) it would be expected that the identity styles would be used fairly consistently as a means of coping with a variety of life events in the areas of personal relationships and job experiences.

A number of other theorists and researchers have also focused on the need to incorporate notions of the self into models of development in adulthood and old age and are converging on the importance of more detailed descriptions of the content of the self in adulthood, its role in influencing behavior, and the processes through which the self changes in response to life experiences. One model that has proved highly testable within this framework is that of "possible selves" (Markus & Nurius, 1986), the elements of the self that represent what the individual could become, would like to become, and is afraid of becoming. Possible selves can include the hoped-for and dreaded self, both of which are internally defined within the context of the self as a whole.

Possible selves are theorized to serve as psychological resources that can both motivate the individual toward future behavior and serve as a defense of the self in the present. The individual is motivated to strive to achieve a hoped-for possible self and will attempt to avoid a dreaded or feared possible self. To the extent that the individual is successful in this process, positive feelings of life satisfaction are theorized to emerge. When the individual is unable to realize a hoped-for possible self or is unable to avoid the dreaded possible self, negative self-evaluations and affect will follow. However, here the defensive function of the possible self construct comes into play. Assuming that most psychologically healthy adults attempt to preserve a positive self-concept, the realization that one is approaching a state of unfulfillment will lead the individual to revise the possible self so that it is more consistent with current experiences.

The possible selves construct is assessed through a questionnaire measure that asks respondents to describe their hoped-for and feared or dreaded possible selves, and to evaluate their capability of, respectively, achieving or avoiding these states. Applications of the possible selves construct to middle-aged and older adults have revealed that the possible selves are accessible to conscious awareness, can be objectively rated into content-based categories, and relate in predicted ways to life satisfaction and self-reports of behavior (Cross & Markus, 1991). For example, having a possible self in the area of health was predictive of health-related behaviors in a sample of middle-aged and older adults (Hooker & Kaus, 1992).

Lacking within the possible selves framework, however, is an overarching umbrella or scheme for defining the content of the many possible selves that the individual might have. A hierarchical structure is not implied within this framework, and as yet the model remains highly descriptive. However, the operationalization of the possible selves construct into a relatively straightforward questionnaire measure provides one viable solution to the problem of testability in the identity process model. It may be fruitful, then, to combine elements of both the possible selves and identity process model into a more comprehensive and operationalizable approach.

The process of identity assimilation, viewed in terms of possible selves, would be regarded as the defensive function of maintaining consistency of the self over time and maintaining positive life satisfaction even in the face of failure to realize desired possible selves or avoid dreaded ones. The process of identity accommodation would be comparable to revisions of possible selves when the realization of positive goals is in jeopardy. Providing context for the possible selves would be the individual's identity as it has evolved through psychosocial development in adolescence and adulthood. Ideas about expected events throughout the life-span and revision in age-specific goals would also be seen as proceeding within the context of the life-span construct. An ordering of possible selves in terms of importance would be an important step in altering the methodology of the possible selves model to conform to the propositions of the identity model with its emphasis on a hierarchical or integrated structure.

THE ROLE OF CONTEXT
IN IDENTITY DEVELOPMENT

Thus far, analysis of identity and the self in midlife has focused on inner psycholog-ical processes, the ways in which individuals come to define and modify their self-views through their interactions with the environment in adulthood. Although the phenomenological perspective implied by this approach is consistent with long-standing tradition in personality psychology, a life-span approach to development in the adult years requires the incorporation of contextual factors related to social and historical influences (Haan, Millsap, & Hartka, 1986; Helson & Moane, 1987; VanManen & Whitbourne, 1997). The social and historical context includes events and experiences of daily life that have a direct bearing on the individual, including relations with family members, work involvements, and community participation. Relationships in these domains are a particularly rich source of stimulation for identity development (Slagle, 1992).

Looking at the "experiences" defined within the identity process model, it is necessary to include not only those that the individual perceives as relevant to identity, but those experiences that have a direct impact on the individual's physical and psychological functioning, regardless of how they are perceived. The available literature on the role of context in stimulating identity development must be limited mainly to speculation, as the available research generally focuses not on identity but on variables relating to personality and well-being. In this section, we will describe a general framework in which experiences in adulthood are seen as influencing the individual in direct ways, through their impact on physical and psychological func-tioning, and in indirect ways, through their interaction with identity assimilation and accommodation.

Long-Term Relationships

The family situation presents a major stimulus for development in the middle years. As marital relationships shift with the passing of the decades, some of them ending, the individual is faced with events that must constantly be integrated into the sense of oneself as a loving partner. At the most concrete and direct level, lifestyle factors such as exercise, diet, and the use of cigarettes, alcohol, and other potentially harm-ful substances are often shared within couples. The behavior of the individual's partner may promote either beneficial or harmful exposure to these lifestyle factors. Psychological well-being can also be affected by the moods, behavior, and overall adjustment of an intimate partner. Socially, the ability of a couple who share re-sources to provide for their material needs in comfort through their work involve-ments directly influences the course of their daily lives.

In addition to these direct effects of an intimate partner on the individual's development through adulthood, experiences within the intimate relationship can influence identity by providing a unique source of highly personal information about the self that can stimulate both identity assimilation and accommodation (Whitbourne & Ebmeyer, 1990). Feedback from one's intimate partner can have the most meaning to the individual because it is based on such a long history of interactions and because over this history, partners share vulnerable aspects of the self with each other. The assimilative individual may resist this information, the accommodative individual may become too reliant on it, but in either case, interactions within this context are likely to have a great deal of emotional power and meaning.

Parenting

Outside the intimate relationship, experiences with children serve as influences on the structure and demands of everyday life that have direct bearing on the adult's psychological functioning. Ample evidence exists documenting the impact of children, both favorable and unfavorable, on the psychological well-being of the individual and the parenting couple (Entwistle & Doering, 1981; Koski & Steinberg, 1990; Silverberg & Steinberg, 1987).

Beyond the impact of children on well-being are the many varied influences on the adult's life connected to raising children. Each new development throughout the childhood and adolescent years leads the middle-aged adult parent into new experiences and influences all of which involve the need to learn new parenting skills. New social experiences are also provided through children and their involvements in, for example, childcare, school, athletic teams, and friends.

In addition to these new and varied experiences, the adult's life is also affected by the way that children reflect on the parent's identity and self-esteem (la-Sorsa & Fodor, 1990; Zayas, 1987). Children provide a unique source of information regarding the individual's identity, reflecting both the favorable and unfavorable qualities of the self back onto the parent. To the middle-aged adult whose identity is that of a competent parent, the constant reminders of one's failings, conservatism, and insensitivity by the average adolescent child may present challenges to long-cherished views of the self as a rational and adaptive individual who is in touch with contemporary society. In an attempt to maintain a favorable identity as a parent, the individual may screen the negative feedback provided by a child through identity assimilation. However, the adult may be stimulated to develop a more realistic identity through the process of accommodation, in which this negative feedback is integrated into an overall view of the self as parent. More general knowledge about the self may also be provided by observing "oneself" in one's children.

Work-Related Experiences

Experiences at work have a direct bearing on the middle-aged adult's development through exposure to job-related stress, levels of physical and intellectual activity, and social relationships formed with co-workers (Bruhn, 1989). The individual's economic well-being is also directly linked to the salary provided by the job, and this salary also sets the parameters for many lifestyle factors.

In terms of identity processes, feedback from supervisors, co-workers, and job contacts provides important sources of stimulation for identity assimilation and accommodation to operate in middle adulthood. In keeping with the assumption that individuals attempt to maintain a favorable identity as a competent worker, occupational experiences that contradict this identity will trigger the identity assimilation process to operate as a defense against this negative information. However, countering this process would be the operation of identity accommodation when experiences such as failure to be promoted, negative performance evaluations, and, in drastic cases, job loss become so disconfirming that they can no longer be perceived as consistent with this favorable identity (Merriam, 1987).

Community Activities

Serving as a constant stimulus to development in the middle years are the events encountered as a result of exposure to one's local community. The specific people within one's neighborhood can have particular effects on individuals, as these contacts often serve as the source of new experiences through, for example, local charitable organizations, religious groups, informal sports teams, or groups that pursue particular artistic interests. Locations and relocations of oneself and one's neighbors ensure that these influences are rarely stable over time. Traveling to new places, making new friends through chance acquaintances, and the opening or closing of opportunities all present potential sources of identity development in the long stretch of years between the 30s and the late 60s.

The experiences within the context of one's community also influence the individual through the interpretive template provided by identity in terms of the treatment and regard received from neighbors, members of one's community, and social acquaintances. Gains in respect for the performance of volunteer and community services or activity in hobbies or on sports teams can enhance the individual's identity as a competent and virtuous person. In contrast to experiences within the realms of family and work, though, experiences that have potentially disconfirming information about one's identity in the volunteer realm can be more easily disregarded. However, should the individual consistently be shunned or excluded from participation in these activities, it is possible that identity accommodation may eventually be stimulated so that the individual develops a more realistic self-appraisal.

Social and Historical Context

Historical factors exert a broad set of influences on the individual's well-being both directly, through the impact of social and political policies of one's government, and indirectly, as influences on the nature of the individual's identity style as it evolves from early through middle adulthood.

In general, social and historical events outside the more immediate realm of the individual's home, workplace, and community provide a broad set of influences that can have an impact on the individual's physical and psychological health. For example, in the case of economic recession, the individual's job stability is threatened, and the quality of life may be severely restricted. As mentioned earlier, the loss of a job provides an experience that is discrepant with one's identity as a competent worker and must be dealt with at that level as well. More dramatically, disasters such as earthquakes or fires threaten the security of one's daily existence, and may stimulate a set of related events that alter completely the course of one's life. The prevalence of crime, particularly violent crime, in one's community is another environmental factor that can have as wide an impact as disasters or war, threatening one's life and the well-being of one's family. Of course, living in a district or country that is ravaged by war, famine, and political unrest has countless effects on the adult's quality of life. Involvement in the military when one's country goes to war can radically alter the entire course of one's life through the effect of wartime mobilization on career opportunities, marriage stability, economic resources, and the development of subsequent psychopathology (Elder, Gimbel, & Ivie, 1991; Elder, Pavalko, & Hastings, 1991; Opp, 1987; Pavalko & Elder, 1990).

With regard to identity, experiences involving natural or politically caused disaster can have profound impact on the individual's assumptions about the self and world (Janoff-Bulman, 1992). Early trauma in the context of the family is particularly damaging to the individual's sense of identity, and can have pathological effects throughout the life course (Nash, Hulsey, Sexton, & Harralson, 1993; Van-der-Kolk, 1989).

The social and political climate is a further influence on the individual in that attitudes toward the individual's particular sex, race, ethnic group, or social class can lead to discrimination and the restriction of opportunities (Carlson & Videka-Sherman, 1990). Not only do such experiences detract from the quality of the individual's life, but they also alter the individual's sense of identity (Megwalu, 1990; Myers, Speight, Highlen, & Cox, 1991). Also responsive to the prevailing social and political climate are qualities such as values (Whitbourne et al., 1992) and even the expression of personality traits, generally regarded as insensitive to environmental input (Helson & Wink, 1992; Wink & Helson, 1993).

For example, older black women, both historically and presently, have had to deal with limitations in their socio-environment (Ralston, 1997). Many African-American women have been forced to enter the workforce, often in low paying domestic service jobs, to help provide for their families. They have also been faced with post-slavery America where the dominant society has both overtly and covertly worked to limit their social involvement and economic opportunities. Consequently, it is likely that they have been faced with the need to accommodate these experiences into their identity. Over time, their involvement in these roles (community, family, and work) has left them with the capacities to compensate for their environment and to become productive citizens. However, as these women age, they will be faced with new challenges to their identity. A review of the literature shows that middle-aged and older black women are at risk for health problems. They are more likely to suffer from strokes, cancer, diabetes, and poor nutrition as compared to black males and whites of both sexes. These health problems will present a challenge to the middle-aged black woman who sees herself as active, virile, and productive.

In considering the effect of social and political factors on development, it is also necessary to incorporate the concept of cohort or period effects. The particular period in which one lives one's life reflects predominant views and expectations regarding age, gender, ethnicity, and racial status. Individuals who became adults in the 1950s may have been more likely to develop an assimilative or stable identity style compared to those whose formative years were in the 1960s. Exposure to changing social and historical trends may have a further influence on identity development, however. Even the stable adults of the 1950s may have found themselves questioning their values and beliefs in the tumultuous period of the late 1960s. The "midlife crisis" may, in this regard, be seen in part as a reaction to social trends in the 1970s and early 1980s that encouraged self-exploration and the shedding of dowdy middle-aged trappings.

In the case of gender expectations, attitudes toward women and their involvement in the workplace versus the home in particular have been a critical influence on current cohorts of middle-aged women. For example, the "empty nest" transition, when the last child leaves the home, was found to be stressful in women who had become young adults during the post–World War II years, a time when women were expected to remain full-time homemakers. By contrast, women who became young adults at a time when women were needed to work outside the home during the Depression and World War II found the empty nest transition to be a positive experience (Adelmann, Antonucci, Crohan, & Coleman, 1989). Similarly, the ability of gifted women to reach their potential for success has varied in accordance with the development of more accepting social attitudes toward women's achievements (Schuster, 1990).

The effects of historical context on development in midlife can also be seen in comparisons of parental satisfaction, comparing men born during the Depression and World War II years with men from the "baby boom" cohort. The older cohort of men, who grew to maturity prior to the feminist movement, report themselves to be less involved and satisfied with parenting than the baby boom men. A possible cause of this cohort difference is the impact of the feminist movement. Men who are part of the baby boom generation may have wanted to become more involved with their children or have been encouraged to do so by their working wives, who demanded a more active parenting role from them. An additional factor contributing to the greater involvement of baby boom men with their children may have been dissatisfaction with the parenting that they received from their fathers, members of the Depression–World War II cohort (Carlson & Videka-Sherman, 1990).

RECIPROCAL INFLUENCES ON DEVELOPMENT

This analysis of the factors affecting identity development in midlife has focused on the role of environmental influences in stimulating change in the adult's life as well as the operation of identity processes. This formulation does not, however, address the reciprocal impact of the individual on the environment throughout adulthood (Caspi, Bem, & Elder, 1989). Individuals are not simply passive participants in the events that occur during the middle years but create situations that in turn have an impact on their future development.

The influence of the individual is by necessity most often limited to impact within the specific area of responsibility and control that exists within the individual's domain. Thus, for example, the middle-aged adult may respond to financial limitations because of the performance of the nation's economy (an area over which the average individual has no control) by conscientious reductions of the family budget, and thereby preserve the security of the individual's family. If the adult behaves irresponsibly, the family and the individual will suffer further deprivations. Individuals also have control over the family circumstances they create by choosing a partner, deciding whether and when to have children, and influencing the way those children are raised. The events within the family, then, reflect and further influence the middle-aged adult's identity and sense of well-being. Responses to disasters may also be mediated by the individual's approach to coping with the stress of the trauma, such that a higher sense of self-efficacy regarding the ability to overcome the disaster may mediate otherwise negative outcomes (Murphy, 1988). Finally, in the area of health, individuals make choices about taking steps to prevent the onset of disease in midlife and old age, and these behavioral choices alter whatever inherited predispositions the individual might have to developing that disease. Similarly, the individual can take steps to attempt to slow down or compensate for the normal effects of the aging process on physical and psychological functioning rather than simply wait for these changes to take place (Whitbourne, 1996b).

In exploring the interactive relationship between the individual and the environment in adulthood, it is clear that development in midlife must be viewed as a continuous process within the context of the entire life course. Decisions made in young adulthood have an impact on the experiences that influence the individual in midlife and, similarly, directions begun in midlife set paths of development into old age. The forces that promote continuity include the overarching framework provided by identity, which maintains the consistency of the self over time, as well as the environmental factors of race, occupational status, and educational background. Counteracting the trends toward stability are the unpredictable forces within the environment that affect nation and community, and the changing social trends as translated into cohort influences and effects of historical period. Within the realm of identity, the reactions of others to the individual present new and constantly changing sources of potential alterations in views of the self.

With the many complexities that exist in identifying reciprocal linkages between identity and experiences in family, work, the community, and the broader society, there are many pieces of the puzzle that will need to be specified in future research and theory. As a developmental psychology of midlife begins to emerge, it is clear that suitable models will require an interdisciplinary perspective. Whatever the outcome of this enterprise, it is also clear that an understanding of midlife will bring together models of early development with perspectives on aging to provide a truly life-span view of development.

SUMMARY

The traditional view of midlife as a period of quiescence has been challenged by popular images in the media of the middle years as a period of psychological turmoil. Personality theorists differ in their conceptualizations of midlife, with Erikson's theory having the most direct applicability. Erikson's proposal that intimacy, generativity, and ego integrity represent distinct phases of personality growth can be challenged in that resolution of these psychosocial issues are more appropriately viewed as developmental phases with identity remaining the central process of the self's evolution through the middle and later years of adulthood. A starting point for examining the development of the self in adulthood is a model in which identity is theorized to form an organizing schema through which the individual's experiences are interpreted. Piagetian-like processes of identity assimilation and identity accommodation are theorized to form the basis for the relationship between the individual and experiences in adulthood. Individuals can be differentiated according to the assimilative identity style, the accommodative identity style, or the balanced identity style. Each of the identity styles has associated with it proposed approaches to life experiences in middle adulthood and characteristic problematic patterns of behavior that cause the individual to seek psychotherapy or counseling. Adding to the focus on identity are social-cognitive models of the self including the "life-span construct" and "possible selves."

Contextual factors in midlife must also be considered in theoretical models of the self. The impact of context on identity development includes family relationships, experiences at work, historical and social phenomena, and the social and political climate, factors that vary further by cohort or period. Reciprocal influences must also be considered in any discussion of the development of the self in midlife.

There remain many pieces of the puzzle that will need to be specified in future research and theory. Through an interdisciplinary perspective that incorporates a view of the middle years in terms of the life course as a whole, conceptualizations of adult development will gain in depth and richness to provide an exciting new understanding of the self in midlife.

REFERENCES

Adelmann, P. K., Antonucci, T. C., Crohan, S. E., & Coleman, L. M. (1989). Empty nest, cohort, and employment in the well-being of midlife women. *Sex Roles, 20,* 173–189.

Bruhn, J. G. (1989). Job stress: An opportunity for professional growth. *Career Development Quarterly, 37,* 306–315.

Carlson, B. E., & Videka-Sherman, L. (1990). An empirical test of androgyny in the middle years: Evidence from a national survey. *Sex Roles, 23,* 305–324.

Caspi, A., Bem, D. J., & Elder, G. H. (1989). Continuities and consequences of interactional styles across the life course. *Journal of Personality, 57,* 375–406.

Cattell, R. B. (1982). *The inheritance of personality and ability.* New York: Academic Press.

Conley, J. J. (1985). Longitudinal stability of personality traits: A multitrait-multimethod-multioccasion analysis. *Journal of Personality and Social Psychology, 49,* 1266–1282.

Cross, S., & Markus, H. (1991). Possible selves across the life span. *Human Development, 34,* 230–255.

Elder, G. H., Gimbel, C., & Ivie, R. (1991). Turning points in life: The case of military service and war. *Military Psychology, 3,* 215–231.

Elder, G. H., Pavalko, E. K., & Hastings, T. J. (1991). Talent, history, and the fulfillment of promise. *Psychiatry, 54,* 251–267.

Entwistle, D. R., & Doering, S. G. (1981). *The first birth: A family turning point.* Baltimore MD: Johns Hopkins Press.

Erikson, E. H. (1963). *Childhood and society* (2nd ed.). New York: Norton.

Eysenck, H. J. (1967). *The biological basis of personality.* Springfield, IL: Charles C. Thomas.

Freud, S. (1906/1942). On psychotherapy. In E. Jones (Ed.), *Collected papers.* London: Hogarth Press.

Gould, R. L. (1978). *Transformations: Growth and change in adult life.* New York: Simon & Schuster.

Grotevant, H. D. (1987). Toward a process model of identity formation. *Journal of Adolescent Research, 2,* 203–222.

Haan, N., Millsap, R., & Hartka, E. (1986). As time goes by: Change and stability in personality over fifty years. *Psychology and Aging, 1,* 230–232.

Havighurst, R. (1972). *Developmental tasks and education* (3rd ed.). New York: McKay.

Helson, R., & Moane, G. (1987). Personality change in women from college to midlife. *Journal of Personality and Social Psychology, 53,* 176–186.

Helson, R., & Wink, P. (1992). Personality change in women from the early 40s to the early 50s. *Psychology and Aging, 7,* 46–55.

Hooker, K., & Kaus, C. R. (1992). Possible selves and health behavior in later life. *Journal of Aging and Health, 4,* 390–411.

Hyman, R. B. (1988). Four stages of adulthood: An exploratory study of growth patterns of inner-direction and time-competence in women. *Journal of Research in Personality, 22,* 117–127.

Janoff-Bulman, R. (1992). *Shattered assumptions: Toward a psychology of trauma and victimization.* New York: Free Press.

Josselson, R. (1987). Identity diffusion: A long-term follow-up. *Adolescent Psychiatry, 14,* 230–258.

Jung, C. G. (1968). *Analytical psychology: Its theory and practice.* New York: Vintage Books.

Kahn, S., Zimmerman, G., Czikszentimihalyi, M., & Getzels, J. W. (1985). Relations between identity in young adulthood and intimacy in midlife. *Journal of Personality and Social Psychology, 49,* 1316–1322.

Koski, K. J., & Steinberg, L. (1990). Parenting satisfaction of mothers during midlife. *Journal of Youth and Adolescence, 19,* 465–474.

Kroger, J., & Haslett, S. J. (1991). A comparison of ego identity status transition pathways and change rates across five identity domains. *International Journal of Aging and Human Development, 32,* 303–330.

la-Sorsa, V. A., & Fodor, I. G. (1990). Adolescent daughter/midlife mother dyad: A new look at separation and self-definition. Special Issue: Women at midlife and beyond. *Psychology of Women Quarterly, 14,* 593–606.

Levinson, D. J., Darrow, C. N., Klein, E. B., Levinson, M. H., & McKee, B. (1978). *The seasons of a man's life.* New York: Knopf.

Marcia, J. E. (1966). Development and validation of ego-identity status. *Journal of Personality and Social Psychology, 3,* 551–558.

Markus, H., & Nurius, P. (1986). Possible selves. *American Psychologist, 41,* 954–969.

Maslow, A. (1962). *Toward a psychology of being.* Princeton, NJ: Van Nostrand Reinhold.

McCrae, R. R., & Costa, P. T. J. (1990). *Personality in adulthood.* New York: Guilford.

Megwalu, H. R. (1990). Black identity development: An international perspective. *Journal of African Psychology, 1,* 9–14.

Merriam, S. B. (1987). Young, middle, and preretirement adults' experiences with retraining after job loss. *Educational Gerontology, 13,* 249–262.

Murphy, S. A. (1988). Mediating effects of intrapersonal and social support on mental health 1 and 3 years after a natural disaster. *Journal of Traumatic Stress, 1,* 155–172.

Myers, L. J., Speight, S. L., Highlen, P. S., & Cox, C. I. (1991). Identity development and worldview toward an optimal conceptualization. Special Issue: Multiculturalism as a fourth force in counseling. *Journal of Counseling and Development, 70,* 54–63.

Nash, M. R., Hulsey, T. L., Sexton, M. C., Harralson, T. L., & Lambert, W. (1993). Long-term sequelae of childhood sexual abuse: Perceived family environment, psychopathology, and dissociation. *Journal of Consulting and Clinical Psychology, 61,* 276–283.

Nemiroff, R. A., & Colarusso, C. A. (1985). *The race against time: Psychotherapy and psychoanalysis in the half of life.* New York: Plenum.

Opp, L. (1987). Normative mid-life concerns among Vietnam veterans with post-traumatic stress disorders: Some preliminary empirical findings. *Journal of Contemporary Psychotherapy, 17,* 174–194.

Pavalko, E. K., & Elder, G. H. (1990). World War II and divorce: A life-course perspective. *American Journal of Sociology, 95,* 1213–1234.

Piaget, J. (1975/1977). *The development of thought* (A. Rosin, Trans.). Oxford: Basil Blackwell.

Ralston, P. A. (1997). Midlife and older black women. In J. M. Coyle (Ed.), *Handbook on Women and Aging* (pp. 273–289). Westport, CT: Greenwood.

Rogers, C. R. (1961). *On becoming a person.* Boston: Houghton Mifflin.

Ryff, C. D. (1991). Possible selves in adulthood and old age: A tale of shifting horizons. *Psychology and Aging, 6,* 286–295.

Sadavoy, J., & Leszcz, M. (1987). *Treating the elderly with psychotherapy: The scope for change in later life.* Madison, CT: International Universities Press.

Schaie, K. W. (1977–1978). Toward a stage theory of adult cognitive development. *Journal of Aging and Human Development, 8,* 129–138.

Schuster, D. T. (1990). Fulfillment of potential, life satisfaction, and competence: Comparing four cohorts of gifted women at midlife. *Journal of Educational Psychology, 82,* 471–478.

Silverberg, S. B., & Steinberg, L. (1987). Adolescent autonomy, parent-adolescent conflict, and parental well-being. *Journal of Youth and Adolescence, 16,* 293–312.

Slagle, S. J. (1992). Critical developments in early and middle adulthood: Implications for psychoanalysis with a case illustration. *Psychoanalysis and Psychotherapy, 10,* 33–57.

Tesch, S. A., & Cameron, K. A. (1987). Openness to experience and development of adult identity. *Journal of Personality, 55,* 615–630.

Tesch, S. A., & Whitbourne, S. K. (1982). Intimacy and identity status in young adults. *Journal of Personality and Social Psychology, 43,* 1041–1051.

Vaillant, G. E. (1977). *Adaptation to life.* Boston: Little, Brown.

Van-der-Kolk, B. A. (1989). The compulsion to repeat the trauma: Re-enactment, revictimization, and masochism. *Psychiatric Clinics of North America, 12,* 389–411.

VanManen, K.-J., & Whitbourne, S. K. (1997). Psychosocial development and life events in adulthood. *Psychology and Aging, 12,* 239–246.

Whitbourne, S. K. (1985). The psychological construction of the life span. In J. E. Birren & K. W. Schaie (Eds.), *Handbook of the psychology of aging* (pp. 594–618). New York: Van Nostrand Reinhold.

Whitbourne, S. K. (1986a). *Adult development.* New York: Praeger.

Whitbourne, S. K. (1986b). *The me I know: A study of adult identity.* New York: Springer Verlag.

Whitbourne, S. K. (1986c). Openness to experience, identity flexibility, and life change in adults. *Journal of Personality and Social Psychology, 50,* 163–168.

Whitbourne, S. K. (1987). Personality development in adulthood and old age: Relationships among identity style, health, and well-being. In K. W. Schaie (Ed.), *Annual Review of Gerontology and Geriatrics* (pp. 189–216). New York: Springer.

Whitbourne, S. K. (1996a). *The aging individual: Physical and psychological perspectives.* New York: Springer.

Whitbourne, S. K., & Dannefer, W. D. (1985–1986). The life drawing as a measure of time perspective in adulthood. *International Journal of Aging and Human Development, 22,* 147–155.

Whitbourne, S. K., & Ebmeyer, J. B. (1990). *Identity and intimacy in marriage: A study of couples.* New York: Springer Verlag.

Whitbourne, S. K., & Powers, C. B. (1994). Older women's constructs about their lives: A quantitative and qualitative exploration. *International Journal of Aging and Human Development, 38,* 293–306.

Whitbourne, S. K. (1996b). Psychological perspectives on the normal aging process. In L. L. Carstensen & B. A. Edelstein (Eds.), *Handbook of the practice of clinical gerontology* (pp. 3–35). Beverly Hills, CA: Sage Publishers.

Whitbourne, S. K., & VanManen, K.-J. (1996). Age differences and predictors of identity status in adulthood. *Journal of Adult Development, 3,* 59–70.

Whitbourne, S. K., Zuschlag, M. K., Elliot, L. B., & Waterman, A. S. (1992). Psychosocial development in adulthood: A 22-year sequential study. *Journal of Personality and Social Psychology, 63,* 260–271.

Wink, P., & Helson, R. (1993). Personality change in women and their partners. *Journal of Personality and Social Psychology, 65,* 597–605.

Zayas, L. H. (1987). Psychodynamic and developmental aspects of expectant and new fatherhood: Clinical derivatives from the literature. *Clinical Social Work Journal, 15,* 8–21.

The Midlife Crisis Revisited

Stanley D. Rosenberg and Harriet J. Rosenberg

Dartmouth Medical School, Lebanon, New Hampshire

Michael P. Farrell

State University of New York at Buffalo, Buffalo, New York

INTRODUCTION

The task of "revisiting the midlife crisis" is a little like being asked to write a ghost story. The phantom has already, for example, had an extensive series of eulogies and postmortem examinations. Susan Whitbourne, in a thorough review, discusses the concept as pure figment, representing it as a sort of collective "fantasy" concocted by middle-aged white males for middle-aged white males (1986). Chapters and reviews by Chiriboga (1989a,b), Hunter and Sundel (1989), McCrae and Costa (1990), and Schaie and Willis (1986), have come to remarkably consistent conclusions: the empirical evidence in support of the concept of a general midlife crisis is so thin as to be absolutely ethereal. Some of these reviews have even credited our group (Farrell & Rosenberg, 1981a, 1981b; Rosenberg & Farrell, 1976) with helping to slay the offending hypothesis, or at least driving some of the nails into its coffin. However, like another famous ghost (Shakespeare's Banquo) the midlife crisis has the disquieting habit of reappearing from time to time, and even still draws an audience. Like most reappearing specters, it seems to have a story that it is attempting to convey, and perhaps a need to correct some misunderstandings. We would like to borrow from another Shakespearean plot and exercise the somewhat perverse

47

option of not coming to bury the corpse, but rather to praise it; that is, we would like to suggest that there is value in relistening to the story of the midlife crisis.

In this chapter, we revisit midlife crisis theory in several different ways. First, we reexamine the concept, particularly as it emerged in the 1960s and 1970s in the social science literature. Second, because the previously cited reviews have been so comprehensive, we discuss only briefly some of the research that called the theory into question. Third, we also revisit a group of men and their families whom we had first studied in the early 1970s in an attempt to assess the impact of the midlife transition. We have continued following trajectories of change in this sample as they have progressed from early to later middle age. This journey has enabled us to revisit our own thinking about midlife processes as represented in *Men at Midlife* (Farrell & Rosenberg, 1981a), and led us to begin reconceptualizing the midlife crisis from the framework of narrative psychology.

Emergent conceptualizations in narrative psychology, and their application to life-span development, appear to offer a compelling way to order the results of 20 years of theorizing and research on midlife crises. The evolving paradigm of narrative psychology, which has been buttressed by developments in the philosophy of science, has helped to underline the centrality of the "story" in shaping scientific theory (Landau, 1991; Suppe, 1974) as well as everyday experience. Like much in psychology, this way of understanding the role of narratives harks back to William James's (1897) observation that scientific theories "proceed from our indomitable desire to cast the world into a more rational shape in our minds than the crude order of our experience." This principle, as current research in memory and cognition shows, is perhaps nowhere more true than in the area of personal history. We develop and express our understandings and explanations of ourselves through stories, those deep structures that organize specific narratives. Despite some important statements in this area, for example, Propp's (1928/1968) *Morphology of the Folktale,* no definitive glossary of story types has yet been specified. However, there is considerable agreement that people utilize a rather limited set of story lines, often drawing on actions and character types from mythology, folktales, and legend, in narrating personal history. At the levels of characterization, ideology, and causal explanation, stories must also fit within culturally shared frames. The midlife crisis can be viewed as one such story, and can become, in Lakoff and Johnson's terminology, one of the "metaphors we live by" (1980).

THE MIDLIFE CRISIS STORY IN THE 1960s AND 1970s

An Identity Crisis

Although it can be difficult to describe a chimera, the midlife crisis once had (or at least seemed to have) fairly recognizable dimensions; that is, like love (another great illusion, according to Freud), people recognized it when they saw it. The midlife crisis was not a professional crisis, nor a marital crisis, nor an economic crisis, although these surface manifestations could certainly signal its presence. "Midlife crisis theory," as it emerged in the 1970s, was less a paradigm than a set of beliefs or assumptions about the relation between the subject's experience of self (generally, although not always explicitly, as conveyed in life story accounts) and correlative attitudes, symptoms, and personality dimensions. The end of young adulthood and the beginning of middle age was thought to produce a reevaluation of the self, and (potentially) accompanying symptoms of depression, anxiety, and manic flight. Although there were many variants represented, a true midlife crisis, circa the 1960s and 1970s literature, was, first and foremost, a crisis of identity, and such crises were almost always attributed to males; that is, midlife was frequently portrayed, in both popular and scholarly literature, as a time of dramatic personality change and life review. As a predictable life stage event, it was thought to include increased introspection, a realization of time passing (mortality, generativity concerns), and focus on opportunities lost (sexual, relational, occupational). Symptomatic changes in behavior including increased substance abuse, divorce, and suicide were alleged and later disproved empirically. It was a concept reflective of the shifting ideological and explanatory frameworks characteristic of the late 1960s and early 1970s: an era that included a culture of alienation, questioning of societal norms, and a burgeoning of alternate lifestyles (Rosenberg, 1976; Rosenberg & Bergen, 1976). The notion of a universal midlife crisis was compelling; it provided a rationale for perceived despair, an opportunity/justification for lifestyle change. It was a notion conceived in an era when much of the popular culture, and most especially the youth culture, questioned the value of living one's life to achieve a socially validated identity. While Erikson (1950) had argued for a psychological ideal whereby the developing adult found authenticity by expressing his or her innermost self through enactment of social roles in a culture that made sense, the "midlife crisis" represented a repudiation of that ideal. In "A Culture of Discontent" (Rosenberg, 1976), the very idea that authenticity could be found, except in opposition to a dehumanizing, irrational society, was seen as absurd. In the midlife crisis of theater, film, and novel (Updike, Heller, Vonnegut), the dramatic action was launched by the protagonist's "awakening" to the perception that his earlier life, structured around the pursuit of identity, was a kind of madness or self-deception (Rosenberg & Farrell, 1976). If the culture was unmasked by the reported atrocities of Vietnam, what internal value could be served by finding a place in that system? At the same time, the crisis concept allowed hope for personal development, for a new synthesis between a reworked personality and a revamped life course. If conventional, conformist approaches to fulfillment and authenticity were bogus, crisis protagonists were still portrayed as finding freedom and rebirth once they dared to throw off the shackles of conventional identity. Of course, this idea evoked fear as well as fascination. The specter loomed: the midlife crisis could lead to catastrophic risk taking or it could offer an opportunity to create a more satisfactory self.

Testing the Midlife Crisis Theory

The problem of translating these ideas into more formal theory was that the core claims associated with, or derivative of, the midlife crisis construct were misunderstood. In the several excellent reviews referred to above, for example, there seems to be less than perfect agreement as to what the "midlife as crisis" model consisted of; what its conceptual roots may have been, and what sort of empirical tests were required to confirm or disconfirm its validity. This is partially due to the fact that midlife crisis theory represents a fuzzy set, with some reviewers, for example, seeing the work of Elliot Jaques (1965) as seminal and others not even referencing it. Various writers have either emphasized or ignored Jung's (1923, 1950/1959) theory of adult developmental change as a point of embarkation for midlife crisis theory. The core group of crisis theorists to whom virtually all reviewers refer consists of Daniel Levinson (Levinson, Darrow, Klein, Levinson, & McKee, 1978), Roger Gould (1978), and George Vaillant (1977). Although all can be characterized as ego psychologists, Levinson's approach was the most singularly rooted in Erikson's (1950) conception of crisis in development. Vaillant, on the other hand, can be seen as an outlier in this group in that he describes multiple paths of development, not all of which involve crisis in the midlife period. Unfortunately, the proponents of crisis theory were neither always terribly explicit nor necessarily in agreement with one another on the major points of the model. Clearly, each of the three writers viewed the male midlife experience through a somewhat different lens. For a fuller explication of each of these theorists, and the differences among them, see Whitbourne and Weinstock (1986, pp. 229–244).

Perhaps most crucially, the domain of validity to which the midlife crisis should be applied was not specified in the 1970s. Was it a unitary phenomenon across time and cultures, genders, classes, kinship structures, and so on? What aspects of personality, psychopathology, or behavior should be affected by the crisis, and in what ways? A central theme in the various crisis theories could, however, be identified. It was that of temporality in Heideger's sense; that is, temporality as being toward death (1979). The intrusion of the awareness of death, of personal finitude, was the triggering mechanism of the midlife crisis not only in Jaques's seminal thesis, but also in the major conceptualizations and empirical studies that followed. This unifying thematic of awareness of death becomes particularly relevant in light of the fact that temporality has also been seen, in a quite different tradition, as the defining property of narrative. Indeed, temporal ordering is an absolute requirement for a coherent text, and for an acceptable autobiographic account. We will return to this point shortly, and it will represent the basis of our attempt to reconstruct the midlife crisis hypothesis in terms more congruent both with current theoretical trends in the study of personality and with the existent data on midlife change.

Crisis Theory as Survivor

Since the 1960s, efforts at empirical verification of the midlife crisis as a universal, or very common, developmental experience, have consistently produced negative results. However, despite this apparently negative evidence, both popular and scientific writers continue to employ the midlife crisis as a descriptive and explanatory construct. The persistence of this ghost is itself a social and psychological phenomenon that must be accounted for. We will argue that it is based on three sets of factors. First, midlife crisis "theory" has spawned more refined, second-generation research on stress and coping in relation to socially conditioned, age grade changes in specific areas such as work and family life. It has survived in the form of the midlife squeeze hypothesis (Chiriboga, 1989b; Farrell & Barnes, 1994; Pearlin, 1985; Silverberg & Steinberg, 1990). Second, the midlife crisis is a social myth, embodying well-established age grade stereotypes, for example, terms like "male menopause," fictional images like those represented in *Death of a Salesman,* or biographically derived examples, like Gauguin running off to the South Seas. The widely believed idea of midlife as crisis may also reflect our attempts to account for general feelings of alienation or strain in the culture. The experiences of loss, stress, or strain and consequent efforts at reorganization, can be fairly ubiquitous throughout the adult life-span and across various historical time periods. Although such events may be randomly distributed in early and middle adulthood, memory functions to organize experience around specific plot lines or markers that carry explanatory value. This is part of the narratory principle (Sarbin, 1986), which we describe below. This principle would predict the propensity of the person, or those in his life space, to cognitively distort a fluctuating pattern of distress or alienation from current roles as constituting a "midlife crisis." Indeed, this sobriquet is glibly applied to moments in the lives of men in their 30s, 40s, and 50s, with little concern for plotting real variations in subjective distress or for matching the symptoms with a specified syndrome.

Third, and most central to this discussion, midlife crisis may be a fairly common experience at one level of psychological development—the level of narrative identity. All three factors that appear to sustain the concept, despite its shortcomings, derive from a common process: the midlife crisis is a good story; that is, it fulfills the basic narrative requirements of "reportability" (Labov, 1972), "dramatic engagement" (Gergen & Gergen, 1989), and utilization of culturally supported explanatory systems. Reportability refers to the fact that crisis is unusual in some way, or that it runs counter to everyday expectations. Dramatic engagement is engendered by nongradual change, or movement away from a stable state narrative. Crisis stories thus engage the audience in a way that a stability story could not. If the subject told his "story" as represented in Costa and McCrae's studies (1976, 1978, 1980a, 1980b), which emphasize trait stability through adulthood, for example, it would not be a tellable narrative: "I really haven't changed at all for years and years and years. My basic personality and way of responding to things is quite stable. While

I've had some minor ups and downs, like backaches and job stagnation, I've never had a real crisis or turning point to talk of. . . ." Although this may well be the modal experience, it lacks a certain dramatic flair. Aside from being an engaging story, the midlife crisis fits well with folk psychologic beliefs about the meaning of aging to men, and their ways of dealing with life events. From Updike's *Rabbit* (1960), to Woody Allen's characters in *Manhattan* and *A Midsummer Night's Sex Comedy,* men's stereotypic responses to the narcissistic losses of middle age make good drama.

MIDLIFE CRISIS AS PERSONAL MYTH: THE EMERGENCE OF NARRATIVE PSYCHOLOGY

The midlife crisis does not pass empirical muster as a psychiatric syndrome, a biologically determined event, nor a developmental inevitability. It is, rather, a socially mediated fantasy, or personal myth that is manifest in what is commonly called a "life story." In other words, the reality of the midlife crisis may reside at the level of a narrative form that provides the person with a way of shaping and understanding the events and experiences that constitute the flux of his or her life. There is increasing evidence that people strive to make sense of who they are and where they fit in the world by organizing their personal histories around story structures (Linde, 1993). The midlife crisis represents a core story or plot line around which the personal narrative might be constructed at a particular point in the adult lifespan. As a deep structure, it is quite flexible, and can be used to organize a broad set of narrative variations.

The midlife crisis narrative(s), which emerged in the works of Levinson, Gould, and Vaillant, draw partially from relatively universal archetypes. They also constitute story lines grounded in a particular time and space in history and the particular understandings of selfhood that reside in that time and place. The post–World War II economy was one filled with economic expansion, unprecedented levels of upward mobility, and an increasingly emphatic view of the person as an autonomous, self-determining entity who could blaze a unique and glorious path through the forest of opportunities that lay waiting for him or her. By the late 1950s and 1960s, Erik Erikson emerged as the most articulate codifier of this view of selfhood and adult development, and the midlife crisis model was cast in Eriksonian (Erikson, 1950, 1959) terms. Although he portrayed the "identity crisis" as an adolescent phenomenon, the term and the concept were clearly exported in both the popular and scholarly literature to other life stages. A variety of disruptions in self-concept and psychological well-being were "explained" in terms of Erikson's ego-psychologic view of the self and the identity struggles he identified with adolescence.

Thus, the Eriksonian concept of the adolescent identity crisis (itself a kind of fantasy or metaphor) was, in much of the midlife crisis literature, extended to midlife developmental processes as well. The midlife crisis was often explicitly described as a kind of second adolescence. In both instances, the fact that the "crisis" was essentially a movement within a narrative, or a shift in narrative tone, was misunderstood. The term "identity crisis" was never meant to refer to a description of an easily operationalized set of behaviors nor to alterations of "personality" as otherwise measured. Rather, it referred to a highly subjective, subtle set of changes in internal organization, object and self representations, and feeling states. This confusion over operationalization was partially attributable to the fact that behavioral scientists had not in the 1970s, by and large, developed the conceptual and methodologic tools to articulate and examine the narrative dimension of personality. Only more recently, led by the efforts of Bruner (1986), Gergen (1977, 1980), Sarbin (1986), and Spence (1982), has the narrative dimension of self-construction, as much as the stability or change of core psychological traits, coping style, or affective state, come to be recognized as a primary dimension of life-span development. McAdams (1993, 1994), following Hogan (1987), McClelland (1951), and others has argued that personality can be conceptualized at three distinct levels: (1) dispositional traits, (2) personal concerns, and (3) life narrative. Midlife crisis theory was a Level 2 model, primarily derived from Level 3 data (life story type interviews), which was largely tested with variables and research designs that tapped Levels 1 and 2. Recent work in lifespan developmental psychology emphasizes the role of narrative in the construction and maintenance of identity (Bruner, 1986; Cohler, 1982; Gergen & Gergen, 1989, McAdams, 1985, Sarbin, 1986). This emergent constructivist paradigm views the development of the self as essentially a process of life story construction (Howard, 1991). Following Ricoeur (1981), these writers have also focused on temporality as the "ultimate referent" of narrativity (p. 165), and concomitantly on employment as the defining characteristic of the "good" life story. Narrative psychology offers us at least three ways of understanding the midlife crisis: (1) the midlife crisis is an archetypal story or plot line that functions as a sort of scaffolding for the construction of the individual life story; (2) midlife may be correlated with systematic changes in dimensions of personal narrative, such as perspective or affective tone; and (3) the midlife crisis may be conceptualized as a narrative crisis in the sense that midlife events or experiences coalesce to render the narrator unable to produce a coherent, continuous life story text. To the extent that the "self" is experienced as or is manifest in the life story, such narrative foreclosure would be a subjective crisis of great intensity.

First, in the most direct application of the narrative framework, we can characterize the midlife crisis as a story genre, one with very deep roots in Western culture. Dante's *Divine Comedy* provides the outline of this story: "In the middle of the journey of our life, I came to myself within a dark wood where the straight way was lost. Ah, how hard it is to tell of that wood, savage and harsh and dense . . . So bitter is it that death is hardly more." Dante's story is an instance of what Propp (1928/ 1968) would call a heroic tale. These always involve a hero embarking on a journey of transformation. In heroic tales, the protagonist is sent on or equipped for his journey by a "helper" or causal agent, and he must undergo tests in which he is either defeated or is able to transcend to a higher state. In Dante's story, the helper is death or its shadow, temporality (awareness of finitude). Although this deep structure can support multiple variations, its defining elements in contemporary life stories appear to include a profound sense of disenchantment, signaling that the previous state of stability or stagnation has been disrupted by the arrival of the helper: awareness of personal mortality. At the surface level of midlife crisis stories, previously chosen commitments come to be experienced as problematic or invalid. This perception is associated with intense psychic pain, but also with a somewhat inchoate sense that the experience cannot be fully described nor understood. Imagery of death and rebirth are common story elements, and these are also tied to visual and spatial metaphors of life as journey/quest played out on a horizon of finite time.

This way of understanding midlife crises is most congruent with the specific narrative psychology perspective articulated by Gergen and Gergen (1987). Gergen and Gergen argue that people must draw on basic narrative forms, such as tragedy, romantic epic, or comedy to understand and represent their lives and, concomitantly, to reflect their identity or moral character. The midlife crisis contains a time-specific (the middle of the journey) plot alteration they would characterize as a precipitant to a regressive movement, that is, movement toward a negative state. Regressive movements may crystallize into more permanent decline, in which case they would represent tragic plots. Alternatively, regression may give way to reversal and progression, the sequence characteristic of romantic or heroic sagas. These two plots were clearly manifest both in the popular and literary representations of midlife crisis, and in the interview (i.e., life story) data on which the work of Levinson, Gould, and Vaillant was largely based.

McAdams (1993) provides an alternative series of observations on the intersect between midlife and what he describes as "personal myths," his term for the deep structures that organize life stories. McAdams argues that "for many . . . adults the forties can be a time of reassessment and revision of the life story . . . [and can] involve significant changes in self-understanding that may have profound implications for mythmaking" (pp. 198–199). Citing a number of studies on aging, he contends that the 40s mark a move from a "youthful, passionate perspective" to a "tempered, refined, philosophical orientation" (p. 199). The contextualization of thought, movement toward postformal thought, confrontation of opposites, and apprehension of a sense of an ending [i.e., temporality] are seen by McAdams as the "four cardinal features" that color personal narrative in the fourth decade. More generally, McAdams argues that identity is not a concern limited to adolescence and young adulthood. Rather, he sees it as an issue of concern throughout the adult life-span that is reflected in continuing efforts at narrative maintenance and narrative revision (1993). He outlines seven features or dimensions along which life stories or personal narratives might be assessed. These include narrative tone (e.g., optimism vs. pessimism); imagery (characteristic symbols or metaphors); themes (e.g., autonomy or intimacy); ideological setting (prevailing values or beliefs in context); nuclear episodes (including climactic or defining moments); character (especially key images that function as idealized self-representations), and ending (1993). Crisis, from the point of view of this model, would appear to involve moments of radical revision or change on one or more of these dimensions. The hypothesis that specific narrative shifts, or change itself, are more probable at midlife than at other moments in the adult life-span has not yet been tested with an adequate longitudinal design.

THE STUDIES

Life story data from our own longitudinal studies of men in middle adulthood (Farrell, Rosenberg, & Rosenberg, 1993; Rosenberg, 1991; Rosenberg, Rosenberg, & Farrell, 1992) suggest still another way in which the perspective of narrative psychology may be useful in examining the concept of midlife crisis. The data for analysis come from a two-part longitudinal study of men and their families prior to and after launching their children.[1] At Time 1 (1971–1974) we surveyed a representative sample of 300 middle-aged men (ages 38–48) and 150 young men (ages 23–33) from both urban and rural New England. Our studies utilized a large cross-sectional design combining survey data and intensive semistructured interviews with both subjects and collaterals to support or disprove the notion of a universal crisis of middle age. Out of the larger sample, 20 men and their families were selected for both extended individual and whole family interviews. In the course of these contacts, a considerable amount of "hard" data was collected about each man (e.g., demographic information, measures of personality, attitudes, and health), as well as lengthy individual and family oral histories, which explored their relationships, beliefs, feelings, and aspirations. The 20 intensive study subjects spanned a broad range in terms of such standard demographic and psychological variables as education, occupation, ethnicity, marital status, and self-reported personality characteristics. They thus exhibited much variation in the nature of their responses to the midlife transition. In our book, *Men at Midlife,* (Farrell & Rosenberg, 1981a), we discussed the many patterns of response to middle adulthood that we found and concluded that there is not a common pattern of midlife crisis in men. Our assumption was that because life circumstances and psychological characteristics differed considerably for individuals, the particular mixture of these two variables would override general life tasks, stresses, and expectations of middle age and result in different response patterns. Indeed, we discovered that the normative reaction of our male subjects was neither despair nor elation, but rather a tendency to deny and avoid pressures and stressors. Rather than painful introspection, or conscious confrontation of negative occurrences, our study subjects attempted to distance and

[1]The authors wish to express thanks to Madelyn Schmitt, Karlana Carpen, Anne Boedecker, Sue Hagerman, and Debra Horowski for help in conducting interviews.

maintain their preferred version of reality as long as possible. A man's response to middle age, as well as his response to other periods of adult life, appeared to depend on the meaning he attributed to personal life events and his experiential understanding of them. This understanding or meaning evolved not only from an internal self that had a personal history and a specific psychological makeup but a self that was also a product of external forces. How a man understands himself and his life is partially dependent on his interactions in an intimate world of significant others, a world that also contains values, attitudes, and expectations about what it is to be an adult male.

Interviews with the 20 men and their families were videotaped and sound recorded in their homes and in our research offices. Families were first interviewed together and asked to tell about the major eras in their family life. Then each family member was interviewed alone. Fathers and mothers were asked to provide an overview of their own life stories and also to tell the story of their lives in their current marriages. Children were asked to tell about personal and familial history, as well as about their relationships to their parents. At Time 2 (1984–1985), 17 of the original group of men were reinterviewed in the standard life story format ("tell me about your life since . . .") and then in a joint session with wives and available children. Family members were also interviewed separately to comment on the group discussion, while grown children who had left the family were later contacted for individual interviews. This design has provided us with two parallel sets of narratives, collected approximately 12 to 13 years apart, permitting us to observe changes in the dominant thematics, style, and structure of these oral texts.

It should be acknowledged that the relationship between identity or sense of self and the oral texts to be examined is surely somewhat problematic. Such variables as defensiveness, dissimulation, or mood-driven variability in self-representation may all influence the form and content of the life story. Even to the extent that one grants some commitment to sincerity, the subject's access to more intimate aspects of self, to intentions and desires, cannot be assumed. The vulnerability of everyday memory to decay and distortion, the mundane and ubiquitous neurotic processes of repression, displacement, and denial, the (perhaps) pervasive proclivity to live through a false self (Lacan, 1977), all render quite problematic any postulated relationship between the life story and the speaker's "self" or "identity." This would be true even in the most ideal situation, where no "noise" is introduced into the discourse by the speaker's perception, beliefs, and feelings about the interviewer as audience. For these reasons, the psychoanalytic situation, particularly the technique of free association, has been privileged, perhaps with some justification, as the only appropriate context for bringing forth an authentic text of identity.

However, the narrative approach to life-span development has questioned this privilege, arguing that: "Not just the dialogue of the clinical situation, but also discourse among persons more generally . . . may be regarded as narrative to be interpreted in a manner analogous to the free associations of the analysand. Application of the psychoanalytic approach to the study of wishes and intents outside of the clinical situation . . . provides event narratives similar in some respects to those of the psychoanalytic interview" (Cohler, 1982, p. 209). While asserting this principle of textual equivalence does not make it so, a number of cogent arguments can be offered for the use of generic life story texts in studying the evolution of self representation over time. On one level, we may question the nature of the psychoanalytic narrative or case history. Schimek (1975), for example, has illustrated that the analyst does not "discover" or "uncover" a latent personal narrative but rather constructs a plausible narrative based on evidence (i.e., transference material), which can be constructed as a plausible life story only through acceptance of the Freudian metatheory and through the authority of the figure of the analyst. Although more reflexive personal narratives, offered in response to requests to describe or explain one's self, may strike us as more or less profound or more or less adequate, they may also have the advantage of adhering more closely to the phenomenology of everyday life. Such textual presentations of self are a constituent part of social life, and we are compelled, for both internal and external reasons, to engage in the sort of meaning making that permits us to (at least potentially) provide answers to the underlying questions the life story must address: Who am I? and How have I become the person I am? Most adult developmental theorists (see Cohler, 1982, pp. 206–207), as well as sociolinguists (e.g., Linde, 1993; Tonkin, 1992) assume that the individual must have viable answers to these questions, as manifested in the narrative intelligibility of his/her accounts.

Time 1 Narratives

We try here to describe some of the changes we have found as our study subjects have moved from early to late middle age, and some of the questions these shifts point to about personal narrative, and the impact of family culture (or collective narratives) on adult identity and crises. It may be helpful to briefly review some major aspects of our subjects' narratives in early middle age (Time 1). As we have already noted, in the analysis of the earlier life stories, as well as more conventional attitudinal, state, and trait measures (Farrell & Rosenberg, 1981a), we found little support for the then prominent "crisis" model. The disruption of identity and life structure at the point of the midlife transition did not appear to be a normative event. While we examined a variety of pathology and change parameters in our large community sample of men, we were particularly interested in testing Elliot Jaques's (1965) hypotheses regarding a variety of depressive reactions evoked in this life stage. Jaques, too, used various forms of narrative (poetry, painting, fiction) in his attempts to understand midlife processes. Studying the life and works of ". . . 310 painters, composers, poets, writers . . . of undoubted greatness or of genius" (p. 502), Jaques speculated that this crisis was a developmental inevitability, triggered by the intruding awareness of mortality and finitude. This confrontation with one's own finitude, he further argued, nullifies the manic defensive posture of early adulthood ("doing" as a defense against feeling), leading also to the resurfacing of the repressed and denied awareness of the destructive, hateful side of human nature. For some, this shift in temporal perspective, experiencing their lives as more than half completed, rendered narrative impossible. Rossini's life is perhaps the exemplar of this pattern: "'His comparative silence during the period 1832–1868 (i.e., from 40 to his death at 74) makes his biography like the narrative of two lives, swift triumph, and a long life of seclusion'" (p. 502). In other cases, themes of unselfconscious optimism and mastery gave way to preoccupation with death, impotence, and despair.

Our first phase study subjects, those in their early 40s, did not provide life stories dominated by depressive thematics, but rather exhibited a variety of affective tones to individual and family life stories. Some portrayed a powerful sense of mastery and gratification. This is not to say that we found stories filled with descriptions of universal satisfaction. Rather, we found that a number of variables, including social class, marital status, and family situation, all affected narrative self-representation, and that crisislike episodes or themes were as common in "young adult" as in "midlife" males.

We also found little confirmation for other hypotheses linking gender to narrative characteristics as related to life stage. The narratives of men in early midlife were not nearly so focused on the "career imperative" (Neugarten, 1968) as had been suggested, nor were women as concerned about empty nest issues. We described an apparent shift in predominant identity issues and the familial story whereby the men exhibited an increased emphasis on the parental role in their personal narratives. Women's life stories in this period contained much more positive assessment about the movement toward a postparental stage, and the opportunity for expanded involvement in extrafamilial roles. The men's increasing emphasis on the importance of the family as the anchor of emotional well-being; their anxious and prideful investment in children's successes and failures; their protective concerns about neighbors and schoolmates as potential threats or contaminants, were quite congruent with the identity structure Gutmann (1987) has called the "parental imperative." He has argued for the universality of an equation between the adult self and parenthood, observing that among unprompted Navajo, Mayan, and Druze informants ". . . the parental theme in the lives of [men] . . . in their thirties and forties is stunningly clear. Time and again . . . male subjects linked their pleasures, complaints, and remedies to their situations as parents and to the welfare of their families" (p. 188).

Large-scale longitudinal studies in our own culture, which can be characterized as relatively contraparental, confirm the significance of these thematics in personal narratives at culturally scripted life stages. Lowenthal, Thurnher, and Chiriboga (1975) report that "family centeredness is a dominant theme" in men's life stories, and that parenthood is a central aspiration in young adulthood.

Gutmann describes this shift to parenthood as the central aspect of identity for most adults across a variety of historical and cultural contexts. In its tone, content, and pervasiveness in self-narrative, it has the quality of a "chronic emergency," which requires no less than a reshaping of self. From the narrative or life story perspective, we would say that cultural scripts require and support this evolution in self-characterization. Preparental men enact a role slot by telling life stories filled with hedonism, aggression, and power; parenthood signals a narrative shift to roles characterized by self control, sense of community, and the weight of responsibility. Both mothers and fathers are observed to relinquish this story emphasis on their own narcissistic strivings: ". . . the conjugal couple routinely and, if things have gone as they should, automatically surrender a large piece of their narcissistic claims to personal omnipotentiality and immortality, conceding these instead to the child" (1987, p. 198). This displacement of narcissistic strivings, as we will see, has profound effects on the family's later rendering of its own history and its own identity; that is, as parenthood comes to be experienced as the central aspect of self, family narratives come increasingly to be built around a particular plot line: "Part of the ethos of this culture is to assume that a more or less favorable outcome in the child's future life is a direct result of the quality of parenting" (Cohler, 1982, p. 221).

We also noted a clear trend in the earlier narratives for description of a power shift in the family group. Families reported a diminution of paternal authority and patterns of alliance and collusion between mothers and children; that is, the father's position of dominance was not openly challenged, nor talked about in his presence. Rather, "secret" hostility or rebellion toward the fathers was indirectly, often gently, expressed. The holes in family narratives these struggles and secrets necessitated did not, however, impair either their coherence or their shared property: the plot line of the family narrative was understood and agreed upon, and the characterization of roles within the family well known.

There was a cohesive, almost rehearsed, quality to these family accounts, with parents and children using many overlapping anecdotes, descriptions, metaphors, and icons. For example, the "damaged sailboat in the garage" was a condensed symbol employed by one of the study families in a manner that was simultaneously self-deprecatory ("What a foolish acquisition"), but also as a means of asserting a collective identity around such traits as adventurousness, action orientation, and broad-ranging capability ("We can and will try almost anything"). The oral histories generated in early middle age appeared to fulfill Ricoeur's (1977) criteria of narrative, displaying the formal characteristics of stories or epics, with clearly demarcated beginning, middle, and end structure, and principles of causality that provided narrative intelligibility. Burgos (1989) finds this same aesthetic quality in the life stories she has collected with older peasant women in France. She describes their discourse as being patterned on the form of the epic novel. She is impressed with ". . . the liveliness of their style, the ease and fluency with which they talked, the strength and accuracy of the images they used, their thematic coherence, the richness and evocation of the world they described" (p. 33). That such effective narrative flow also characterized our own family sagas is somewhat surprising, in that we violated one of the procedural conventions that supports such unconflicted discourse; that is, oral history research generally avoids ". . . references to the sub-ject's private life: sexuality, dreams and fantasies, suffering, and so on" (p. 31). In contrast, such intimate material, personal and familial, was pervasive and crucial to the understanding of the narratives collected in our study of adult development.

The identity attributions within the earlier family narratives may not always have felt positive, but they did seem to have a quality of mutual acceptance and perma-nence. For example, the scapegoated child in one of the families studied, Debbie (Farrell & Rosenberg, 1981a, pp. 159–160), is referred to as "hopeless" by the rest of the family because ". . . she acts like a little biddy . . . . She gets the house in an uproar." Parents described Debbie as being intrusive: "She sleeps with her eyes and ears open." Undergoing surgery for a hand injury, this late adolescent was under general anesthesia. During the operation, one eye popped open and couldn't be closed. This incident became both a joke and a central part of the fabric of the family narrative: "Debbie couldn't even mind her own business during surgery." Although these identity attributions often seemed extreme and cruel, ignoring, for example, Debbie's competence and generosity, they fit well into a coherent plot line that organized family practices and collective self-concept. Debbie herself was as much caught up in the concept of herself as a "hopeless little biddy" as her siblings and parents.

Narrative theory (Polkinghorne, 1988; Ricoeur, 1981; Toolan, 1988) argues that oral histories, which function as "texts of identity," will strive to fulfill more formal criteria for narrative intelligibility, including adherence to a clear linear sense of time. To the extent that life stories may lack such narrative coherence and consis-tency, identity formation or maintenance can be seen as pathologic. This potentially problematic, triangular relationship between narrative, temporality, and the con-structed self at midlife is exemplified in the set of life story texts gathered in our longitudinal study of middle-aged men. More specifically, comparing our Time 1 and Time 2 data has provided us with a preliminary basis for examining the condi-tions under which a person's life story may achieve narrative coherence and tem-porality, or fail to maintain such integration.

These boundary conditions appear to relate not only to the vagaries of disruptive life events, but also to the content and structure of earlier mythologies of self, to the dynamics of parenthood, and to changing ideologies in the broader culture; that is to say, shifts in frame may require modification of personal narratives that go beyond the narrator's ability to edit and reconstruct a recognizable, continuous story line, particularly one that provides a valued identity.

Time 2 Narratives

A basic structural property of narrative, the plural unity of past, present, and future, could not be assumed in late middle age. Many of our subjects at Time 2 became essentially unable to render the events of their lives into coherent stories at this life stage. As later life events served to discredit elements of the subjects' earlier narrative claims, the possibility of constructing a viable future, of maintaining a sense of narrative anticipation, became increasingly problematic. The ensuing loss of temporality and narrative intelligibility was associated with other dimensions of personal disorganization and subjective distress, at least at the level of representation in personal narratives. This cluster of alterations in narrative, losses of narrative intelligibility, temporal clarity, and future hope can be seen as one type of male "midlife crisis" at the level of narrative identity. Although not universal nor disconnected from familial or social circumstance, this particular form of narrative derailment may represent a particular vulnerability for midlife males in our culture.

The life stories presented at the second stage interviews of these same men and their families in later middle age were often markedly dissimilar in these dimensions. The loss of coherence, narrative continuity, and collaborative agreement between family members was striking; more consonant with Hareven's characterization of typical oral history accounts than that of Burgos (1989). Hareven (1978) describes a proclivity for confusion, digression, and loss of narrative frame in her study of life history and social change in industrial New England. This loss of narrative coherence, Hareven observes, is related to the recounting of difficult experiences, or to attempts to narrate portions of the life story in which highly negative, identity-disrupting events may have occurred. She finds that respondents repress events, misrepresent and reinterpret history and in so doing become confused about past and present and other aspects of temporal order. Two temporal tracks appear to underlie life stories, one organizing experience before the life traumas, and one after, when "things were not the same anymore" (p. 142).

For our subjects, a certain event or set of life changes, often involving their children, was associated with similar feelings of "things not being the same." It was as if the earlier life story had been disrupted or discredited, and a new version could not be satisfactorily patched together. Hareven's mill workers, in losing their careers, seemed to have lost the foundations of their assumptive world and narrative frame. So, too, did some of the later midlife men in our study, in losing their careers as fathers, also lose the organizing axis of their life stories and narrative identities.

Clearly, the integration of trauma, or the desire to suppress unpleasant or discrediting material from the life story, need not disrupt narrative flow. Greenwald (1980), for example, has described the powerful capacity for "fabrication and revision of [personal] history" (p. 615), which he likens to a totalitarian regime's freedom to recast national history. The literature on narrative identity has generally assumed the subject's overriding capacity to find narrative coherence in a wide assortment of "events." Sarbin summarizes a series of experiments demonstrating this "narratory principle" (1986, pp. 12–15). In one, Michotte (1963) constructed an apparatus that allowed the subjects to view two colored rectangles in motion. The experimenter moved the rectangles at various speeds and directions. Asked for descriptions, the subjects anthropomorphized freely, and attributed causality to the movement observed. If rectangle A, for example, moved toward rectangle B and B began to move, the observers would say, "B got out of the way." Subjects created "stories" in which the "characters" manifest motives, interpretive thoughts, and complex interactions. The stories subjects imputed to the movement of the shapes even produced frequent laughter.

A similar experiment by Heider and Simmel (1944), involving a film showing random movements of a triangle, a circle, and a rectangle, was also transformed by subjects into a narrative of complex human actions:

> A man has planned to meet a girl and the girl comes along with another man. The first man tells the second to go; the second tells the first, and he shakes his head. Then the two men have a fight and the girl starts to go into the room. . . . She apparently does not want to be with the first man. The first man follows her into the room after having left the second in a rather weakened condition leaning on the wall outside the room. . . . The girl gets worried and races from one corner to the other in the far part of the room. . . . The first man goes back and tries to open his door, but he is so blinded by rage and frustration that he cannot open it. . . . (p. 13)

Clearly, the story does not, as the subjects believe, derive from observed events. Rather, a stereotypic plot line (a love triangle involving rivalry, male combat, and female flight/rescue) is used by the subject to organize random or meaningless events. The story creates the experience rather than being determined by it. In an extension of this principle, Spence (1982) describes the ubiquity of "narrative smoothing" in the psychoanalytic process: the systematic omission, selective reporting, and evocation of "privileged competence," which allows the analyst to render a case both a "good story" and a "proof" of certain theoretical assertions. Freud was himself guilty of some rather dramatic smoothing, as Steele (1982, 1986) has demonstrated. In his own autobiographical accounts, Freud consistently claimed that, prior to 1907, his work was rejected, ignored, and scorned, a claim reinforced by his biographers. However, later historians demonstrated, by going back to the original texts, that in fact Freud's "early works were widely reviewed and that all the reviews were respectful of his efforts and most were positive in their evaluation of his work" (Steele, 1986, p. 263). Thus, Freud, and later Jung, were able to shape their personal narrative in the form of the myth of the hero: early defeat or rejection followed by ennobling struggle and eventual victory.

In the realm of life stories generally, we consistently find an impressive degree of "narrative competence" (Mandler, 1984), the capacity to impose narrative coherence on inherently random events and to emplot a largely unpredictable life course (Gergen, 1977, 1980). How then do we understand the limiting conditions of emplotment in the personal narrative? Although the literature we have cited emphasizes the subject's power to bind and gloss, there are also very real limits to this power. As Roos (1989) observes, "A coherent narrative is not something which can be created by the narrator at will, but something which is only possible in certain circumstances" (p. 28). It is also evident that evaluating narrative intelligibility is itself problematic, the lower limit of narrative coherence being difficult to specify. As Toolan (1988) argues, "Perceiving non-random connectedness in a sequence of events is the prerogative of the addressee . . . the ultimate authority for ratifying a text as a narrative rests . . . with the perceiver . . ." (p. 8).

However, comparison between the recorded life stories from the 1970s and those from the 1980s clearly demonstrates a marked shift in the quality of coherence in the texts. Understanding sequence, characterization, and plot requires considerably more expansion and cross-referencing of surrounding texts at the later time, and many more misunderstandings between interviewer and respondents occur. The loss of time frame, for example, is illustrated in the following segment. One of our study subjects, Arthur, is a highly educated, articulate man now in his late 50s. The interviews with him in the previous decade are a model of the sort of clarity and skill described by Burgos (1989): they carried a compelling and coherent portrait of his life. In the later interview, Arthur describes a series of vivid "dreams" during a recent illness. He tells us that they have helped him to better recollect what he has previously described as a very unpleasant, even tragic childhood in a rather enmeshed family. The context of the later interview involves intense conflict with his wife, and considerable alienation from his daughter, over long-standing issues of control and mutual anger. These problems threaten to undermine earlier narrative claims of being an extraordinarily close, committed, and caring family. (For a fuller description of this family narrative, see Rosenberg, Rosenberg, & Farrell, 1992.) He suddenly sounds confused and irritable when talking about these dreams:

> Arthur: The dream memories I have are very pleasant for some reason. I remember people in the kindergarten, Frankie McDougall, Larry Blankin, Sarah Blankin. . . . All these people who I'd totally forgotten for 40 years suddenly come back in one dream. It was like I was actually back in my childhood again!
>
> Rosenberg: Was it hard for you to feel like you were back in your childhood?
>
> Arthur: Pardon? [This is the first time in a long discussion he has had trouble hearing me.]
>
> Rosenberg: Was it hard for you?
>
> Arthur: Yes, I guess so. It was a very vivid picture. I saw my father very clearly [father has been deceased for many years], I knew he wasn't there. It must have brought me back before the crash in 1929. That puts me before two years old, or maybe I was reconstructing from a photograph I saw of him in the 1930s. But it was definitely him in the twenties, when he was quite happy. I know that being in the 80s, he was in his thirties then, or maybe the twenties, but quite happy.

Arthur's story thus becomes difficult to comprehend around these descriptions, failing in the narrative requirement for coherence or "followability." It also contradicts, or at least radically revises, earlier representations of his father as a depressed, angry, cruel man who abused both alcohol and his son, a representation that motivates much of the subject's autobiographic narrative. It is also filled with ambiguity about then and now, chronology, fantasy, and reality. Space does not permit full illustration of the varieties of narrative disruption found in the later interviews. However, they are in many ways similar to the discourse frequently encountered in the initial or middle phases of the psychoanalytic situation, where

> The subject is in effect caught in the morass of a certain temporal stagnation, block-
> age, a battle of past and present that refuses to admit authentic futurity into its midst . . .
> the force of past experience is such that it perpetually intrudes, the present often seeming
> to be little more than an awkward and painful epiphenomenon. (Freeman, 1985, p. 138)

Along with this tendency toward fractionation of narrative, both as presented and in relation to previous life story plots and representations, we also found two other thematic shifts in many of both the men's and the couples' narratives. The first was an increased emphasis on the parental imperative, despite the fact that children were generally no longer living in the parental home. In a significant number of the late midlife narratives, adult children took on the role of signifying the parents' (especially father's) moral failings. This was dramatized either by the child "failing" (abusing alcohol, getting divorced, career instability) or by conflict in the relationship with parents. The second, often associated, shift was a sharp increase in depressive thematics and death imagery as compared to the earlier midlife narratives. The most pronounced change could be seen in the discourse of several of the men who were the least depressed in early middle age, in those who had been the most successful and most involved in marriages, families, and occupations. As Jaques's work (1965) suggests, this depressive experience as expressed through references to finitude, death, and hate, is more pronounced in the men than in the women.

Another study subject, a 55-year-old skilled worker who we will call Jack, ex-emplifies a rather different pattern in a number of respects, yet still interweaves the thematics of death and the centrality of fatherhood in his highly conflicted account of the changes in his life over the past 12 years. Jack became a father for the first time only ten years earlier. He describes the transformation brought about by the unexpected conception and birth of their son, long after he and his wife had assumed that such an event was biologically impossible for them:

> Jack: I wasted my life before. . . . I never even thought before. I fired from the hip.
> My marriage is much closer now than it was before. . . . My dreams are all for Steven
> [son] now. It's too late for me. . . . I have no regrets about the past ten years. I can honestly
> say it is the first time in my life I'm doing anything worthwhile.

His testimony about parenthood as rebirth takes place in the context of Jack's continual coughing, and frequent smoking, during the day of interviewing. He admits to the fear that he ". . . will not be around to see Steven grow up." Jack quickly reveals that he has emphysema, for which he has been recently hospitalized. His wife reports the warning recently received from the family doctor: ". . . he will be dead in five years if he doesn't give it up." Jack insists, however, that "Smoking is my only pleasure left," since he has given up drinking. He also expresses puzzlement at his own behavior, saying that he has twice before ". . . given up smoking just like that," but now finds himself unable to do so. Jack remarks ruefully at one point, "The family might be better off if I die. It would let Steven go to college on my life insurance." Death and hatred also saturate this telling of the family history in its emphasis on the loss of grandparents, and in Jack's description of his mother as ". . . a mean, miserable person . . . she hated me."

In trying to understand the significance of these shifts in life story thematics and style, we are forced to confront what Burgos has recently referred to as ". . . the fundamental ambiguity which characterizes the understanding of a life story, especially when it is a question not of a 'spontaneous' autobiography but of one that has been elicited by a researcher. . . ." (1989, p. 29) Not only are the texts themselves ambiguous, but the interpretive frames, assumptions, and techniques available for analyzing life story texts still lack, in certain key respects, conceptual clarity. There is little consensus in the narrative school of life-span development concerning several particularly salient issues. These include ambiguity about the processes by which personal narrative is generated and sustained; about the relation between life story and identity; and about the limits of revisionism in the construction of these stories.

First, there is considerable variation in the balance attributed to more internal, personal desire and creativity, as opposed to general cultural scripts and primary group dynamics, in shaping life stories. The most traditional view, and probably most widely held in the adult development literature, holds that the personal narrative reflects a search for truth whereby as the subject ". . . strains for order, continuity and coherence of what he has experienced, so will he strive for coherence in his own self, between his subjective past, his present and a possible desirable future . . ." (Wyatt, 1986, p. 203). In this view, the narrative must ". . . continue to make sense over time, preserving the sense of self-consistency" (Cohler, 1982, p. 206). Even this relatively essentialist perspective, closely linked to Erikson's concept of ego identity, also acknowledges the interpersonal dimension of life story narrative as it reflects self-understanding. Erikson writes:

> It is this identity of something in the individual's core, with an essential aspect of a group's inner coherence, which is under consideration here: for the young individual must learn to be most himself where he means most to others; those others, to be sure, who have come to mean most to him. The term identity expresses such a mutual relation in that it connotes both a persistent sameness within oneself (self-sameness) and a persistent sharing of some kind of essential character with others. (1956, p. 61)

At the other end of this particular spectrum, we see recent attempts to deconstruct this ego-psychological view of identity (Sampson, 1989). Geertz's characterization (caricature?) of the North American version of the self attempts to underline its assumptions:

> The Western conception of the person as a bounded, unique, more or less integrated motivational and cognitive universe, a dynamic center of awareness, emotion, judgment and action, organized into a distinctive whole and set contrastively against other such wholes and against a social and natural background is, however incorrigible it may seem to us, a rather peculiar idea within the context of the world's cultures. (1979, p. 229)

Drawing from social constructionism, cross-cultural psychology, critical theory, and deconstructionism, this approach argues that the Eriksonian concept of self or identity ". . . describes a fictitious character, the bourgeois individual, whose integrated wholeness, unique individuality and status as a subject . . . has become null and void" (Sampson, 1989, p. 3). Extending this perspective, Slugoski and Ginsburg (1989) have gone so far as to suggest that what has been called "ego identity" is really no more than a reflection of the explanatory speech from which it is inferred. Identity, as manifest in the personal narrative, can be seen ". . . as a model of culturally sanctioned ways of talking about oneself and others during a certain stage of life in Western societies" (p. 51), a mode of speech that society makes differentially available and then associates with psychic maturity and health.

Both the Eriksonian and the deconstructionist schools concur on the necessity for social validation of the personal narrative if it is to serve its function of providing a sense of integration and continuity, fictional or authentic. Ricoeur's general formulation in which accounts must have the formal characteristics of stories and epics and must be "'followable' and, in this sense, self explanatory" (1977, p. 869) is probably the most widely cited in this literature, but is itself ambiguous. The audience that must be satisfied, the degree of adherence to a particular narrative form required, and the salience of different dimensions of the narrative in creating a viable personhood remain to be specified.

One attempt at this specification has been offered by Plath (1980). With the deconstructionists, he is critical of the "ballistic missile imagery of maturity and aging" implied in such language as "life trajectory." He argues that we reject such "entity" models, and reconceptualize the process of construction of personal narrative "as a problem of co-biography." Plath observes that most life stories are shaped in collaboration with "consociates," intimate others with whom the subject interacts consistently and over long spans of time. He differentiates consociates from others in the life space along a number of dimensions: a sense of mutual dependence, concern, shared fate, and belief that "my consociates know the 'real me'" (p. 289).

Plath appears to be accurate in the assertion that this "convoy" of consociates has "the power to certify which version of [my] life's narrative is 'authoritative'" (1980, p. 289). This is simply a specification of the more general demand that the personal narrative be followable, be in accord with cultural scripts that define allowable representations of self. We encounter and respond to such criteria primarily in as much as they are mediated in face-to-face discourse with intimate others. Plath defines the convoy as consisting of "an array of kin, friends, lovers, colleagues, classmates . . ." (p. 289), a description that appears too general if we look at the life stories offered by our study subjects. There appears to be considerable ethnographic data supporting the notion that it is the clan or family unit that is the basic frame for self-identification (Jacobson-Widding, 1983). Narrative representations of self appear generally to be constructed and confirmed in intimate, bounded, enduring, face-to-face relationships. Gergen and Gergen (1989) comment that, "Narratives typically require the interweaving of identities and thus the support of others within the social sphere of interaction." It is not some generalized language community or some objective others that define the boundaries of good life stories. Rather, the spouse and the nuclear family are the most salient and the most common audience involved in hearing and validating personal narrative. In many crucial respects everyday life stories depend on the clan or family: they are most commonly interwoven with family history, they are mutually constructed in collaboration with a family, and they are most frequently and fully articulated in front of the family.

Like Berger and Kellner (1964) we find that the "marital conversation" takes primacy over other discourse in shaping conceptions of self, of group identity, and of personal history. They argue that marriage in contemporary American culture represents a watershed, not only in status and role relationships, but also in the very process by which the explanatory language and structure of the subject's narrative are selected and refined. The early years of marriage, Berger and Kellner observe, are characterized by an intense pulling away from many others in the convoy as previously constituted (friends, siblings) and an investment in the construction of a shared reality that specifies the couple's individual and common identities. Our earlier findings (Farrell & Rosenberg, 1981a, 1981b) are quite congruent with this analysis. Couples displayed a convergence in imagery, and accounts of complex situations, which could have been brought about only by collaborative effort. This dynamic is very apparent, for example, in the narratives offered by husband and wife, separately and conjointly, to justify the idealization of some children in the family and the scapegoating of others. Similarly, the midlife crisis story, although generally considered as a male plot, was also a story narrated by all family members. Although the voices might have spoken different parts (e.g., blaming vs. self-recrimination or justifying), the couples interviewed appeared to have come to some joint agreement as to the plot outline and narrative tone.

CONCLUSIONS

We conclude by offering some tentative observations about the evolution of personal narrative from early to late middle age. It is at this level of experience or organization of self that the "midlife crisis" appears to be a meaningful construct. We would hypothesize that it is still a meaningful concept for organizing the life stories of men in advanced Western societies. Extrapolating primarily from our own longitudinal studies, we would locate this narrative shift more in late (fifth decade) rather than early (fourth decade) middle age. When it does surface, the midlife crisis story can be manifest in personal narratives, or life stories, in several different ways. At the level of plot, the midlife crisis is a kind of archetypal form. As a dramatic device, the crisis undoes stability narratives, and marks a turning point in either a romantic/heroic saga or a tragic decline. The crisis, that is, represents a demand for a radical revision of the ongoing narrative of earlier adulthood. The crisis is manifest, in McAdams's terminology (1993), in change of narrative tone, perspective, and sense of delimited future. Unlike McAdams (1993), we do not find it common for midlife narratives, early or late, to exemplify greater contextualization of thought, use of postformal operations, nor the confrontation of oppositions within the personality. However, it is necessary to increase our database to systematically test these hypotheses.

The findings from our study do leave us especially interested in understanding why, at midlife, many of our subjects were no longer able to construct narratives conveying a sense of "plural unity of future, past and present" (Ricoeur, 1981, p. 167). In the life stories we have elicited, late middle age is frequently associated with discourse that no longer manifests the emplotment characteristic of most personal narrative. Ellipses, evasions, confusion of sequence, silences, empty speech, and dissimulation are far more prevalent in the later interviews, and appear to be related to three processes. The first of these is the shift in family power structure, which, as we have argued elsewhere (Rosenberg et al., 1992), both reflects and mitigates toward radical revisions in family ideology and family narrative. As the paternalistic ethos that characterized these families shifted, under the weight of both internal developmental changes and shifts in the broader culture, the narratives that embodied these ideologies become insupportable. Although the changes in patterns of authority and control were evident in earlier middle age, their full ideological impact, and effect on family narrative, were not manifest until the later period of family development. For the men particularly, the identity-sustaining function of the earlier family narrative, and the tensions that this politicized discourse concealed, became dramatically evident. Many of our subjects seemed unable to recover from the negation of their identity claims of earlier adulthood and the revisions of family history that occurred in later middle age. These assaults appeared to result, in turn, in the loss of temporality and emplotment in their life stories.

This loss of narrative coherence also appeared to be linked to the emphasis on the parental imperative found so frequently in the men's earlier narratives. By committing to stories in which their futures relied on their children, allowing evasion of personal mortality and finitude in their narratives, they may have escaped direct confrontation with depressive issues in earlier middle age. At the same time, their narratives failed to articulate certain aspects of self, and created a need for story lines that required domination of and emotional reliance on their children. Their "investment" in this particular version of fatherhood was frequently described by the spouses and offspring as oppressive. Rather than being willing actors and actresses in their fathers' stories, the adult children of these men were frequently engaged in struggles to find their own narrative voices. This often required the negation of the earlier family narrative and the identities it framed. Jaques described a significant proportion of men who were able to complete the heroic quest, working through the earlier midlife crisis by confrontation with fears of loss and death. Having understood and accepted the idea of their own mortality, and having felt the associated grief of this and other losses, ". . . the last half of life can be lived with conscious knowledge of eventual death. . . . The gain is in the deepening of awareness, understanding and self realization" (1965, pp. 512–513). This would represent one type of ending or final chapter, one of transcendence, as narrated in the heroic midlife crisis myth. For the men in our longitudinal studies, this ideal change in narrative content and structure was not particularly in evidence. A substantial proportion described journeys that appeared to be mired in defeat and humiliation rather than ones exemplifying the hero's victory.

In certain respects, the particular version of midlife crisis we are describing may be unique to a particular generation or cohort of men, those who came of age during World War II and the Korean War. These men, as Elder (1974) and others have found, were particularly focused on familial and security issues during their formative years, and faced the midlife transition during a period of marked change in ideology regarding gender roles and authority relations. In a concurrent study of a younger cohort drawn from the same population described above, and in a separate longitudinal study of another Vietnam-era sample (Rosenberg, 1993; Schnurr, Friedman, and Rosenberg, 1993; Schnurr, Rosenberg, & Friedman, 1993), we gathered life story narratives from several hundred "baby-boomers." Their midlife narratives differed from those of their fathers' generation in several dimensions. First, rather than the adult narratives describing an early commitment to standard identities, many of these men discussed a persistent sense of skepticism and partial alienation from conventional social roles, even if this alienation was subtle. The 1960s midlife crisis, in which a man moved suddenly to a sense of questioning himself, his relationships, and his culture, could not occur in the narratives of this group simply because the alienated stance was a characteristic of their narratives from adolescence on. When marked midlife change was reported in the life stories of the Vietnam-era men, it was frequently in the direction of attempts to better ground themselves in standard religions (which they had previously rejected), or in the achievement of more stable marriages and careers, work seen in the "classic" models as the focus of earlier adulthood. These men were also noticeably less focused on family involvement and identification with children as defining aspects of self. Vietnam-era respondents were much more likely to fill their narratives with accounts of their own search for fulfillment, their ambivalence over ideologic and life style choices, and with the pain associated with more contemporary problems like divorce, blended families, and their own substance-use difficulties. If the midlife crisis story of the 1960s and 1970s focused on the desire to escape an oppressive identity that foreclosed a sense of self (Rosenberg & Farrell, 1976), the crisis story of the 1980s and 1990s involved a quest to finally occupy an adult identity. There was also frequent mention, in the baby-boomer narratives (those of men reaching their 40s in the 1980s and 1990s), of occupation-related issues like "burnout," "downsizing," the diminution of autonomy in the professions, and the impact of corporate mergers and acquisitions on work life. Terms like "midlife crisis" and "male menopause" were used (often in a rueful, self-deprecatory tone) by the baby-boomers, but they were used to describe rather different narratives than those reported by Levinson and others in the 1960s and 1970s. Again, it is not at all clear that midlife (i.e., the age 40 transition) was a point of particular stress in these life stories, but rather that the term midlife crisis was a commonly used organizing device for narrating a wide variety of possible setbacks, regrets, negative feeling states, and role changes whether or not these events and sentiments are tightly linked to age or life stage.

Finally, we were impressed, in listening to the later-middle-aged subjects, with the limits of revisionist freedom they seemed able to exercise. Having committed themselves to a particular narrative strategy in the early and middle stages of adulthood, they were left in later middle age without a coherent account of the past that justified present realities and pointed to a viable future. Like Rossini, some of our subjects seem to lose their narrative voice, finding it painful or impossible to articulate any life story texts. More commonly, they provided strangulated texts, in which the protection of "secrets" became the major work of the discourse, only to intermittently give way to the need to confess and be granted expiation. For many of these subjects, having grown up in the disruption of the Depression and World War II, the personal narrative typically embodied themes of struggle for survival or transcendence rather than continuity. Experiencing disconfirmation of key aspects of their central adult identity, these men exhibited heightened vulnerability to a sense of regressive malaise, which was reflected in narrative tone, self attribution, and future orientation. Future research may help us to clarify the personal, familial, cultural, and historical circumstances under which such changes in narrative are characteristic of that portion of life-span development known as midlife.

REFERENCES

Berger, B., & Kellner, H. (1964). Marriage and the construction of reality: An exercise in the micro-sociology of knowledge. *Diogenes, 46,* 1–23.

Bruner, J. (1986). *Actual minds, possible worlds.* Cambridge, MA: Harvard University Press.

Burgos, M. (1989). Life stories, narrativity and the search for the self. *Life Stories, 5,* 29–37.

Chiriboga, D. A. (1989a). Mental health at the midpoint: Crisis, challenge, or relief? In K. Hunter & M. Sundel (Eds.), *Midlife myths: Issues, findings, and practical implications* (pp. 116–141). Newberry Park, CA: Sage.

Chiriboga, David A., (1989b). Stress and loss in middle age. In R. A. Kalish (Ed.), *Midlife loss: Coping strategies* (pp. 42–86). Newberry Park, CA: Sage.

Cohler, B. J. (1982). Personal narrative and life course. In P. B. Baltes & O. G. Brim (Eds.), *Life span development and behavior* (pp. 205–241). New York: Academic Press.

Costa, P. T., Jr., & McCrae, R. R. (1976). Age differences in personality structure: A cluster analytic approach. *Journal of Gerontology, 31,* 564–670.

Costa, P. T., Jr., & McCrae, R. R. (1978). Objective personality assessment. In M. Storandt, I. C. Siegler, & M. F. Elias (Eds.), *The clinical psychology of aging* (pp. 119–143). New York: Plenum Press.

Costa, P. T., Jr., & McCrae, R. R. (1980a). Still stable after all these years: Personality as a key to some issues in adulthood and old age. In P. Baltes (Ed.), *Life-span development and behavior* (Vol. 3, pp. 65–102). New York: Academic Press.

Costa, P. T., Jr., & McCrae, R. R. (1980b). Set like plaster? Evidence for the stability of adult personality. In T. Heatherton & J. Weinberger (Eds.), *Can personality change?* (pp. 299–314). Washington, DC: American Psychological Association.

Elder, G. H., Jr. (1974). *Children of the Great Depression.* Chicago: University of Chicago Press.

Erikson, E. (1950). *Childhood and society* (2nd ed.). New York: Norton.

Erikson, E. (1956). The problem of ego identity. *Journal of the American Psychoanalytic Association, 4*(1), 56–121.

Erikson, E. (1959). Identity and the life cycle: Selected papers. *Psychological Issues Monograph, 1,* 1–177.

Farrell, M. P., & Barnes, G. (1994, March). *The interrelationship of the well-being of parents and their adolescent children.* Paper presented at Groves Conference on Families, San Jose, CA.

Farrell, M. P., & Rosenberg, S. D. (1981a). *Men at midlife.* Dover, MA: Auburn House.

Farrell, M., & Rosenberg, S. (1981b). Parents and children at mid-life. In C. Getty & W. Humphreys (Eds.), *Perspectives on the family.* New York: Appleton Century, Crofts.

Farrell, M., Rosenberg, S., & Rosenberg, H. (1993). Changing texts of identity from early to late middle age. In J. Demick, K. Bursik, & R. DiBiase (Eds.), *Parental development* (pp. 203–224). Hillsdale, NJ: Erlbaum.

Freeman, M. (1985). Psychoanalytic narration and the problem of historical knowledge. *Psychoanalysis and Contemporary Thought, 8*[$](2), 133–181.

Geertz, C. (1979). From the native's point of view: On the nature of anthropological understanding. In P. Rabinow & W. M. Sullivan (Eds.), *Interpretive social science* (pp. 225–241). Berkeley: University of California Press.

Gergen, K. J. (1977). Social exchange theory in a world of transient fact. In E. Hamblin & J. Kunkel (Eds.), *Behavioral theory in sociology.* New Brunswick, NJ: Transaction Books.

Gergen, K. J. (1980). The emerging crisis in theory of life-span development. In P. B. Baltes & O. G. Brim (Eds.), *Life span development and behavior* (pp. 32–63). New York: Academic Press.

Gergen, M. M., & Gergen, K. J. (1987). The self in temporal perspective. In R. Abeles (Ed.), *Life span perspectives and social psychology* (pp. 121–137). Hillsdale, NJ: Erlbaum.

Gergen, M. M., & Gergen, K. J. (1989). The self in temporal perspective. In R. Abeles (Ed.), *Life-span social psychology.* Hillsdale, NJ: Erlbaum.

Gould, R. L. (1978). *Transformations.* New York: Simon & Schuster.

Greenwald, A. G. (1980). The totalitarian ego: Fabrication and revision of personal history. *American Psychologist, 35*(7), 603–618.

Gutmann, D. L. (1987). *Reclaimed powers: Toward a new psychology of men and women in later life.* New York: Basic Books.

Hareven, T. K. (1978). The search for generational memory: Tribal rites in industrial society. *Dædalus: Journal of the American Academy of Arts and Sciences, 107,* 137–149.

Heideger, M. (1979). *Being and time* (15th ed.). Tubingen: Max Niemeyer Verlag.

Heider, F., & Simmel, M. (1944). An experimental study of apparent behavior. *American Journal of Psychology, 57,* 243–259.

Hogan, R. (1987). Personality psychology: Back to basics. In J. Aronoff, A. I. Rabin, & R. A. Zucker (Eds.), *The emergence of personality* (pp. 79–104). New York: Springer Verlag.

Howard, G. S. (1991). Culture tales: A narrative approach to thinking, cross-cultural psychology, and psychotherapy. *American Psychologist, 46*(3), 187–197.

Hunter, K., & Sundel, M. (1989). *Midlife myths: Issues, findings, and practical implications.* Newberry Park, CA: Sage.

Jacobson-Widding, A. (Ed.). (1983). *Identity: Personal and socio-cultural.* Atlantic Highlands, NJ: Humanities Press, Inc.

James, W. (1897). *The dilemma of determinism in the will to believe and other essays in popular philosophy* (pp. 145–183). New York: Dover.

Jaques, E. (1965). Death and the mid-life crisis. *International Journal of Psychoanalysis, 46,* 502–514.

Jung, C. G. (1923). *Psychological types.* New York: Harcourt Brace.

Jung, C. G. (1950/1959). A study in the process of individuation. In *Collected works* (Vol. 9, Pt. I). Princeton, NJ: Princeton University Press.

Labov, W. (1972). *Socio-linguistic patterns.* Philadelphia: University of Pennsylvania Press.

Lacan, J. (1977). *Ecrits: A selection* (A. Sheridan, Trans.). New York: W. W. Norton & Company. (Original work published 1966)

Lakoff, G., & Johnson, M. (1980). *Metaphors we live by.* Chicago: University of Chicago Press.

Landau, M. (1991). *Narratives of human evolution.* New Haven: Yale University Press.

Levinson, D. J., Darrow, C. N., Klein, E. B., Levinson, M. H., & McKee, B. (1978). *The seasons of a man's life.* New York: Knopf.

Linde, C. (1993). *Life stories: The creation of coherence.* New York: Oxford University Press.

Lowenthal, M., Thurnher, M., & Chiriboga, D. (1975). *Four stages of life.* San Francisco: Jossey-Bass.

Mandler, J. M. (1983, August). *Stories: The function of structure.* Paper presented at the annual meeting of the American Psychological Association, Anaheim, CA.

Mandler, J. M. (1984). *Stories, scripts and scenes: Aspects of a schema theory.* Hillsdale, NJ: Erlbaum.

McAdams, D. (1985). *Power, intimacy, and the life story.* Homewood, IL: Dorsey Press.

McAdams, D. (1993). *The stories we live by.* New York: William Morrow and Company.

McAdams, D. (1994). Can personality change? Levels of stability and growth in personality areas across the life span. In T. Heatherton & J. Weinberger (Eds.), *Can personality change?* (pp. 299–314). Washington, DC: American Psychological Association.

McClelland, D. C. (1951). *Personality.* New York: Holt, Rinehart & Winston.

McCrae, R. R., & Costa, P. T., Jr. (1990). *Personality in adulthood.* New York: Gilford Press.

Michotte, A. E. (1963). The perception of causality. London: Methuen. Trans. (T. R. Miles & E. Miles, Trans.). (Original work published 1946.)

Neugarten, B. L. (Ed.). (1968). *Middle age and aging.* Chicago: University of Chicago Press.

Pearlin, L. I. (1985). Life strains and psychological distress among adults. In A. Monat & R. S. Lazarus (Eds.), *Stress and coping: An anthology* (pp. 192–207). New York: Columbia University Press.

Plath, D. W. (1980). Contours of consocation: Lessons from a Japanese narrative. In P. B. Baltes & O. G. Brim (Eds.), *Life-span development and behavior* (pp. 287–305). New York: Academic Press.

Polkinghorne, D. (1988). *Narrative knowing and the human sciences.* Albany, NY: SUNY Press.

Propp, V. (1928/1968). *The morphology of the folktale,* Austin: University of Texas Press.

Ricoeur, P. (1977). The question of proof in Freud's psychoanalytic writings. *Journal of the American Psychoanalytic Association, 25,* 835–872.

Ricoeur, P. (1981). Narrative time. In W. J. T. Mitchell (Ed.), *On narrative* (pp. 165–186). Chicago: University of Chicago Press.

Roos, J. P. (1989). The text and life: An introduction to Martine Burgos' research. *Life Stories, 5,* 27–28.

Rosenberg, S. (1976). A culture of discontent. In C. Thomas and R. Bryne-Laport, (Eds.), *Contemporary alienation.* New York, NY: Praeger.

Rosenberg, S. (1991, February). *Family albums: Ideology and identity in representing the past.* Paper presented at the University of California at Santa Barbara Interdisciplinary Humanities Center program on "Human Temporality," a conference on *Memory, Story, History.*

Rosenberg, S. (1993). Threshhold of thrill: Life stories in the skies over Southeast Asia. In M. Cooke and A. Woolacott (Eds.), *Gendering war talk* (pp. 43–66). Princeton, NJ: Princeton University Press.

Rosenberg, S., & Bergen, B. (1976). *The cold fire.* Hanover, NH: University Press of New England.

Rosenberg, S., & Farrell, M. (1976). Identity and crisis in middle aged men. *International Journal of Aging and Human Development, 7*(2), 153–170.

Rosenberg, S., & Farrell, M. (1981). The mid-life transition. In Robert Lewis (Ed.), *Men in difficult times.* Englewood Cliffs, NJ: Prentice Hall.

Rosenberg, S., & Rosenberg, H. (1981). Identity concerns in early motherhood. In C. Getty and W. Humphreys (Eds.), *Perspectives on the Family.* New York: Appleton Century, Crofts.

Rosenberg, S., Rosenberg, H., & Farrell, M. (1992). In the name of the father. In G. Rosenwald and R. Ochberg (Eds.), *Storied lives* (pp. 41–59). New Haven: Yale University Press.

Sampson, E. E. (1989). The deconstruction of the self. In J. Shotter & K. J. Gergen (Eds.), *Texts of identity* (pp. 1–19). Newberry Park, CA: Sage.

Sarbin, T. R. (Ed.). (1986). *Narrative psychology: The storied nature of human conduct.* New York: Praeger.

Schaie, K. W., & Willis, S. L. (1986). *Adult development and aging* (2nd. ed.). Boston: Little, Brown.

Schimek, J. (1975). The interpretations of the past: Childhood trauma, psychic reality, and historical truth. *Journal of the American Psychoanalytic Association, 23,* 845–865.

Schnurr, P., Friedman, M., & Rosenberg, S. (1993). Premilitary MMPI scores as predictors of combat-related PTSD symptomatology. *American Journal of Psychiatry, 150*(3), 479–483.

Schnurr, P., Rosenberg, S., & Friedman, M. (1993). Change in MMPI scores from college to adulthood as a function of military service. *Journal of Abnormal Psychology, 102*(2), 288–296.

Silverberg, S. B., & Steinberg, L. (1990). Psychological well-being of parents with early adolescent children. *Developmental Psychology, 26*(4), 658–666.

Slugoski, B. R., & Ginsburg, G. P. (1989). Ego identity and explanatory speech. In J. Shotter & K. J. Gergen (Eds.), *Texts of identity* (pp. 36–55). Newberry Park, CA: Sage.

Spence, D. P. (1982). *Narrative truth and historical truth: Meaning and interpretation in psychoanalysis.* New York: W. W. Norton.

Steele, R. S. (1982). *Freud and Jung: Conflicts of interpretation* (with Consulting Editor S. V. Swinney). London: Routledge & Kegan Paul.

Steele, R. S. (1986). Deconstructing histories: Toward a systematic criticism of psychological narratives. In T. R. Sarbin (Ed.), *Narrative psychology: The storied nature of human conduct* (pp. 256–275). New York: Praeger.

Suppe, F. (1974). *The structure of scientific theories.* Chicago: University of Illinois Press.

Tonkin, E. (1992). Narrating our pasts: The social construction of oral history. In *Studies in oral and literate culture, N22.* Cambridge: Cambridge University Press.

Toolan, M. J. (1988). *Narrative: A critical linguistic introduction.* New York: Routledge.

Updike, J. (1960). *Rabbit run.* New York: Knopf.

Vaillant, G. (1977). *Adaptation to life.* Boston: Little, Brown.

Whitbourne, S. K. (1986). *The me I know: A study of adult identity.* New York: Springer Verlag.

Whitbourne, S. K., & Weinstock, C. S. (1986). *Adult development* (2nd ed.). New York: Praeger.

Wyatt, F. (1986). The narrative in psychoanalysis: Psychoanalytic notes on storytelling, listening, and interpreting. In T. R. Sarbin (Ed.), *Narrative psychology: The storied nature of human conduct* (pp. 193–210). New York: Praeger.

PART II

Biological Functioning and Physical Health at Midlife

This part of the book investigates more closely specific issues that relate to biological functioning and physical health during midlife. These chapters include important contributions by Susan S. Merrill and Lois M. Verbrugge in their review of "Health and Disease in Midlife." Nancy E. Avis provides a fresh look at an area of critical importance for women in her chapter, "Women's Health at Midlife." Finally, Ilene C. Siegler, Berton H. Kaplan, Dean D. Von Dras, and Daniel B. Mark review and extend the literature on cardiovascular functioning in their chapter, "Cardiovascular Health: A Challenge for Midlife."

CHAPTER 4

Health and Disease in Midlife

Susan S. Merrill

California Medical Review Incorporated (CMRI), San Francisco, California

Lois M. Verbrugge

Institute of Gerontology, University of Michigan, Ann Arbor, Michigan

"How old would you be if you didn't know how old you was?"

Satchel Paige

Not so very long ago the age of 45 was considered old. Today, it marks the beginning of the period we call midlife (ages 45–64). Even so, some individuals younger than 45 or older than 64 consider themselves to be in their middle years. Subjective evaluation of one's age is based on internal and external clues. Changes in health and appearance are often the most salient cues for triggering reevaluations of how old one feels. Rather than relying on chronologic age, many people examine their positions within different life contexts (body, family, career) when considering their place in the life-span and deciding whether or not they have reached, are in, or are beyond midlife.

The period we call midlife is a recent phenomenon. Although there have always been people who lived to and through what we now consider midlife, it is only in the last few decades that we have seen dramatic changes in the numbers of adults who enjoy healthy, active lives through their middle years and well into older age. Although midlife is a time of good health and productive activity, it is also the time when noticeable changes in physical and mental abilities begin to occur. Unlike the peak performance of youth and the often abrupt decline in old age, the changes to health in midlife are usually gradual; some are biologically determined, some accompany the demands of social roles, others are the result of lifestyle choices.

Though everyone experiences some physical change due to aging processes, rates of aging vary greatly from one individual to another and within the same person.

In midlife roles, people often find themselves at a peak period, in charge of themselves and others, with a sense of competence and purpose. Notwithstanding the rewards that numerous busy roles may confer, their combined demands of time and energy are often quite draining. Midlife also sees the termination of some roles and the emergence of others. For example, fecundity declines for men and ceases for women with the advent of menopause. The proportion of individuals entering retirement grows, as does the proportion of those becoming grandparents.

Despite incipient physical changes and changing role demands that occur during midlife, there are many individual differences in health. Genetic makeup and life-style factors play an important part in whether chronic disease will emerge, and when. Health habits and abilities to cope with physical change and role transitions have a direct effect on health. Health-related behaviors in youth affect midlife health, just as health habits in midlife affect health and well-being in old age. Women, who must attend to the biologic cycle of menses, gain some experience coping with physiologic change. This experience may help women adjust to physical changes in midlife, and that, in turn, helps them to cope with changes in late life.

In sum, midlife is a relatively recent phenomenon, marked by generally good health and multiple demanding roles, though also accompanied by gradual physical changes and the beginnings of chronic illness and disability. This chapter explores some of these aspects of health in middle age, beginning with physiologic changes occurring during the aging process and the growing prevalence of chronic diseases. A discussion of some of the modifiable factors associated with health and chronic disease follows, illustrating health habits and lifestyle choices that maintain health in midlife. Symptoms and disabilities that occur in middle age are described, and the importance of social roles to health is illustrated. Finally, the advent of what we now consider middle age is discussed, including the increase in life expectancy, decrease in mortality, and the factors that contributed to these phenomena. Differences in the health of men and women are noted where applicable throughout the chapter.

AGING PROCESSES

From birth to death, the body undergoes physiologic changes; these are normal processes of aging rather than pathological changes incurred by disease. Many take place in childhood, such as the complete formation and growth of organs and achieving maximum height; others take place in adulthood, such as the decline in systemic function and the decrease in bone mineral density. In midlife, there are few markers of physical change as dramatic as those that occur in childhood and youth (walking, talking, puberty) or in old age (rapid decline, death). The most distinct physiologic change in midlife is probably menopause. Other physical changes are usually very gradual, without distinctive onset or finale. Some start in early adulthood and become apparent in midlife; others do not begin until late in the middle years.

Most bodily functions reach peak functional capacity by the mid-20s; over the next 20–30 years, a significant amount of physical and physiologic deviation occurs. These declines are usually very gradual, increasing silently through the middle years. Though some changes affect virtually everyone (menopause, presbyopia), there are enormous individual differences in the rate of physiologic change. A person's genetic makeup, health practices, and behavior can increase or delay both the rate and signs of aging and physical decline. However, by age 50 there is usually enough change that it becomes physically noticeable.

One of the most visible signs of physiologic change is in physical appearance. The first outwardly noticeable signs of aging usually become evident by the fifth or sixth decade. The skin begins to wrinkle and sag due to a loss of fat and collagen in the underlying tissues. Small, localized areas of pigmentation in the skin give rise to "age spots," especially in areas exposed to sunlight (e.g., hands and face). Hair becomes thinner and grayer because of a decline in replacement rate and a decrease in melanin production. The number of sweat glands begins to decrease so persons in midlife perspire less than in youth. Fingernails and toenails develop ridges and become thicker and more brittle (Memmler & Wood, 1987; Whitbourne, 1985).

In midlife, people begin to lose height and gain weight. Due to thinning of intervertebral disks in the vertebral column, adults lose about one-half inch of height per decade beginning in their 40s (Memmler & Wood, 1987). From about age 20 onward, people tend to gain weight throughout young and middle adulthood (Katchadourian, 1987). Abdominal girth shows increases of 6–16% in men and 25–35% in women (Whitbourne, 1985). Where body fat accounts for about 10% of body weight in adolescence, it comprises at least 20% by the middle years of adulthood. In late middle and older ages, there is a tendency to lose lean body mass (muscle and bone mineral) and gain body fat.

Maximum strength and peak joint function are attained in early adulthood. Muscle strength begins to decrease noticeably by age 45. A gradual loss of muscle cells results in the smaller size of each individual muscle, and loss of strength becomes most apparent in legs and back. About 10–15% of maximum strength is lost between ages 35 and 60. The cushions for movement of bones (e.g., collagen, tendons, ligaments, synovial fluid) become less efficient throughout adulthood, and persons in midlife often begin to experience joint stiffness and decreased ease of movement.

Maximum bone density is achieved by the mid- to late 30s; from this point forward, there is a progressive loss of bone due to bone resorption rate (tearing down of bone) increasing and new bone apposition rate (building of bone) decreasing (Memmler & Wood, 1987; Whitbourne 1985). The rate of bone loss begins slowly and accelerates in the 50s. Women experience approximately twice the rate of bone loss as men. By the end of midlife, bones will be less strong, more brittle, break more easily, and heal more slowly.

Beginning at age 40, the basal metabolic rate gradually declines, decreasing the efficiency of oxygen consumption and making it more difficult to sustain physical efforts of endurance for as long as in youth. Vital capacity (the volume of air moved into and out of the lungs when ventilating maximally) begins to decline in the early 40s, and results in a loss in capacity of 30–40% by age 70 (Katchadourian, 1987; Lynne-Davies, 1977).

Though the heart muscle itself does not seem to change significantly, especially if a person is physically active, by the mid-50s heart rate is slower and more irregular (Katchadourian, 1987). The heart continuously loses its effectiveness as a pumping device, primarily because of a linear decline in the body's maximum oxygen consumption and a steady decrease in the maximum heart rate attained during utmost levels of exertion. Arterial walls become more rigid and thicken, there is an increase in aortic stiffness (Lakatta, 1990), and there is an increase of lipids in the arteries (Whitbourne, 1985). The incidence of cardiovascular disease escalates in the late 40s and early 50s, and this is especially true for men. There is a 30–40% loss in aerobic power of the heart by age 65 (Shepard, 1978).

Several other systemic changes begin to take place in midlife. As early as age 40, the body begins to lose the ability to increase body heat production and decrease heat loss when necessary. As individuals enter their fifth decade, there begins a decrease in the number and size of nephrons in the kidneys. Immune response becomes weaker as we grow older (Miller, 1990), though there is some evidence that immune response for women is less affected by age (Smith, 1992).

Sensory changes take place and become noticeable in midlife. A decrease in olfactory cells begins in the fourth decade and continues through life. This decline contributes to a lesser sense of smell and a diminished sense of taste.

Gradual hearing loss begins in the 30s and continues progressively over the life-span, with sensitivity to high-frequency tones impaired earlier and more severely than sensitivity to low-frequency tones. Young adults normally can hear frequencies ranging from 20 to 20,000 Hz. The inability to hear high frequencies becomes common near age 50; by the end of midlife and into old age approximately 25% of the population has a clinically significant hearing loss (Horvath & Davis, 1990). Men tend to experience greater hearing loss than women; beginning about age 40, men have poorer hearing than women at frequencies greater than 4000 Hz. By age 60, it is difficult for men to hear frequencies greater than 2000 Hz (Whitbourne, 1985).

The ability of the eye to accommodate (the lens shift in focus from far to near objects) reaches its peak at age 8. A gradual decline in accommodative capacity occurs over the life-span, with a 50% reduction achieved by age 35 (Horvath & Davis, 1990; Whitbourne, 1985). Presbyopia, the lessened ability to focus on near objects, is the most common physiologic change in the eyes. Although some are presbyopic by age 35, particularly individuals living in warmer climates (Weale, 1981), this condition will affect virtually everyone by mid- to late midlife, typically between ages 45 and 55 (Abrahamson, 1984; Katchadourian, 1987), and will result in the need for corrective lenses. About 32% of people ages 36–45 are myopic (unable to focus on far objects), and the proportion of individuals with myopia increases through midlife (Grosvenor, 1987; Horvath & Davis, 1990).

Some aspects of sleep become more problematic for the middle-aged. The total number of hours slept and amount of REM (rapid eye movement) sleep remains stable; however, beginning in the 40s, wakeful periods become more frequent and there is progressively less of the deepest kind of sleep (stage 4). The amount of time spent lying awake in bed at night begins to increase (Dement, Miles, & Bliwise, 1982; Katchadourian, 1987; Webb, 1982), resulting in feeling less rested in the mornings.

Both men and women experience reproductive changes in adulthood. For men, a gradual decrease in testosterone begins in early adulthood and continues through life. Although there are cases of men in their 80s fathering children, the quantity of viable sperm usually begins to decrease in the late 40s or 50s. For women, the inability to conceive children is marked by menopause. In her 40s, a woman's capacity to conceive and bear children gradually declines until menopause, which usually occurs between ages 45 and 55. At this point the ovaries become chiefly scar tissue, which no longer produce ova or much estrogen (Memmler & Wood, 1987). Though many women experience symptoms because of the hormonal imbalances that accompany menopause (e.g., dizzy spells, rapid increases in body temperature or "hot flashes," sudden mood changes), menopause is not a traumatic event for most women. Rather, it is the marker of a certain distance in life and the knowledge that they are no longer able to conceive and bear children (Siegal, 1992). The chapter by Avis in this book provides more discussion on menopause and fertility.

DISEASE PREVALENCE AND INCIDENCE

In midlife the frequency of chronic illnesses, persistent symptoms, and disability begins to rise. However, all changes in health during midlife are not negative. The frequency of accidents declines, and individuals become less susceptible to colds and the allergies of their youth. Indeed, many people live through their middle years without knowing what it is to be sick or incapacitated. Nevertheless, increasingly more people develop chronic diseases and persistent health problems.

The increasing rates of disease can be seen when examining prevalence and incidence data. Prevalence measures the number or proportion of people in a population who have a disease or condition at a point in time. Incidence measures the number of new cases of an illness or condition over a period of time (e.g., a year).

Prevalence of chronic conditions rises with each decade from midlife on. This includes an increase in both potentially fatal conditions (e.g., coronary heart disease, cancer, stroke) and nonfatal ones (e.g., arthritis, varicose veins, bursitis). Men have higher prevalence of fatal diseases and women have higher prevalence of nonfatal ones (Kandrack, Grant, & Segall, 1991; Verbrugge, 1985; Verbrugge & Wingard,

1987; Wingard, 1984). The most prevalent conditions in midlife are primarily nonfatal.

These points are illustrated in Table I, which shows prevalence of chronic conditions in the noninstitutionalized United States population ages 45–64 (Adams & Benson, 1992). The rates are based on self-reports from the 1991 National Health Interview Survey. Only 3 of the top 30 most prevalent conditions are potentially fatal (heart disease, diabetes, and some diseases of the prostate or female genital organs). Men have a higher prevalence of 8 conditions, including heart disease. Of the remaining 22, women have a greater prevalence of 19 conditions, all nonfatal (e.g., arthritis, sinusitis, varicose veins, cataracts, bunions, corns, and calluses). The rates for diabetes and ingrown nails are virtually the same for men and women.

Although national interview surveys give us an estimate of the prevalence of diseases in the entire population, epidemiologic research studies generally focus on one particular disease or condition. These often provide prevalence and incidence rates based on physiological or clinical measures of disease in addition to self-reports, and fatal or disabling conditions tend to be studied more than nonfatal ones. Table II presents a number of recent studies that provide prevalence rates for diseases that become more common in midlife.

Prevalence rates for these diseases are generally higher for men than for women, and higher for the later rather than earlier years of midlife. Men have higher prevalence of fatal conditions (coronary heart disease, most cancers, stroke). Rates of psychiatric disorders are also greater for men. Women have higher prevalence of diabetes (until late midlife), osteoarthritis of hand and knee, and a major depressive episode. Dementia, including Alzheimer's disease, is uncommon in middle age, but becomes more widespread after midlife.

Only a few studies estimate incidence rates of conditions for men and women in midlife (see Table III). With the exception of breast cancer, men have higher incidence of all fatal conditions than do women. Women have higher incidence rates of breast cancer and osteoporotic fracture of the hip. Incidence rates increase over the course of midlife, lowest rates are in the early years of midlife, and highest rates in the later years. This means that the risk of acquiring a chronic condition increases with age. Over time, gender differences increase for some conditions (stroke, cancer, osteoporotic fracture) and decrease for others (heart attack, diabetes).

In sum, the conditions most common in midlife are nonfatal, though the prevalence of both fatal and nonfatal conditions increases. This indicates that growing numbers of people are experiencing persistent conditions. Incidence rates for chronic diseases also increase, indicating the growing risk of developing those diseases. Women experience more nonfatal chronic conditions than men do; arthritis is the leading chronic condition for women in midlife. Men have the same repertoire of conditions as women, but a higher prevalence of fatal chronic diseases.

TABLE I   Prevalence of Leading Chronic Conditions in the Noninstitutionalized United States Population Aged 45–64 by Gender, 1991

Rank order[a]	Condition	Number of conditions per 1000 population	
		Men	Women
1	Arthritis	193.2 [2]	284.7 [1]
2	Hypertension	242.4 [1]	245.4 [2]
3	Chronic sinusitis	148.0 [6]	192.5 [3]
4	Deformities or other orthopedic impairments	159.6 [4]	149.5 [4]
5	Hearing impairments	178.5 [3]	107.0 [7]
6	Heart disease	152.7 [5]	116.9 [5]
7	Hayfever and allergies	98.0 [7]	115.5 [6]
8	Hemorrhoids	72.0 [8]	64.6[11]
9	Diabetes	57.9[10]	57.0[12]
10	Varicose veins of lower extremities	26.1	88.7 [8]
11	Chronic bronchitis	41.6[13]	65.2[10]
12	Tinnitus	57.5[11]	43.4[17]
13	Visual impairment	63.5 [9]	32.7
14	Migraine headache	26.4[19]	66.3 [9]
15	Intervertebral disk disorders	47.4[12]	40.6[19]
16	Bursitis	38.0[15]	43.9[16]
17	Abdominal hernia	41.1[14]	39.9[20]
18	Asthma	33.7[17]	47.2[13]
19	Dermatitis	33.6[18]	46.7[15]
20	Diseases of prostate	25.5	
	Diseases of female genital organs		46.8[14]
21	Frequent indigestion	37.7[16]	32.3
22	Corns and calluses	23.2	42.4[18]
23	Ingrown nails	26.3[20]	26.8
24	Ulcers	25.2	27.1
25	Dry, itching skin	21.7	24.6
26	Bone spurs or tendonitis	18.3	24.4
27	Cataracts	16.1	23.9
28	Gastritis or duodenitis	12.7	27.2
29	Frequent constipation	8.1	29.3
30	Bunions	4.5	29.1

Note. From Adams and Benson (1992). Superscript indicates 20 leading conditions for each gender.
[a] Rank ordered for total population.

TABLE II   Prevalence of Selected Diseases in Midlife, by Gender

Reference	Study disease or condition	Years of data collection	Age ranges	Men	Women
National Heart Lung and Blood Institute, 1992	Coronary heart disease (% population)	1988	45–64	9.1	4.1
Collins, 1993	Breast cancer, malignant (per 1000)	1986–88	45–64		9.6
	Lung cancer, malignant (per 1000)	1986–88	45–64	1.7	1.3
	Prostate cancer, malignant (per 1000)	1986–88	45–64	2.9	
	Colon, rectal, and stomach cancers, malignant (per 1000)	1986–88	45–64	2.4	1.7
	Skin cancer, malignant (per 1000)	1986–88	45–64	20.4	10.5
Wolf et al., 1992	Stroke (% Framingham cohort)	1953–62	55–64	1.4	1.1
		1963–72	55–64	2.3	1.3
		1973–82	55–64	3.1	1.7
Cowie et al., 1993	Non-insulin-dependent diabetes mellitus (% population)	1976–80	45–59	11.1[a] 7.1[b]	20.6[a] 10.8[b]
			60–74	26.0[a] 16.4[b]	21.9[a] 16.5[b]
Lawrence et al., 1989	Osteoarthritis, hand diagnosis based on history (per 100)	1960–82	40–59 60+	3.4 17.0	8.4 29.6
	Osteoarthritis, hand diagnosis based on exam (per 100)	1960–82	40–59 60+	4.0 20.3	8.9 40.8
	Osteoarthritis, knee diagnosis based on x ray (per 100)		45–54 55–64	2.3 4.1	3.6 7.3
Kessler et al., 1993	Major depressive episode: Lifetime (% population) Past 12 months (% population)	1990–92	45–54	11.8 4.0	21.8 11.0
Robins et al., 1991	Any psychiatric disorder (% ECA[d] cohort)	1980s	45–64	47.0[a] 28.0[b] 33.0[c]	33.0[a] 24.0[b] 32.0[c]
Bachman et al., 1992	Dementia (per 1000)	1982–83	61–64 65–69 70–74 75–79	7.8 7.0 31.6 31.3	0.0 10.4 9.6 38.6
	Alzheimer's disease (per 1000)	1982–83	61–64 65–69 70–74 75–79	0.0 3.5 10.5 7.8	0.0 7.8 0.0 29.0

[a] African-American.

[b] Caucasian.

[c] Hispanic.

[d] ECA, epidemiologic catchment area.

TABLE III   Incidence of Selected Diseases in Midlife, by Gender

Reference	Disease or condition	Years of data collection	Age ranges	Men	Women
Kannel & Belanger, 1991	Heart failure (per 1000)		45–54	2.0	1.0
			55–64	4.0	3.0
Havas, 1992	Heart attack (% Maryland population)	1988	40–49	7.9	1.8
			50–59	12.7	4.8
			60–69	17.6	10.3
	Stroke (% Maryland population)		40–49	2.5	2.5
			50–59	6.1	4.2
			60–69	13.4	12.3
Wolf et al., 1992	Stroke (% Framingham cohort)	1953–62	55–64	5.6	5.5
		1963–72	55–64	7.2	4.5
		1973–82	55–64	8.0	5.1
Bamford et al., 1990	Stroke (per 1000):	1981–86			
	Cerebral infarct		45–54	1.1	0.6
			55–64	5.4	3.3
	Primary intracerebral hemorrhage		45–54	0.3	0.1
			55–64	1.0	0.4
	Subarachnoid hemorrhage		45–54	0.1	0.3
			55–64	0.2	0.7
National Cancer Institute, 1993	Breast cancer, malignant (per 100,000)	1990	45–49	0.9	191.4
			50–54	1.1	225.0
			55–59	2.1	273.9
			60–64	2.8	347.1
	Lung cancer, malignant (per 100,000)		45–49	16.7	13.2
			50–54	47.9	32.5
			55–59	107.8	67.3
			60–64	192.4	113.2
	Prostate cancer, malignant (per 100,000)		45–49	7.6	
			50–54	37.5	
			55–59	114.4	
			60–64	287.6	
	Colorectal Cancer, malignant (per 100,000)		45–49	29.0	23.0
			50–54	56.9	47.3
			55–59	108.7	76.9
			60–64	184.3	121.6
Persson et al., 1993	Breast cancer (per 100,000)	1964–68	45–49		122.1
			50–54		127.7
			55–59		140.3
			60–64		158.1
		1974–78	45–49		149.5
			50–54		152.0
			55–59		164.0
			60–64		193.0

(continues)

TABLE III   *(continued)*

Reference	Disease or condition	Years of data collection	Age ranges	Men	Women
Persson et al., 1993	Breast cancer (per 100,000)	1984–88	45–49		157.4
			50–54		162.5
			55–59		184.7
			60–64		229.3
National Institute of Arthritis, Diabetes, & Digestive & Kidney Diseases, 1985	Non-insulin-dependent diabetes mellitus (per 10,000)	1979–81	45–54	61.9	27.1
			55–64	61.9	55.5
Owen, et al., 1980	Osteoporotic fracture of the hip (per 100,000 person years)	1956–74	40–49	4.1	11.1
			50–59	37.4	62.0
			60–69	92.3	250.3

RISK FACTORS FOR DISEASE

There are many factors that contribute to disease and injury, including biologic predispositions, risks encountered in work and leisure activities, health habits, and lifestyle. All of these are called risk factors.

Genetic makeup determines many of our attributes and provides protection from, or increased risk for, disease over the course of a lifetime. Family history of disease also may put an individual at increased risk for that particular disease.

But for most conditions and diseases, it is the way we live our lives that has the greatest influence on delaying and preventing physiologic decline and disease. Individuals who engage in occupations, household chores, or leisure activities that may be considered risky or dangerous (e.g., mining, skyscraper construction, roof repair, mountain climbing, drag racing) are more likely to be injured while engaging in such activities. Certain occupations expose workers to toxins that contribute to disease (e.g., asbestos workers, textile workers). Men usually engage in more of these kinds of activities than women.

Both men and women in midlife engage in deleterious health habits; men generally smoke and drink more than women, but more women tend to be overweight, consume higher levels of dietary fat, and are physically inactive. Just as health habits in youth affect health in midlife, prevailing habits contribute to current and future well-being. Studies of disease often examine the risks and benefits to health incurred by behaviors such as cigarette smoking, alcohol use, dietary habits, and physical activity.

Many risk factors are modifiable; that is, individuals can diminish their exposure to toxins or change behaviors to delay the onset of disease and promote good health. Table IV presents a summary of some known or possible modifiable risk factors for

TABLE IV   Modifiable Risk Factors for Selected Diseases

Risk factor	CHD	STR	NIDDM	BRE	LUNG	PRO	COLRE	MEL	OSPOR	OA
Cigarette smoking	X[a]	X	X	X	X	X	X	X	X	X
Alcohol	?		?						X	
Dietary factors										
Cholesterol	X	X								
Calories			X							
Fat intake	X	X	?	?		X	?			
Salt intake		X								
Fiber			0				0			
Calcium									0	
Potassium	0									
Overweight	X	X	X						X	?
Physical inactivity	0	0	0						0	0
Exposure to toxins				X	X	X	X			
Exposure to ultraviolet rays								X		
Hypertension	X	X								
Diabetes	X	X							X	
Hormone replacement	0			?					0	

Note. CHD, Coronary heart disease; STR, stroke; NIDDM, non-insulin-dependent diabetes mellitus; BRE, breast cancer; LUNG, lung cancer; PRO, prostate cancer; COLRE, colorectal cancer; MEL, melanoma; OSPOR, osteoporosis; OA, osteoarthritis.

[a]X, Positive effect; 0, inverse effect; ?, possible positive effect.

a number of conditions and diseases. The majority of these risk factors involve health habits and lifestyle. Most findings about risks pertain to fatal conditions; there is much less work on the risks for nonfatal conditions.

Cigarette smoking has been studied as a risk factor for most diseases and conditions (Bartecchi, MacKenzie, & Schrier, 1994). It has been found to be a risk for many cancers (American Cancer Society, 1994), predominantly lung cancer (Freedman & Navidi, 1990; Knekt, 1993; Kunst, Looman, & Mackenbach, 1993). The American Cancer Society (1994) estimates that cigarette smoking is responsible for 90% and 79% of lung cancers among men and women, respectively. Those who smoke are also at increased risk of coronary heart disease (American Heart Association, 1994; Hein, Suadicani, & Gyntelberg, 1992b; Wilson, Anderson, & Castelli,

1991), stroke (American Heart Association, 1994; Rosengren, Tsipogianni, & Wilhelmsen, Harmsen, 1990), diabetes, and osteoporosis (Cooper 1991). Smoking increases the risk of coronary heart disease and stroke by 70% (Katchadourian, 1987). Women who smoke are at increased risk of earlier menopause (Brambilla & McKinlay, 1989; S. M. McKinlay, Bifano, & McKinlay, 1985; S. M. McKinlay, Brambilla, & Posner, 1992). Among persons aged 45–64, 28.6% of men and 26.1% of women currently smoke (National Center for Health Statistics, 1994). There is evidence that cessation of smoking decreases risk for lung cancer, coronary heart disease, and stroke almost immediately (Freedman & Navidi, 1990; Kawachi et al., 1993, 1994; Sobue et al., 1993).

Drinking too much alcohol impairs judgment and coordination, elevating the risk for accidents. Indeed, alcohol is involved in a large proportion of motor vehicle accidents. Consumption of too much alcohol has been associated with various cancers (American Cancer Society, 1994) and osteoporosis (Cooper, 1991; Hernandez-Avila et al., 1991). Abuse of alcohol has been linked to coronary heart disease (American Heart Association, 1994), though there is some evidence that moderate amounts may protect against heart disease. In the United States, 68.4% of men and 47.6% of women aged 45–64 drink alcohol. Of these, 14.4% of men and 4.1% of women classify themselves as heavy drinkers, consuming 14 or more alcoholic drinks per week (National Center for Health Statistics, 1994).

A number of dietary factors have been associated with a host of diseases and conditions. Too many calories, high amounts of dietary fat (especially animal fat), too much dietary cholesterol, obesity, and low potassium are associated with coronary heart disease (American Heart Association, 1994). Clinical evidence suggests that cholesterol levels below 200 are optimal for good health. Over a quarter of those in middle age have elevated cholesterol (>200): 26.1% of men and 25.2% of women aged 45–54, and 31.4% of men and 40.4% of women aged 55–64 (National Center for Health Statistics, 1994). Consuming high amounts of fat, a high number of calories, low amounts of fiber, not enough fruits and vegetables, and being overweight are risk factors for many kinds of cancer, such as colorectal and breast cancers (American Cancer Society, 1994; Barrett-Conner & Friedlander, 1993). A diet high in fat and salt and being overweight put individuals at higher risk for stroke (American Heart Association, 1994), and low calcium intake and obesity contribute to osteoporosis (Cooper, 1991; Torgerson, Garton, & Reid, 1993). Obesity also contributes to osteoarthritis (Carman, et al., 1994) and diabetes (Cassano, Rosner, Vokonas, & Weiss, 1992; Haffner, Mitchell, Hazuda, & Stern, 1991). People with abdominal adiposity tend to be at higher risk of diabetes than those with a different adipose distribution.

Though more individuals are dieting, the prevalence of obesity and overweight is growing. Over the past three decades the average weight for individuals in middle age (and other ages) has steadily increased (Kuczmarski, Flegal, Campbell, & Johnson, 1994). There are more people in later midlife who are overweight than in the early years of midlife, and more women than men are overweight. Among those aged 45–54, 35.6% of men and 41.6% of women are overweight or obese, and 40.1% of men and 48.5% of women aged 55–64 are overweight (National Center for Health Statistics, 1994).

Physical activity can help to prevent or delay the onset of disease and disability. Physical inactivity has been linked to coronary heart disease and stroke (American Heart Association, 1994), diabetes (Manson et al., 1991), and osteoporosis (Cooper, 1991; Kelsey, Browner, Seeleyu, Nevitt, & Cummings, 1992). Exercise also benefits the immune system and prevents the risk for premature death. As individuals move through midlife, there is a tendency to decrease physical activity and exercise. Activity levels for men drop more than those for women by the early 60s. However, until age 60, men are substantially more active than women; hence, the larger observed decline in activity level for men is a product of their initially greater activity levels (Shepard & Montelpore, 1988).

People exposed to toxins at work or at home are at greater risk of developing some types of cancer and lung disease (e.g., asbestos workers, persons who use strong toxic pesticides on their yards or gardens, radon gas trapped in the home). Those who work without protection in the sun or who sunbathe, particularly persons with fair skin, are at increased risk of developing melanoma and other skin cancers.

There are some conditions and diseases that are risk factors themselves for other conditions. For example, people with hypertension and diabetes are at greater risk for coronary heart disease and stroke (American Heart Association, 1994). People with hypertension have five times the risk of developing coronary heart disease than those with normal blood pressure (Katchadourian, 1987). Control of these diseases by diet and exercise will reduce the risk for these conditions as well as decrease the risk for heart disease and stroke. Medication is also beneficial in controlling some chronic conditions, such as hypertension.

Hormone replacement therapy, initially used to mediate symptoms experienced by women going through menopause, is prescribed for longer periods of time to reduce the risk of osteoporosis, stroke, and heart disease (Falkeborn et al., 1993; Spector & Brennan, 1992; Torgerson et al., 1993). All of these diseases increase in prevalence and incidence after menopause. For women with a personal or family history of breast or endometrial cancer, hormone replacement therapy is not recommended, as it may promote these types of cancer.

Health habits can not only reduce disease risks but also positively influence some aging processes. Weight gain that often occurs during midlife can be offset by a low-calorie, low-fat diet and regular exercise. Exercise is also beneficial in compensating for muscular deterioration and bone loss. Smoking cessation and exercise can combat and sometimes reverse cardiovascular system changes and increase vital lung capacity. Good health habits can even delay the decrease in vital capacity until the seventh decade (Whitbourne, 1985).

In sum, eating a balanced diet low in fat, maintaining a desirable weight, exercising, not smoking, drinking in moderation (or abstention), and avoiding too much exposure to ultraviolet rays in youth will prevent or delay disease and deleterious conditions and also delay some of the aging changes that take place in midlife. Benefits are often accrued soon after modifying behavior. Further, practicing these healthy behaviors can benefit individuals who are diseased or disabled. Even individuals who had poor health habits in youth can improve their health in midlife by adjusting behaviors.

SYMPTOMS

There are a variety of symptoms that people in midlife often experience more frequently than in youth, including diminished energy, pain, tiredness, and fatigue. These symptoms may or may not be related to a detectable illness, but contribute to both disability and decreased satisfaction with life. Severe or prolonged symptoms may induce people to change their regular activities for a few days or sometimes permanently. For the majority of those in midlife, symptoms are not constant, but come and go; occasionally they interfere with daily activities, but usually they do not.

Sometimes rather vague symptoms indicate subterranean pathologic changes. More often, they are transitory and reflect aging processes or stresses of daily life. Wear and tear on joints can result in stiffness, particularly in the mornings, and occasional pain. More time is needed to recuperate from illness or fatigue. Periods of high-level physical exertion require lengthier and more frequent rest intervals. People find themselves unable to stay up as late at night as in youth.

Much of our information on symptoms is anecdotal in nature; symptoms are the stuff of life, not of surveys. There are few national data for symptoms and discomforts of daily life in middle age, though these symptoms are the majority of the ill-health experience. It is difficult to measure symptoms that are ambiguous or vague, but questions about general pain and tiredness can certainly be asked. Symptom information is necessarily self-reported.

Symptoms most experienced by people in midlife are musculoskeletal in nature, and respiratory symptoms rank second. Other groups of symptoms are much less prevalent. The most common symptoms from these groups are headache, pain and stiffness in many body sites, cold symptoms, tiredness, and tension or nervousness (Verbrugge, 1986b). Whether mild or serious, symptoms can contribute to a diminished sense of well-being.

Although the majority of individuals who experience these symptoms suffer from relatively mild ones, some individuals endure chronic pain and chronic fatigue syndrome, which are serious and debilitating ailments. Chronic pain is relatively widespread in the population. Croft, Rigby, Boswell, Schollum, and Silman (1993) found that 9.3% of men and 25% of women aged 45–54 reported chronic pain lasting more than 3 months. For those aged 55–64, 17.2% of the men and 17.4% of the women experienced chronic pain. Because the cause for pain is often not found, treatment is usually focused on pain management. However, relapse following initial successful treatment of chronic pain ranges from 30 to 60% (Turk & Rudy, 1991). Associated with chronic pain are numbers of somatic syndromes such as swollen joints, dry eyes and mouth, numb arms and legs, and tiredness or fatigue. Fatigue is one of the most common complaints issued in general medical practice (Calabrese, Danao, Camara, & Wilke, 1992). Chronic fatigue syndrome, disabling fatigue for at least 6 months (Shafran, 1991), affects more people in the first years of midlife than in the latter years, and it affects more women than men.

DISABILITY

As disease becomes more prevalent and symptoms a more familiar occurrence in midlife, functional limitation and disability become more common. Trouble with functioning is prompted by both aging and pathological changes. Individuals may begin to find themselves restricted in physical, cognitive, and emotional abilities, thus making daily activities more difficult to perform. The primary cause of functional limitations and disability in midlife is chronic disease, and limitations due to chronic conditions increase with age.

The process of disablement follows the scheme initially introduced by Nagi (1979, 1991) and elaborated by Verbrugge and Jette (1994). The initial pathway begins with active pathology (disease or decline resulting in interference with normal physiologic processes), which leads to impairment (abnormalities or loss in a body system), followed by functional limitation (limitation in performance of fundamental physical and mental actions used in daily life), and results in disability (limitation of socially defined roles and tasks). The aging changes that occur in midlife, and the growing prevalence of chronic disease, can result in a gradual increase in functional limitation and disability in the middle years. Predisposing risk factors (lifestyle, health habits), medical care, and other therapeutic regimens can affect this trajectory at any stage, either promoting, delaying, or preventing disability.

The prevalence of disability in personal care and household chores is quite low for middle-aged individuals, unlike for those of older age. Disability in midlife is usually measured by restriction in major roles, bed-days, and work-loss days. Restriction in activity is usually divided into major (job, keeping house) and secondary (recreation, leisure) activities, and is measured by inability or limitation doing these, rather than by limitation in personal care (e.g., activities of daily living) and household management (e.g., instrumental activities of daily living). Bed-days refer to the number of days spent in bed because of illness or injury; work-loss days refer to the number of days lost from work because of a health problem.

Three quarters of the middle-aged population experience no activity limitation of any kind (Table V). The percent of limited women is just 1.3% more than men. Of those who experience activity limitation, two-thirds are limited in a major activity. Men are more likely to be restricted in a major activity than women (16.9% vs. 15.8%). Women are more likely to be limited in moderate or secondary activities

TABLE V   Activity Limitations Because of Chronic Conditions
in Population Aged 45–64, by Gender

Degree of limitation	Men (%)	Women (%)
No activity limitation	78.5	77.2
Activity limitation	21.5	22.8
Limitation in major activity[a]	16.9	15.8
Unable to carry on major activity	10.2	7.3
Limited in amount or kind of major activity	6.6	8.6
Limited, but not in major activity	4.6	7.0
Bed disability (days per person)	6.6	9.2
Work disability (days per person)	5.9	6.6

Note. From Adams and Benson (1992).

[a]Major activity: job, keeping house, going to school.

than men (7.0% vs. 4.4%). Women in midlife spend more days in bed and miss more work days because of chronic illness. Acute conditions also result in more activity limitation, days in bed, and days lost from work for women.

In recent decades, disability levels have been increasing (Waldron, 1983; Wingard, 1984). Restricted activity because of both acute and chronic conditions has risen sharply, and is primarily due to cutting back on activities rather than an increase in staying in bed (Verbrugge, 1984). In addition, the proportion of persons in midlife who are limited in both major and secondary activities has increased steadily over time. Both acute and chronic conditions are responsible for the increases in disability, though it is primarily the growing prevalence of chronic disease that contributes to greater disability.

SOCIAL ROLES AND HEALTH

The pace of role change is swift in early adulthood, but midlife sees more stability of roles and less transition. Generally, people are reaching the pinnacles of careers, launching children into adulthood, and enjoying a varied array of social roles and activities. However, there have been a number of shifts in the roles occupied in midlife such that they are more varied than ever. Couples who had children early in life may begin a second family; these persons may find themselves occupying the simultaneous roles of parent to young children and grandparent. More couples are delaying marriage and parenthood; more women are having children later in life, increasingly without a spouse. Some persons abandon one career in midlife to pursue another, entirely different career path. As businesses increasingly offer early retirement packages to older employees, more people retire early from one job and begin a new job. As more people live well into old age, more persons in midlife find themselves the caretakers of elderly parents or relatives.

Some of these shifts in roles have been thought to affect health, particularly women's health and well-being. The average age of marriage has increased and more women are postponing childbirth until late in their reproductive life (Knaub, Eversoll, & Voss, 1983). This means more adults are entering midlife with young children, who demand great quantities of time and energy. At the same time, more women are employed at a job outside the home. An additional role, that of caretaker for an elderly parent or relative, is encountered in midlife, and is a role primarily occupied by women. Women continue to carry the majority of the child care and household duties, so their free time is severely restricted; with the added responsibility of caring for an aging adult, stress and fatigue may escalate.

Scholarly interest in women's health when considering the responsibilities and burdens of multiple roles has led to a number of interesting findings. Employment is generally beneficial to women's physical and mental health (Nathanson, 1980); and the combined roles of employment, marriage, and parenthood are associated with good physical health for both men and women (Verbrugge, 1983). The rewards and stresses experienced by women in their roles as mothers is more strongly related to well-being than the rewards and stresses in the caregiver roles (Stephens, Franks, & Townsend, 1994). The quality and context of roles are as important to health and well-being as the roles themselves. Low-quality roles may jeopardize health, whereas high-quality roles may have positive effects on mental (Stephens et al., 1994) and physical health (Verbrugge, 1986a). Persons able to manage many roles successfully may receive beneficial effects (Sieber, 1974; Thoits, 1983), and those, in turn, may help delay the onset of disability and disease.

MORTALITY

Until the middle of the nineteenth century, life expectancy was less than what we now consider the beginning years of midlife. Infectious diseases were the primary cause of mortality; lack of accurate knowledge of disease pathogens and well-intentioned but improper medical interventions made matters worse. The advent of public health interventions in the mid-1800s decreased infectious disease rates substantially. By 1900, life expectancies for newborn males and females were 48.2 and 51.1 years, respectively. The average age of death for males and females in 1900 was 46.3 and 48.3 years, respectively (National Center for Health Statistics, 1991).

Infectious disease was the primary cause of death until the mid-1900s. Though still deadly (one can think of AIDS and new antibiotic-resistant strains of tuberculosis), it is not the scourge it once was. The large decline in mortality in the second half of the nineteenth century was due wholly to a decrease in deaths from infectious diseases; there is no evidence of a decline from other causes (McKeown, Record, & Turner, 1975). The factors that helped bring about this decline were an improvement in standards of living, of which the most salient feature was a better diet, and improvements in hygiene. Better nutrition improved ability to withstand airborne infections; better hygiene and community sanitation decreased exposure to water and food-borne diseases. As infectious disease rates declined and more people lived through midlife, chronic diseases became more prevalent.

Increasing public knowledge about health, growing prosperity, and the introduction of antibiotics improved life expectancy and reduced mortality rates further in the 1900s. These advances in health paved the way for the largest birth cohort in recorded history, the "baby boom" generation. Born between 1946 and 1964, this group will be the largest ever in the United States to enter into and live through midlife to old age. Children and grandchildren of this cohort can expect even longer lives. Life expectancy for infants born late in the twentieth century is 72.3 years for males (72.9 years for white males, 64.6 years for black males) and 78.9 years for females (79.6 years for white females, 73.8 years for black females) (National Center for Health Statistics, 1994).

Underlying the increase in life expectancy are declining mortality rates, steadily dropping since the mid–nineteenth century (McKinlay & McKinlay, 1977). Rates have consistently declined by an average of 1.3% per year in the twentieth century (Brock, Guralnik, & Brody, 1990). Population mortality early in the twentieth century was 16.1 per 1000 men and 13.7 per 1000 women. Currently, among those aged 45–54, mortality rates are 6.3 per 1000 for men (5.5 for white men, 12.6 for black men) and 3.5 per 1000 for women (3.1 for white women, 6.4 for black women). Rates for those aged 55–64 are 16.1 per 1000 for men (14.7 for white men, 26.2 for black men) and 9.1 per 1000 women (8.2 for white women, 14.5 for black women) (National Center for Health Statistics, 1991).

Chronic diseases are now the principal causes of death for individuals from the middle years on. Table VI shows the mortality rates for the 15 leading causes of death among men and women in early and late midlife (National Center for Health Statistics, 1991). Heart disease and malignant neoplasms are the leading causes of death at those ages. In the first half of midlife, cancer claims more lives than heart disease, while the reverse is true in the latter half of midlife. The mortality rate from heart disease for men is double that for women. The gender difference is largest at ages 45–54 and decreases in later years. For cancer, it is much smaller in early midlife, but increases with age. Men experience higher mortality than women for all 15 leading causes of death.

Women's mortality advantage is new to the twentieth century. In the nineteenth century infectious diseases claimed lives without favoring either gender, and for women, mortality during childbirth was exceptionally high. The female advantage in mortality began in the late nineteenth century with the curbing of infectious disease and the introduction of aseptic methods in childbirth. This gender gap in mortality grew from the early twentieth century until the 1970s. The consensus of

TABLE VI   Midlife Mortality Rates from 15 Leading Causes of Death

Rank order[a]	Cause	Deaths per 100,000 population			
		45–54 yrs		55–64 yrs	
		Men	Women	Men	Women
	All causes	629.0	350.9	1606.9	904.7
1	Diseases of the heart	199.8[1]	66.7[2]	584.7[1]	237.0[2]
2	Malignant neoplasms	166.3[2]	154.9[1]	526.7[2]	376.6[1]
3	Cerebrovascular disease	21.0[8]	17.4[3]	59.5[3]	44.0[3]
4	Accidents and adverse effects	47.0[3]	16.0[4]	51.2[5]	20.7[6]
	Motor vehicle accidents	22.5[6]	9.5[6]	21.5	10.5[9]
	All other accidents	24.5[5]	6.6[10]	29.7[7]	10.2[10]
5	Chronic obstructive pulmonary disease and allied conditions	10.2[10]	8.5[8]	59.5[4]	39.0[4]
6	Pneumonia and influenza	10.0	4.8	25.1[9]	13.3[8]
7	Diabetes mellitus	11.5	9.2[7]	28.6[8]	27.5[5]
8	Suicide	21.7[7]	7.9[9]	25.0[10]	7.2
9	Chronic liver disease and cirrhosis	29.1[4]	11.0[5]	45.7[6]	19.8[7]
10	Nephritis, nephrotic syndrome, and nephrosis	3.9	2.7	10.9	8.1
11	Atherosclerosis	1.0	0.5	4.9	2.5
12	Homicide and legal intervention	11.4[9]	3.1	8.2	2.5
13	Septicemia	3.7	2.8	10.4	7.7
14	Emphysema	1.9	1.5	13.5	7.9
15	Congenital abnormalities	1.5	1.3	2.0	1.9
	All other causes	71.1	26.5	99.4	68.3

Notes. From National Center for Health Statistics (1991). Superscript indicates 10 leading causes of death for specific age-gender categories.

[a]Leading causes of death for total population.

researchers (Wingard, 1984) is that this steady increase in the gender difference can be attributed to decreasing mortality rates for diseases affecting only women (i.e., maternal mortality and cancer of the uterus) and increasing mortality rates for diseases affecting primarily men (e.g., lung cancer and cardiovascular disease).

After 1980, the gender difference in mortality began to narrow. For example, mortality from lung cancer has increased for both men and women, but more rapidly for women; therefore, the gender gap for lung cancer mortality has decreased. Late in the twentieth century, women have a mortality advantage of 7 years. Recent gains in life expectancy, however, are accompanied by a higher prevalence of chronic illness and disability (Verbrugge, 1989). Thus, more people will live longer but increasingly be in worse health; women will bear the brunt of this burden as they live longer and experience more disability than men, meaning more of their lives are spent with disability.

CONCLUSION

The period we call midlife is a relatively new phenomenon in human history. Until the beginning of the twentieth century, infectious diseases were the primary cause of death. Chronic diseases were also implicated, but were relatively rare. With the advent of better nutrition and sanitation, and the discovery of antibiotics, mortality rates were dramatically reduced such that the vast majority of individuals live not only to but through midlife and into old age. Still, as people move through the middle years, they observe increasing mortality among their peers, though not nearly to the extent that was observed only a few decades ago. During this century, each subsequent generation has seen improvements in life expectancy and health.

One product of the prosperity and improved health conditions of the twentieth century is the baby boom generation. The largest birth cohort in United States history, it is in the nascence of midlife. Health statistics indicate that this group is healthier than any of its predecessors, with greater life expectancy and lower mortality. Some health habits are better than those of their predecessors (e.g., lower smoking rates, higher levels of physical activity), which bodes well for good health as the group moves through midlife. However, some lifestyle factors are worse than those of previous generations (e.g., more people are overweight, consumption of illicit drugs is greater), which may negate the benefits of healthful habits and healthy legacy. As the baby-boomers move through midlife, they will likely encounter the same markers of aging that previous generations have experienced, including gradual physical change and more chronic health problems.

In midlife individuals begin to see the first signs of their own physical decline. Appearance noticeably changes, marked by indelible lines in the skin and more gray hair. Some of the gradual physiologic changes that have been taking place can no longer be ignored: corrective lenses are needed for reading, more time is needed to recover from strenuous exertion, and belts may need to be loosened a notch. The prevalence of chronic disease and disability begins to climb, and women experience more adverse health conditions and disability than men through the middle years. Individuals begin to know more peers who are ill or impaired. For many, especially those who enjoyed good health through youth, the onset of chronic disease is a shock. What does one do when the realization strikes that the disease will not get better? Others, having faced illness earlier in life, may have better coping mechanisms to deal with new conditions.

There are vast individual differences in the rates of aging and pathological changes. Genetic predisposition, health habits, and lifestyle all contribute significantly to health. The lifestyle and behaviors engaged in during youth and young adulthood can dramatically affect health in midlife, just as middle-aged individuals' health habits and ways of life will affect their journey through midlife and into older age. Individuals do have some control over their health; not only will healthful lifestyle choices improve future health, they can also alleviate or reduce the prevailing effects of symptoms, disability, and disease in daily life.

Midlife is just that, the midstream time of adult life. Beyond youth's constant newness, and not yet at that place in older years where remembered times exceed dreams of the future, midlife is a mix of new opportunities and expanding resources accompanied by incipient declines in physical abilities and some distinct losses. Some dreams have been realized, and others abandoned. While there are new experiences and milestones at every age, midlife sees fewer than youth did. Time seems to pass more quickly, birthdays seem to be celebrated at an accelerated rate. There are new challenges and many satisfying overlapping roles, but less energy with which to meet them. As individuals take stock of their lives, recalling youthful abilities and planning for old age, they find themselves squarely in the middle.

REFERENCES

Abrahamson, I. A., Jr. (1984). Eye changes after forty. *American Family Physician, 29,* 171–181.

Adams, P. F., & Benson, V. (1992). Current estimates form the National Health Interview Survey, 1991. *Vital and health statistics,* Series 10, No. 184 (DHHS Publication No. (PHS) 93-1512). Hyattsville, MD: National Center for Health Statistics.

American Cancer Society. (1994). *Cancer facts and figures—1994.* Atlanta, GA: American Cancer Society National Headquarters.

American Chronic Pain Association. (1994). *Facts about chronic pain fact sheet.* Rocklin, CA: Author.

American Heart Association. (1994). *Heart and stroke facts: 1994 statistical supplement.* Dallas, TX: American Heart Association National Center.

Antman, K. H. (1993). Natural history and epidemiology of malignant mesothelioma. *Chest, 103,* 373S–376S.

Bachman, D. L., Wolf, P. A., Linn, R., Knoefel, J. E., Cobb, J., Belanger, A., D'Agostino, R. B., & White, L. R. (1992). Prevalence of dementia and probable senile dementia of the Alzheimer type in the Framingham study. *Neurology, 42,* 115–119.

Bamford, J., Sandercock, P., Dennis, M., Burn, J., & Warlow, C. (1990). A prospective study of acute cerebrovascular disease in the community: the Oxfordshire Community Stroke Project—1981–86. 2. Incidence, case fatality rates and overall outcome at one year of cerebral infarction, primary intercerebral and subarachnoid haemorrhage. *Journal of Neurology, Neurosurgery, and Psychiatry, 53,* 16–22.

Barrett-Conner, E., & Friedlander, N. J. (1993). Dietary fat, calories, and the risk of breast cancer in postmenopausal women: a prospective population-based study. *Journal of the American College of Nutrition, 12,* 390–399.

Bartecchi, C. E., MacKenzie, T. D., & Schrier, R. W. (1994). The human costs of tobacco use (1). *New England Journal of Medicine, 330,* 907–912.

Bonita, R. (1992). Epidemiology of stroke. *Lancet, 339,* 342–344.

Brambilla, D. J., & McKinlay, S. M. (1989). A prospective study of factors affecting age at menopause. *Journal of Clinical Epidemiology, 42,* 1031–1039.

Brock, D. B., Guralnik, J. M., & Brody, J. A. (1990). Demography and epidemiology of aging in the United States. In E. L. Schneider & J. W. Rowe (Eds.), *The handbook of the biology of aging* (3rd ed., pp. 3–23). San Diego: Academic Press.

Burckhardt, C. S. (1990). Chronic pain. *Nursing Clinics of North America, 25,* 863–870.

Calabrese, L., Danao, T., Camara, E., & Wilke, W. (1992). Chronic fatigue syndrome. *American Family Physician, 45,* 1205–1213.

Carman, W. J., Sowers, M., Hawthorne, V. M., & Weissfeld, L. A. (1994). Obesity as a risk factor for osteoarthritis of the hand and wrist: a prospective study. *American Journal of Epidemiology, 139,* 119–129.

Cassano, P. A., Rosner, B., Vokonas, P. S., & Weiss, S. T. (1992). Obesity and body fat distribution in relation to the incidence of non-insulin-dependent diabetes mellitus. A prospective cohort study of men in the normative aging study. *American Journal of Epidemiology, 136,* 1474–1486.

Chidgey, L. K. (1992). Chronic wrist pain. *Orthopedic Clinics of North America, 23,* 49–64.

Colditz, G. A., Rimm, E. B., Giovanucci, E., Stampfer, M. J., Rosner, B., & Willett, W. C. (1991). A prospective study of parental history of myocardial infarction and coronary artery disease in men. *American Journal of Cardiology, 67,* 933–938.

Colditz, G. A., Willett, W. C., Hunter, D. J., Stampfer, M. J., Manson, J. E., Hennekens, C. H., & Rosner, B. A. (1993). Family history, age, and risk of breast cancer. Prospective data from the Nurses' Health Study. *Journal of the American Medical Association, 270,* 338–343.

Collins, J. G. (1993). *Prevalence of selected chronic conditions: United States, 1986–1988. Vital and Health Statistics.* Series 10, No. 182. (DHHS Publication No. (PHS) 93–1510). Hyattsville, MD: National Center for Health Statistics.

Compston, J. E. (1990). Osteoporosis. *Clinical Endocrinology, 33,* 653-682.

Compston, J. E. (1992). Risk factors for osteoporosis. *Clinical Endocrinology, 36,* 223–224.

Cooper, C. (1991). Review of UK data on the rheumatic diseases—6. Osteoporosis. *British Journal of Rheumatology, 30,* 135–137.

Cowie, C. C., Harris, M. I., Silverman, R. E., Johnson, E. W., & Rust, K. F. (1993). Effect of multiple risk factors on differences between blacks and whites in the prevalence of non-insulin-dependent diabetes mellitus in the United States. *American Journal of Epidemiology, 137,* 719–732.

Croft, P., Rigby, A. S., Boswell, R., Schollum, J., & Silman, A. (1993). The prevalence of chronic widespread pain in the general population. *Journal of Rheumatology, 20,* 710–713.

Cummings, S. R., Kelsey, J. L., Nevitt, M. C., & O'Dowd, J. (1985). Epidemiology of osteoporosis and osteoporotic fractures. *Epidemiologic Reviews, 7,* 178–208.

Dement, W. C., Miles, L. E., & Bliwise, D. L. (1982). Physiologic markers of aging: Human sleep pattern changes. In M. E. Reff & E. L. Schneider (Eds.), *Biological markers of aging.* National Institutes of Health Publication No. 82-2221. Bethesda, MD; National Institutes of Health.

Donald, J. J., & Burhenne, H. G. (1993). Colorectal cancer. Can we lower the death rate in the 1990s? *Canadian Family Physician, 39,* 107–114.

Evans, D. A., Funkenstein, H. H., Albert, M. S., Scherr, P. A., Cook, N. R., Chown, M. J., Hebert, L. E., Hennekens, C. H., & Taylor, J. O. (1989). Prevalence of Alzheimer's disease in a community population of older persons. Higher than previously reported. *Journal of the American Medical Association, 262,* 2551–2556.

Fain, J. A. (1993). National trends in diabetes. An epidemiologic perspective. *Nursing Clinics of North America, 28,* 1–7.

Falkeborn, M., Persson, I., Terent, A., Adami, H. O., Lithell, H., & Bergstrom, R. (1993). Hormone replacement therapy and the risk of stroke. Follow-up of a population-based cohort in Sweden. *Archives of Internal Medicine, 153,* 1201–1209.

Felson, D. T. (1988). Epidemiology of hip and knee osteoarthritis. *Epidemiologic Reviews, 10,* 1–28.

Fleming, L. A. (1991). Osteoporosis: Clinical features, prevention and treatment. *Journal of General Internal Medicine, 7,* 554–562.

Follick, M. J., Smith, T. W., & Ahern, D. K. (1985). The sickness impact profile: a global measure of disability in chronic low back pain. *Pain, 21,* 67–76.

Fraser, G. E., Strahan, T. M., Sabate, J., Beeson, W. L., & Kissinger, D. (1992). Effects of traditional coronary risk factors on rates of incident coronary events in a low-risk population. The Adventist Health Study. *Circulation, 86,* 406–413.

Freedman, D. A., & Navidi, W. C. (1990). Ex-smokers and the multistage model for lung cancer. *Epidemiology, 1,* 21–29.

Garcia-Valdecasas, J. C., Llovera, J. M., deLacy, A. M., Reverter, J. C., Grande, L., Fuster, J., Cugat, E., Visa, J., & Pera, C. (1991). Obstructing colorectal carcinomas. Prospective study. *Diseases of the Colon and Rectum, 34,* 759–762.

Giovannucci, E., Ascherio, A., Rimm, E. B., Colditz, G. A., Stampfer, M. J., & Willett, W. C. (1993). A prospective cohort study of vasectomy and prostate cancer in US men. *Journal of the American Medical Association, 269,* 873–877.

Goldenberg, D. L., Simms, R. W., Geiger, A., & Komaroff, A. L. (1990). High frequency of fibromyalgia in patients with chronic fatigue seen in a primary care practice. *Arthritis and Rheumatism, 33,* 381–387.

Grech, E. D., Ramsdale, D. R., Bray, C. L., & Faragher, E. B. (1992). Family history as an independent risk factor of coronary artery disease. *European Heart Journal, 13,* 1311–1315.

Grosvenor, T. (1987). A review and a suggested classification system for myopia on the basis of age-related prevalence and age of onset. *American Journal of Optometry and Physiological Optics, 64,* 545–554.

Haffner, S. M., Mitchell, B. D., Hazuda, H. P., & Stern, M. P. (1991). Greater influence of central distribution of adipose tissue on incidence of non-insulin-dependent diabetes in women than men. *American Journal of Clinical Nutrition, 53,* 1312–1317.

Hamman, R. F. (1992). Genetic and environmental determinants of non-insulin-dependent diabetes mellitus (NIDDM). *Diabetes and Metabolism Review, 8,* 287–338.

Harmsen, P., Rosengren, A., Tsipogianni, A., & Wilhelmsen, L. (1990). Risk factors for stroke in middle-aged men in Goteborg, Sweden. *Stroke, 21,* 223–229.

Havas, S. (1992). Heart disease, cancer, and stroke in Maryland. *Southern Medical Journal, 85,* 599–607.

Hein, H. O., Suadicani, P., & Gyntelberg, F. (1992a). Lung cancer risk and social class. The Copenhagen Male Study—17 year follow up. *Danish Medical Bulletin, 39,* 173–176.

Hein, H. O., Suadicani, P., & Gyntelberg, F. (1992b). Ischaemic heart disease incidence by social class and form of smoking: the Copenhagen Male Study—17 years' follow-up. *Journal of Internal Medicine, 231,* 477–483.

Helzer, J. E., Burnam, A., & McEvoy, L. T. (1991). Alcohol abuse and dependence. In L. N. Robins & D. A. Regier (Eds.), *Psychiatric disorders in America: The epidemiologic catchment area study* (pp. 81–115). New York: The Free Press.

Hernandez-Avila, M., Colditz, G. A., Stampfer, M. J., Rosner, B., Speizer, F. E., & Willett, W. C. (1991). Caffeine, moderate alcohol intake, and risk of fractures of the hip and forearm in middle aged women. *American Journal of Clinical Nutrition, 54,* 157–163.

Holzman, A. D., Rudy, T. E., Gerber, K. E., Turk, D. C., Sanders, S. H., Zimmerman, J., & Kerns, R. D. (1985). Chronic pain: a multiple-setting comparison of patient characteristics. *Journal of Behavioral Medicine, 8,* 411–422.

Horvath, T. B., & Davis, K. L. (1990). Central nervous system disorders in aging. In E. L. Schneider & J. W. Rowe (Eds.), *The handbook of the biology of aging* (3rd ed., pp. 306–329). San Diego: Academic Press.

Kandrack, M. A., Grant, K. R., & Segall, A. (1991). Gender differences in health related behaviour: some unanswered questions. *Social Science Medicine, 32,* 579–590.

Kannel, W. B., & Belanger, A. J. (1991). Epidemiology of heart failure. *American Heart Journal, 121,* 951–957.

Kaplan, G. A., & Keil, J. E. (1993). Socioeconomic factors and cardiovascular disease: a review of the literature. *Circulation, 88,* 1973–1998.

Katchadourian, H. (1987). *Fifty: Midlife in perspective.* New York: W. H. Freeman.

Katzman, R. (1993). Education and the prevalence of dementia and Alzheimer's disease. *Neurology, 43,* 13–20.

Kawachi, I., Colditz, G. A., Stampfer, M. J., Willett, W. C., Manson, J. E., Rosner, B., Speizer, F. E., & Hennekens, C. H. (1993). Smoking cessation and decreased risk of stroke in women. *Journal of the American Medical Association, 269,* 232–236.

Kawachi, I., Colditz, G. A., Stampfer, M. J., Willett, W. C., Manson, J. E., Rosner, B., Speizer, F. E., & Hennekens, C. H. (1994). Smoking cessation and time course of decreased risks of coronary heart disease in middle-aged women. *Archives of Internal Medicine, 154,* 169–175.

Kelsey, J. L., Browner, W. S., Seeleyu, D. G., Nevitt, M. C., & Cummings, S. R. (1992). Risk factors for fractures of the distal forearm and proximal humerus. The Study of Osteoporotic Fractures Research Group. *American Journal of Epidemiology, 135,* 477–489.

Kessler, R. C., McGonagle, K. A., Swartz, M., Blazer, D. G., & Nelson, C. B. (1993). Sex and depression in the National Comorbidity Survey. I: Lifetime prevalence, chronicity and recurrence. *Journal of Affective Disorders, 29,* 85–96.

Kizilay, P. E. (1992). Predictors of depression in women. *Nursing Clinics of North America, 27,* 983–993.

Knaub, P. K., Eversoll, D. B., & Voss, J. H. (1983). Is parenthood a desirable adult role? An assessment of attitudes held by contemporary women. *Sex Roles, 9,* 355–362.

Knekt, P. (1993). Vitamin E and smoking and the risk of lung cancer. *Annals of the New York Academy of Sciences, 686,* 280–287.

Kohn, G. J., & Lawson, M. J. (1992). Colorectal cancer. Identifying and screening high-risk patients. *Postgraduate Medicine, 91,* 241–253.

Kuczmarski, R. J., Flegal, K. M., Campbell, S. M., & Johnson, C. L. (1994). Increasing prevalence of overweight among U.S. adults. The National Health and Nutrition Surveys, 1960–1991. *Journal of the American Medical Association, 272,* 205–211.

Kunst, A. E., Looman, C. W., & Mackenbach, J. P. (1993). Determinants of regional differences in lung cancer mortality in The Netherlands. *Social Science and Medicine, 37,* 623–631.

Kvale, G., & Heuch, I. (1991). Is the incidence of colorectal cancer related to reproduction? A prospective study of 63,000 women. *International Journal of Cancer, 47,* 390–395.

Kvale, G., Heuch, I., & Nilssen, S. (1991). Reproductive factors and cancers of the breast and genital organs—are the different cancer sites similarly affected? *Cancer Detection and Prevention, 15,* 369–377.

Kyle, D. V., & deShazo, R. D. (1992). Chronic fatigue syndrome: a conundrum. *American Journal of Medical Science, 303,* 28–34.

Lakatta, E. G. (1990). The heart and circulation. In E. L. Schneider & J. W. Rowe (Eds.), *The handbook of the biology of aging* (3rd ed., pp. 181–216). San Diego: Academic Press.

Lakier, J. B. (1992). Smoking and cardiovascular disease. *American Journal of Medicine, 93,* 8S–12S.

Lane, T. J., Matthews, D. A., & Manu, P. (1990). The low yield of physical examinations and laboratory investigations of patients with chronic fatigue. *American Journal of Medical Science, 299,* 313–318.

Large, R., Butler, M., James, F., & Peters, J. (1990). A systems model of chronic musculoskeletal pain. *Australia and North America Journal of Psychiatry, 24,* 529–536.

Larsson, B., Bengtsson, C., Bjorntorp, P., Lapidus, L., Sjorstrom, L., Svardsudd, K., Tibblin, G., Wedel, H., Welin, L., & Wilhelmsen, L. (1992). Is abdominal body fat distribution a major explanation for the sex difference in the incidence of myocardial infarction? The study of men born in 1913 and the study of women, Goteborg, Sweden. *American Journal of Epidemiology, 135,* 266–273.

Lawrence, R. C., Hochberg, M. C., Kelsey, J. L., McDuffie, F. C., Medsger, T. A., Jr., Felts, W. R., & Shulman, L. E. (1989). Estimates of the prevalence of selected arthritic and musculoskeletal diseases in the United States. *Journal of Rheumatology, 16,* 427–441.

Levin, B. (1993). Colorectal cancer screening. *Cancer, 72,* 1056–1060.

Linet, M. S., & Stewart, W. F. (1984). Migraine headache: Epidemiologic perspectives. *Epidemiologic Reviews, 6,* 100–139.

Lipowski, Z. J. (1990). Chronic idiopathic pain syndrome. *Annals of Medicine, 22,* 213–217.

Lordi, G. M., & Reichman, L. B. (1993). Pulmonary complications of asbestos exposure. *American Family Physician, 48,* 1471–1477.

Lynne-Davies, P. (1977). Influence of age on the respiratory system. *Geriatrics, 32,* 57–60.

Manson, J. E., Colditz, G. A., Stampfer, M. J., Willett, W. C., Krolewski, A. S., Rosner, B., Arky, R. A., Speizer, F. E., & Hennekens, C. H. (1991). A prospective study of maturity-onset diabetes mellitus and risk of coronary heart disease and stroke in women. *Archives of Internal Medicine, 151,* 1141–1147.

Manson, J. E., Rimm, E. B., Colditz, G. A., Stampfer, M. J., Willett, W. C., Arky, R. A., Rosner, B., Hennekens, C. H., & Speizer, F. E. (1992). Parity and incidence of non-insulin-dependent diabetes mellitus. *American Journal of Medicine, 93,* 13–18.

Manson, J. E., Rimm, E. B., Stampfer, M. J., Colditz, G. A., Willett, W. C., Krolewski, A. S., Rosner, B., Hennekens, C. H., & Speizer, F. E. (1991). Physical activity and incidence of non-insulin-dependent diabetes mellitus in women. *Lancet, 338,* 774–778.

Mas, J. L., & Zuber, M. (1993). Epidemiology of stroke. *Journal of Neuroradiology, 20(2),* 85–101.

McBride, P. E. (1992). The health consequences of smoking. Cardiovascular diseases. *Medical Clinics of North America, 76,* 333–353.

McKeag, D. B. (1992). The relationship of osteoarthritis and exercise. *Clinics of Sports Medicine, 11,* 471–487.

McKeown, T., Record, R. G., & Turner, R. D. (1975). An interpretation of the decline in mortality in England and Wales during the twentieth century. *Population Studies, 29,* 391–422.

McKinlay, J. B., & McKinlay, S. M. (1977). The questionable contribution of medical measures to the decline of mortality in the United States in the twentieth century. *Milbank Memorial Fund Quarterly, 55,* 405–428.

McKinlay, S. M., Bifano, N. L., & McKinlay, J. B. (1985). Smoking and age at menopause in women. *Annals of Internal Medicine, 103,* 350–356.

McKinlay, S. M., Brambilla, D. J., & Posner, J. G. (1992). The normal menopause transition. *Maturitas, 14,* 103–115.

Memmler, R. L., & Wood, D. L. (1987). *The human body in health and disease* (6th ed.). Philadelphia: JB Lippincott Company.

Miller, R. (1990). Aging and the immune response. In E. L. Schneider & J. W. Rowe (Eds.), *The handbook of the biology of aging* (3rd ed., pp. 157–180). San Diego: Academic Press.

Murtagh, J. (1990). Common problems. Tiredness. *Australian Family Physician, 19,* 909–910.

Nagi, S. Z. (1979). The concept and measurement of disability. In E. D. Berkowitz (Ed.), *Disability policies and government programs.* New York: Praeger.

Nagi, S. Z. (1991). Disability concepts revisited: implications for prevention. In A. M. Pope & A. R. Tarlov (Eds.), in *Disability in America: Toward a national agenda for prevention* (pp. 309–327). Washington, DC: Division of Health Promotion and Disability Prevention, Institute of Medicine, National Academy Press.

Nathanson, C. (1980). Social roles and health status among women: The significance of employment. *Social Science and Medicine, 14,* 463–471.

National Cancer Institute. (1993). *Cancer statistics review, 1973–1990.* (DHHS Publication No. (PHS) 93-2789). Bethesda, MD: National Institutes of Health.

National Center for Health Statistics. (1991). *Vital statistics of the U.S., 1988, Vol. II. Mortality,* Pt. A (DHHS Publication No. (PHS) 91–1101). Hyattsville, MD: Author.

National Center for Health Statistics. (1994). *Health, United States, 1993* (DHHS Publication No. (PHS) 94-1232). Hyattsville, MD: Author.

National Heart, Lung, and Blood Institute. (1992). *National Heart, Lung, and Blood Institute data fact sheet: CHD morbidity.* U.S. Dept. of Health and Human Services. Bethesda, MD: National Institutes of Health.

National Institute of Arthritis, Diabetes, and Digestive and Kidney Diseases. (1985). *Diabetes in America: Diabetes data compiled* (DHHS Publication No. 85-1468). U.S. Department of Health and Human Services. Bethesda, MD: National Institutes of Health.

Nomura, A., Stemmermann, G. N., Chyou, P. H., Marcus, E. B., & Buist, A. S. (1991). Prospective study of pulmonary function and lung cancer. *American Review of Respiratory Disease, 149,* 307–311.

Owen, R. A., Melton, J. L., III, Gallagher, J. C., & Riggs, L. B. (1980). The national cost of acute care of hip fractures associated with osteoporosis. *Clinical Orthopaedics, 150,* 172–176.

Persson, I., Bergstrom, R., Sparen, P., Thorn, M., & Adami, H. O. (1993). Trends in breast cancer incidence in Sweden 1958–1988 by time period and birth cohort. *British Journal of Cancer, 68,* 1247–1253.

Pienta, K. J., & Esper, P. S. (1993). Risk factors for prostate cancer. *Annals of Internal Medicine, 118,* 793–803.

Purdie, D. W. (1992). Screening for osteoporosis. *British Journal of Hospital Medicine, 47,* 605–608.

Reilly, P. A., & Littlejohn, G. O. (1990). Fibrositis/fibromyalgia syndrome: The key to the puzzle of chronic pain. *Medical Journal of Australia, 152,* 226–228.

Robins, L. N., Locke, B. Z., & Regier, D. A. (1991). An overview of psychiatric disorders in America. In L. N. Robins & D. A. Regier (Eds.), *Psychiatric disorders in America: The Epidemiologic Catchment Area Study* (pp. 328–366). New York: The Free Press.

Robinson, J. G., & Leon, A. S. (1994). The prevention of cardiovascular disease. Emphasis on secondary prevention. *Medical Clinics of North America, 78,* 69–98.

Rocca, W. A., Hofman, A., Brayne, C., Breteler, M. M. B., Clarke, M., & Copeland, J. R. M. (1991). Frequency and distribution of Alzheimer's disease in Europe: A collaborative study of 1980–1990 prevalence findings. *Annals of Neurology, 30,* 381–390.

Rudy, T. E., Turk, D. C., Brena, S. F., Stieg, R. L., & Brody, M. C. (1990). Quantification of biomedical findings of chronic pain patients: development of an index of pathology. *Pain, 42,* 167–182.

Samet, J. M. (1992a). The health benefits of smoking cessation. *Medical Clinics of North America, 76,* 399–414.

Samet, J. M. (1992b). Indoor radon and lung cancer. Estimating the risks. *Western Journal of Medicine, 156,* 25–29.

Shafran, S. D. (1991). The chronic fatigue syndrome. *American Journal of Medicine, 90,* 730–739.

Shepard, R. J. (1978). *Physical activity and aging.* Chicago: Yearbook Medical.

Shepard, R. J., & Montelpore, W. (1988). Geriatric benefits of exercise as an adult. *Journal of Gerontology, 43,* M86-M90.

Sieber, S. D. (1974). Toward a theory of role accumulation. *American Sociological Reviews, 39,* 567–578.

Siegal, D. L. (1992). Women's reproductive changes: A marker, not a turning point. In L. Glass & J. Hendricks (Eds.), *Gender and aging* (pp. 53–58). Amityville, NY: Baywood Publishing Company.

Smith, D. W. E. (1992). The biology of gender and aging. In L. Glass & J. Hendricks (Eds.), *Gender and aging* (pp. 5–14). Amityville, NY: Baywood Publishing Company.

Sobue, T., Yamaguchi, N., Suzuki, T., Fujimoto, I., Matsuda, M., Doi, O., Mori, T., Furuse, K., Fukuoka, M., & Yasumitsu, T. (1993). Lung cancer incidence rate for male ex-smokers according to age at cessation of smoking. *Japanese Journal of Cancer Research, 84,* 601–607.

Sorkin, B. A., Rudy, T. E., Hanlon, R. B., Turk, D. C., & Stieg, R. L. (1990). Chronic pain in old and young patients: Differences appear less important than similarities. *Journal of Gerontology, 45,* P64–P68.

Spector, T. D., Brennan, P., Harris, P. A., Studd, J. W., & Silman, A. J. (1992). Do current regimes of hormone replacement therapy protect against subsequent fractures? *Osteoporosis International, 2,* 219–224.

Stamler, J., Stamler, R., & Neaton, J. D. (1993). Blood pressure, systolic and diastolic, and cardiovascular risks. U.S. population data. *Archives of Internal Medicine, 143,* 598–615.

Stephens, M. A. P., Franks, M. M., & Townsend, A. L. (1994). Stress and rewards in women's multiple roles: The case of women in the middle. *Psychology and Aging, 9,* 45–52.

Stolk, R. P., van Splunder, I. P., Schouten, J. S., Witteman, J. C., Hofman, A., & Brobbee, D. E. (1993). High blood pressure and the incidence of non-insulin dependent diabetes mellitus: Findings in a 11.5 year follow-up study in The Netherlands. *European Journal of Epidemiology, 9,* 134–139.

Tepper, S., & Hochberg, M. C. (1993). Factors associated with hip osteoarthritis: Data from the First National Health and Nutrition Examination Survey (NHANES-I). *American Journal of Epidemiology, 137,* 1081–1088.

Thoits, P. A. (1983). Multiple identities and psychological well-being: A reformulation and test of the social isolation hypothesis. *American Sociological Reviews, 48,* 174–187.

Tierney, D., Romito, P., & Messing, K. (1990). She ate not the bread of idleness: Exhaustion is related to domestic and salaried working conditions among 539 Quebec hospital workers. *Women and Health, 16,* 21–42.

Torgerson, D. J., Garton, M. J., & Reid, D. M. (1993). Falling and perimenopausal women. *Age and Ageing, 22,* 59–64.

Tuomilehto, J., Knowler, W. C., & Zimmet, P. (1992). Primary prevention of non-insulin-dependent diabetes mellitus. *Diabetes Metabolism Review, 8,* 339–353.

Turk, D. C., & Rudy, T. E. (1991). Neglected topics in the treatment of chronic pain patients—relapse, noncompliance, and adherence enhancement. *Pain, 44,* 5–28.

Turk, D. C., Rudy, T. E., & Stieg, R. L. (1988). The disability determination dilemma: Toward a multiaxial solution. *Pain, 34,* 217–229.

Verbrugge, L. M. (1976). Sex differentials in morbidity and mortality in the United States. *Social Biology, 23,* 275–296.

Verbrugge, L. M. (1983). Multiple roles and physical health of women and men. *Journal of Health and Social Behavior, 24,* 16–30.

Verbrugge, L. M. (1984). Longer life but worsening health? Trends in health and mortality of middle-aged and older persons. *Milbank Memorial Fund Quarterly, 62,* 475–519.

Verbrugge, L. M. (1985). Gender and health: An update on hypotheses and evidence. *Journal of Health and Social Behavior, 26,* 156–182.

Verbrugge, L. M. (1986a). Role burdens and physical health of women and men. *Women's Health, 11,* 47–77.

Verbrugge, L. M. (1986b). From sneezes to adieux: Stages of health for American men and women. *Social Science and Medicine, 22,* 1195–1212.

Verbrugge, L. M. (1989). Gender, aging and health. In K. S. Markides (Ed.), *Aging and health: Perspectives on gender, ethnicity and class* (pp. 23–87). Newbury Park, CA: Sage.

Verbrugge, L. M., & Jette, A. M. (1994). The disablement process. *Social Science and Medicine, 38,* 1–14.

Verbrugge, L. M., & Wingard, D. L. (1987). Sex differentials in health and mortality. *Women and Health, 12,* 103–145.

Von Korff, M., Dworkin, S. F., & Resche, L. L. (1990). Graded chronic pain status: An epidemiologic evaluation. *Pain, 40,* 279–291.

Waldron, I. (1983). Sex differences in illness incidence, prognosis and mortality: Issues and evidence. *Social Science and Medicine, 17,* 1107–1123.

Weale, R. A. (1981). Human ocular aging and ambient temperature. *British Journal of Opthalmology, 65,* 869–870.

Webb, W. B. (1982). Sleep in older persons. Sleep structures of 50- to 60-year-old men and women. *Journal of Gerontology, 37,* 581–586.

Weissman, M. M., Gland, R., Joyce, P. R., Newman, S., Wells, J. E., & Wittchen, H. U. (1993). Sex differences in rates of depression: Cross-national perspectives. *Journal of Affective Disorder, 29,* 77–84.

Westerfield, B. T. (1992). Asbestos-related lung disease. *Southern Medical Journal, 85,* 616–620.

Whitbourne, S. K. (1985). *The aging body: Physiological changes and psychological consequences.* New York: Springer Verlag.

Wilson, M. G., Michet, C. J., Jr., Ilstrup, D. M., & Melton, L. J., III. (1990). Idiopathic symptomatic osteoarthritis of the hip and knee: A population-based incidence study. *Mayo Clinic Proceedings, 65,* 1214–1221.

Wilson, P. W., Anderson, K. M., & Castelli, W. P. (1991). Twelve-year incidence of coronary heart disease in middle-aged adults during the era of hypertensive therapy: The Framingham offspring study. *American Journal of Medicine, 90,* 11–16.

Wingard, D. L. (1982). The sex differences in mortality rates. *American Journal of Epidemiology, 115,* 205–216.

Wingard, D. L. (1984). The sex differential in morbidity, mortality and lifestyle. In L. Breslow, J. E. Fielding, & L. B. Lave (Eds.), *Annual review of public health* (pp. 433–458). Palo Alto, CA: Annual Reviews, Inc.

Wolf, P. A., D'Agostino, R. B., O'Neal, M. A., Sytkowski, P., Kase, C. S., Belanger, A. J., & Kannel, W. B. (1992). Secular trends in stroke incidence and mortality. The Framingham Study. *Stroke, 23,* 1551–1555.

Zhu, H., & Wang, Z. (1993). Study of occupational lung cancer in asbestos factories in China. *British Journal of Industrial Medicine, 50,* 1039–1042.

CHAPTER 5

Women's Health at Midlife

Nancy E. Avis

Institute for Women's Research, New England Research Institutes, Watertown, Massachusetts

INTRODUCTION

Middle age is often seen as a marker in the aging process for women's health. Physiologically, the most notable event for most women is the cessation of menses—menopause—and the associated hormonal changes. It is unclear whether other physiological changes thought to occur at this time (e.g., changes in weight and body composition, bone density, and lipids) are tied directly to changes in hormones or are independently part of the aging process. In Western societies, middle age is often seen in terms of losses—loss of reproductive capacity, attractiveness, bone density, sexual functioning—the beginning of the eventual decline. Menopause and other physiological changes may also have a psychological effect, as they serve as concrete reminders of aging. Yet, this universal event is experienced quite differently among women and across societies. Cross-cultural studies reveal wide variation in the menopause experience. Psychosocial factors have also been found to influence how menopause and related physiological changes are experienced. This interaction of the biological, psychological, and sociocultural influences determines how women experience menopause.

As the predominant event in women's health at middle age, menopause is largely the subject of this chapter. The last section reviews the long-term health changes thought to be associated with menopause (e.g., bone density, cardiovascular functioning, urogenital functioning) and the implications of menopause for increased risk of cardiovascular disease, osteoporosis, and urogenital changes.

MENOPAUSE

According to popular view and many experts, the menopause, or so-called change of life, is thought to represent a major cultural, psychological, and physiological milestone for women during the middle years. It signifies the end of reproduction and is a prominent biological marker for an aging process in cultures that extol youthfulness. Menopause has been viewed through the ages as a sign of sin and decay, psychological loss, and more recently as a deficiency disease (Kaufert & McKinlay, 1985; McCrea, 1983).

Victorian physicians in the nineteenth century inevitably "blamed the frequency and seriousness of menopause on indiscretions of earlier life" (Stearns, 1975). Twentieth century psychoanalytic writers typically regarded menopause as a critical event in the life of a middle-aged woman that was a threat to her adjustment and self-concept, as exemplified by Helen Deutsch who referred to loss of reproductive life as a partial death (Deutsch, 1945). Since the middle of this century, the medical community in general has often viewed menopause as a deficiency disease in which the postmenopausal woman is in an "estrogen deficient" state due to "ovarian failure" (Kaufert & McKinlay, 1985; McCrea, 1983).

Robert Wilson (1966) has written that "the menopausal woman is not normal; she suffers from a deficiency disease with serious sequelae and needs treatment." Women experiencing this normal end of reproduction are thought to experience regret, to evidence signs of clinical depression (involutional melancholia), to present with a broad range of accompanying symptoms, to be high utilizers of physicians' services, and generally to consume a disproportionate share of medical resources (Reuben, 1969; Wilson, 1966). Such a characterization would appear to receive reinforcement both from pharmaceutical advertisements in professional medical journals (Chapman, 1979; Prather & Fidell, 1975) and from patient images used and developed during the course of medical education (Howell, 1974; Lock, 1985; Scully & Bart, 1973). Those who approach menopause from a life-span perspective, however, are more apt to view menopause as an opportunity for positive growth and development (Neugarten, 1968; Notman, 1990).

Menopause occurs at a time when women are also experiencing other life changes and responsibilities associated with aging. Children are getting older and may be leaving or returning home. Parents are aging and may cause increased worry or caretaking responsibility. For some women this may be a time of increased independence and positive growth. It is often difficult to disentangle the effects of menopause per se from other events associated with middle-age. Because of the complex interaction of this physiological change with a society's views and a woman's own life situation, to understand what menopause means to women, it must be viewed in a biopsychosocial context in women's lives. This chapter reviews the physiological changes associated with menopause, how individuals and societies view menopause, and the interaction among these factors.

Historical Perspective

Menopause was discussed in medical writings as early as A.D. 600. At this time, cessation of menses was described as occurring between the ages of 35 and 50 and linked to a woman's lifestyle. Over the centuries, our understanding of menopause has been influenced by social norms and attitudes as well as the understanding of menstruation and physiology. In 1777 John Leake proposed in his book *Chronic or Slow Diseases Peculiar to Women,* a link between menopause and the development of "various diseases of the chronic kind." Leake further went on to state that menopause led to "pain and giddiness of the head, hysteric disorders, colic pain and a mid-life female weakness." In 1882 Tilt referred to menopause as an event bearing "evil effects." Menopause was viewed as a physiological and psychological crisis. It was thought that the way to prevent symptoms was to avoid being too educated, fashionable, or sexually active and to provide adequate care for husbands and children (Smith-Rosenberg, 1973). In the twentieth century, with increasing understanding of physiology, menopause was defined as a deficiency disease and its symptoms attributed to estrogen deficiency (Kaufert & McKinlay, 1985).

For many years there was little scientific research on menopause. The study of a normal physiologic event did not generate much interest among scientists or the National Institutes of Health (which was largely disease focused). Much of the information about menopause was based on clinical samples of women who sought treatment for menopause-related problems. Until quite recently the focus of developmental psychologists was generally on childhood. While several theorists such as Erikson (1950) and Levinson (1978) discussed stages of life beyond adolescence, there was little research on adult development. Further, some have argued that the theories of Erikson and Levinson are more relevant for men than for women (Barnett & Baruch, 1978; Gilligan, 1979, 1982). Men's experience places an emphasis on chronological development, as men tend to experience continuous uninterrupted events in their occupation and families. Women, on the other hand, have more varying patterns of career, marriage, and childbearing. Thus, the psychological changes and development occurring among midlife women were generally neglected.

In the 1980s, as menopause became increasingly implicated as a risk factor for osteoporosis and cardiovascular disease, it aroused the interest of epidemiologists. With the development of estrogen replacement therapy, medical scientists became more interested in studying menopause. Menopause was now something that was treatable and warranted medical intervention. Thus, this normal physiological process became viewed as a risk factor for disease or a condition warranting treatment, leading to what some see as the increasing medicalization of menopause (Bell, 1990).

During the past several years, the interest in menopause has skyrocketed. Certainly much of this newfound interest is due to the current "baby boom" generation of women, which is approaching menopause. This large cohort of women grew up asserting more control over their reproductive lives and encouraged frank and open discussion of previously taboo topics. Furthermore, with the increased attention to and promotion of hormone replacement therapy (HRT), menopausal women are faced with making a decision that could ultimately affect the rest of their lives. In the past, menopause was something one had little control over and required little active involvement. Now, with menopause increasingly implicated as a risk factor for subsequent disease, and estrogen replacement therapy touted as the panacea for these diseases, menopause has become a time requiring active decision making by women. Women must decide whether to take HRT and possibly increase their risk for breast cancer, suffer various side effects, and worry about the unknown long-term consequences of HRT, or not to take HRT and worry about subsequent osteoporosis and disability. For most women, neither of these options is very appealing.

Methodological Issues

Prior to reviewing research on menopause, it is useful to point out several important methodological issues in studying this life transition. These include (1) patient versus community-based samples, (2) cross-sectional versus longitudinal designs, and (3) measurement issues.

Patient- versus Community-Based Samples

Much of the early research on menopause (as well as some research today) was based on clinical samples of women who sought treatment for menopause-related problems. These patient samples provide a distorted view of the natural menopause transition and have been the source of many myths and stereotypes about menopause. Data are based only on women who are having problems or self-select into seeking medical care. We now know that less than 50 percent of menopausal women seek menopause-related treatment (Avis, Crawford, & McKinlay, 1997; Brown & Brown, 1976; Morse et al., 1994; Rose, 1977; Weideger, 1977). Patient samples are also biased in terms of education, socioeconomic status, other health problems, and general depression (Avis et al., 1997). Although patients provide data on how some women experience menopause, they do not inform us of the "normal" menopausal transition or range of responses to menopause. As data from community-based samples become available, it is apparent that community-based research presents a very different picture than patient-based research and these community-based studies are challenging many of our long-held stereotypes about menopause.

Cross-Sectional versus Longitudinal Studies

Although community-based studies provide data on the general population, rather than populations of only women who self-select into treatment, the majority of these studies have been cross-sectional. Such cross-sectional studies are limited by problems of inference to apparent associations (S. M. McKinlay & McKinlay, 1973). Cross-sectional studies can neither control for premenopausal characteristics of women nor separate effects of aging from those of menopause. Cross-sectional designs can only identify associations (real or spurious). Longitudinal cohort designs can facilitate identification of those associations that are most likely to reflect a cause–effect relationship, through observation of temporal sequences in events or rate changes.

Measurement Issues

Accurate assessment of a woman's menopause status becomes important in determining age of menopause, symptoms associated with menopause, and psychosocial aspects of menopause. Some studies use age as a surrogate for menopause status, which, given the wide distribution in age of menopause, is highly imprecise. Other studies base a woman's menopause status on her retrospective recall of last menstrual period. However, studies that have used retrospective data on age on reproductive history or age of menopause are particularly subject to biased or inaccurate recall (Bean et al., 1979; S. M. McKinlay, Jefferys, & Thompson, 1972; Paganini-Hill, Krailo, & Pike, 1984). Accurate measure of status can be assessed only in a prospectively followed cohort.

Menopause is defined as the permanent cessation of menses. The standard epidemiological definition of natural menopause is 12 consecutive months of amenorrhea, in the absence of surgery or other pathological or physiological cause (e.g., pregnancy, lactation) that would terminate menstruation. Twelve months of amenorrhea is the widely accepted definition used in European studies since the 1950s (Magursky, Mesko, & Sokolik, 1975) and is recommended by Treloar on the basis of his prospective study of normal menstrual patterns (Treloar, 1974). This definition was further agreed upon for population-based epidemiologic studies by an international study group of researchers in Korpilampi Finland (Kaufert et al., 1986) and the World Health Organization (WHO, 1996). The point at which a woman experiences her final menstrual period (FMP) can be determined only retrospectively.

Perimenopause is that period of time immediately prior to menopause, when the endocrinological, biological, and clinical features of approaching menopause begin through the first year after the final menstrual period (WHO, 1996). It is characterized by increased variability in menstrual cycles, skipped menstrual cycles, and changes in hormone levels. Because perimenopause has not been intensively studied, it has been less consistently defined in medical and epidemiological research, thus making cross-study comparisons of this important transition difficult. Brambilla, McKinlay, and Johannes (1994) have shown that the reporting of irregular menses is the best predictor of subsequent menopause. Current epidemiologic studies classify a woman as perimenopausal if she has had a menstrual cycle within the past 3 months and reports changes in cycle regularity, or if she has not had a menstrual period in the past 3–11 months.

In any discussion of menopause, it is crucial to distinguish between natural and surgical menopause. Surgical menopause is defined as menopause induced by a surgical procedure that stops menstruation. Women who have both ovaries or the uterus with or without removal of the ovaries are generally included in this category. Women who have a surgical menopause tend to be younger, of poorer health, and use health care more frequently (S. M. McKinlay, Brambilla, Avis, & McKinlay, 1991). Their menopause experience is also quite different (with more sudden hormonal changes), and is confounded by having a surgical procedure. For research purposes, women who experience a surgical menopause must be considered separately from those experiencing a natural menopause. In describing the menopause experience, this chapter refers to the experience of natural menopause.

Description of the Massachusetts Women's Health Study

In response to these methodological issues, several population-based prospective studies were begun in the 1980s. The largest and most comprehensive prospective cohort study sampled from a general population to date is the Massachusetts Women's Health Study (MWHS) (see Avis & S. M. McKinlay, 1995, J. B. McKinlay, McKinlay, & Brambilla, 1987a, and S. M. McKinlay et al., 1991, for a detailed description of this study). Begun in 1981, the MWHS prospectively studied a cohort of middle-aged women as they approached and experienced menopause. As a significant source of data regarding menopause among the general population of women, results of this study are cited throughout this chapter and a brief study description is provided here.

The MWHS began with a baseline cross-sectional survey in 1981–1982 that employed a two-stage cluster sampling design. First, 38 Massachusetts towns and cities were selected, with probabilities proportional to size, within twelve strata defined by city/town size, per capita income, and percent black. Women born in the years 1926–1936 inclusive were then randomly selected from annually compiled census lists in the selected towns/cities to provide an approximately self-weighting sample. Baseline survey information was gathered through brief mailed questionnaires or in telephone interviews, if no response to two mailings was obtained. A total of 8050 completed responses were obtained, yielding an overall response rate of 77%.

From this cross-sectional sample, a cohort of 2565 women was identified, consisting of women who had menstruated in the preceding 3 months and who had a uterus and at least one ovary intact. Prospective study of the cohort consisted of six telephone contacts that were 9 months apart in the period 1982–1987. Retention of the cohort was excellent with response rates ranging from 94% to 99% over the six contacts, among those who responded at the previous contact. The response rate at the sixth interview was 91.5% of the original cohort.

At each contact, an interview was conducted, including questions related to current health status, current symptoms and medication use, current menstrual status, health service utilization, employment, and any changes in selected socio-demographic variables. Additional information was collected on social support, lifestyle behaviors (e.g., smoking, alcohol consumption, exercise), depression, and attitudes toward menopause.

Beginning in 1986, a sub-cohort of pre and early perimenopausal women was recruited into a follow-up study called MWHS II. The cohort for this study began with a sub-sample of 427 women from the MWHS who had completed all six interviews of the MWHS, lived within an hour of Boston, and were still menstruating at the end of the initial cohort study in 1986. This study involved seven in-person interviews and measurements of reproductive hormones, lipids, bone density at three sites, blood pressure, height, weight, and a range of psychosocial assessments including depression and sexual function over a 10-year period. Measures were taken annually except during a three-year period corresponding to a gap in funding. This cohort was followed until 1996.

Menopause Transition—Physiological Process

The Menopausal Process

At birth, a girl's ovaries contain approximately 500,000 eggs. Only 400 to 500 of these eggs will ever fully ripen and be released during menstruation. The egg and surrounding cells, called follicles, produce the hormones estrogen and progesterone. At the beginning of the menstrual cycle, the pituitary gland releases follicle stimulating hormone (FSH), which targets the ovaries and causes follicles to develop. Typically, one follicle begins to mature and releases increasing amounts of estrogen. The uterine lining begins to thicken. The follicle eventually grows large enough and ruptures, thus releasing the ovum. The ruptured follicle forms the *corpus luteum* and under the influence of luteinizing hormone (LH) produces estrogen and progesterone. These high circulating levels of estrogen and progesterone inhibit the release of FSH. If fertilization does not occur, the *corpus luteum* degenerates and thus stops producing estrogen and progesterone. With the decline in these two hormones, FSH is no longer inhibited, begins to rise again, and the menstrual cycle begins anew.

Menopause is a gradual process that starts long before a woman even notices. Beginning in her 30s, a woman has an increasing number of anovulatory cycles (without eggs) as the number of ovarian follicles declines. Women are generally unaware of these anovulatory cycles. As women approach age 50, the follicles begin to deplete, ovarian hormone production slows, and more and more cycles become anovulatory. The menstrual cycle becomes irregular and at longer intervals, and estrogen levels drop. Greater amounts of FSH are released in an attempt to stimulate the follicles, but eventually the follicles do not respond and menstruation stops altogether. Increased FSH is generally seen as a hormonal indicator of impending menopause. During perimenopause, individual FSH measurements may fluctuate widely. However, if repeated measurements are taken, average levels will show an upward trend. There is accumulating evidence that a single FSH measurement is not a reliable indicator of a woman's final menstrual period (Stellato, Crawford, McKinlay, & Longcope, 1998).

It is important to point out that following menopause, estrogen production does not stop altogether. Although the ovary accounts for more than 90% of the body's total production of estradiol, the most potent naturally occurring estrogen, other forms of estrogen, such as estrone, are produced by other glands such as the adrenal and by peripheral conversion of circulating hormones, such as testosterone. Peripheral aromatization (conversion) of androgens in tissues such as blood, liver, and adipose tissue continues to provide a source of estrone to postmenopausal women.

Factors Related to Age of Menopause

The median age of last menstrual period is between 50 and 52 years (Brambilla & McKinlay, 1989; S. M. McKinlay, Bifano, & McKinlay, 1985) and 80% of women experience their last menstrual period between 45 and 55. There is wide variability among women in the age of menopause. It has been hypothesized that menopause occurs after sufficient depletion of oocytes and that factors that delay or suppress ovulation (e.g., late menarche, multiple pregnancies) might delay onset of menopause. Results of these studies are highly inconsistent, which may result from differences in populations studied, definitions, methods of data collection, and analysis. As previously mentioned, studies that have used retrospective data on age on reproductive history or age of menopause are particularly subject to biased or inaccurate recall (Bean et al., 1979; S. M. McKinlay et al., 1972; Paganini-Hill et al., 1984). Using data from a prospective study of menstrual and reproductive health, Whelan, Sandler, McConnaughey, and Weinberg (1990) reported that women who had short menstrual cycles (<26 days) between ages 20 and 36 were more likely to have an earlier menopause. Women who had ever been pregnant reached menopause slightly later than women who had never been pregnant. They found no association between age of menarche and age of menopause.

The most well established factor related to age of menopause is cigarette smoking. Using prospective data from the Massachusetts Women's Health Study, Brambilla and McKinlay (1989) found that women who smoke cigarettes experience menopause 1–2 years earlier than those who do not. This finding is remarkably consistent across populations (e.g., Adena & Gallagher, 1982; Jick and Porter, 1977; Kaufman, 1980; Willet et al., 1983). Cigarette smoking is thought to affect ovarian function by decreasing production of estrogens, and enhancing rates of metabolism and utilization. Brambilla and McKinlay found no relation between body mass, parity, and use of oral contraceptives and age of menopause.

Using longitudinal data from the MWHS, S. M. McKinlay et al. (1992) were able to determine that the median age for the inception of the perimenopause is 47.5 years. Smokers began perimenopause earlier and nulliparous women were also slightly more likely to begin perimenopause earlier. S. M. McKinlay et al. reported that the median length of the perimenopause state was 3.8 years, with age and smoking related to a shorter perimenopause. Nearly 10% of the premenopausal cohort in this study ceased menstruating abruptly.

Signs and Symptoms Associated with Menopause

It is commonly assumed that because menopause is a physiologically observable or measurable event in humans, the signs or symptoms surrounding this event are also universal in the human female. It is assumed that menopause is inevitably accompanied (to a greater or lesser extent) by hot flushes, sweats, prolonged menstrual irregularities, vaginal dryness, and a host of other "symptoms," including depression, irritability, weight gain, insomnia, and dizziness. Earlier analyses of primarily cross-sectional data in Caucasian populations have provided evidence that these signs and symptoms of menopause are far from ubiquitous (Greene, 1976; Greene & Cooke, 1980; S. M. McKinlay & Jefferys, 1974; Neugarten & Kraines, 1965). These same studies have also suggested that, with the exception of hot flushes and accompanying sweats, other supposed menopausal symptoms are not directly related to this physiological change.

These assumptions regarding menopausal symptoms or stereotypical views of menopause become perpetuated with the use of menopausal checklists that ask women to retrospectively report symptoms they experienced during menopause. Parlee (1974) argues with respect to menstrual symptom reporting that recollected symptom data are more vulnerable to the influence of stereotypical beliefs about the psychological concomitants of menstruation. The time lapse leads women to substitute the symptoms they "believe" to be associated with a particular phase for the symptoms they actually had but do not recall with accuracy.

The following is a review of the primary symptoms thought to be associated with menopause through the impact of hormonal changes on the central nervous system: vasomotor symptoms (hot flashes/flushes and night sweats), mood changes, sleep disturbances, and memory problems.

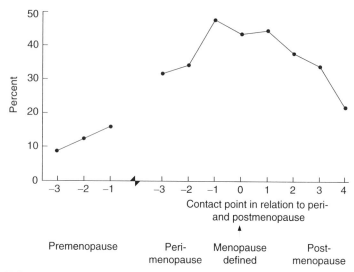

FIGURE 1   Hot flashes reported in previous 2 weeks by contact points pre- and postmenopause (*n* = 1178). Originally adapted by permission of John Wiley & Sons, Inc. from McKinlay, S. M., et al. (1992). The normal menopause transition. *American Journal of Human Biology, 4(1)*, 37–46. Copyright © 1992 by John Wiley & Sons, Inc.; reprinted from Avis, N. E., & McKinlay, S. M. (1995). The Massachusetts Women's Health Study: A longitudinal investigation of the menopause. *Journal of the American Women's Medical Association, 50*, 45–63.

Vasomotor Symptoms

Vasomotor symptoms (hot flashes/flushes and night sweats) are the primary symptoms associated with menopause. Estimates of the incidence of hot flashes from population studies in the United States and worldwide have ranged from 24 to 93% (Kronenberg, 1990). Some discrepancies in the prevalence of hot flash reporting reflect inconsistencies in research methodology as well as study populations. Age ranges and menopause status of women studied differ; some studies are based on patient samples, others on general population samples; and the specific symptom questions and the frame also differ. However, even within study or controlling for methodology, a high degree of variability of symptom reporting is found among women, suggesting considerable individual variation in symptom experience.

   Although cross-sectional studies often report the highest prevalence of hot flashes postmenopause, there are sparse longitudinal data on the age and menopause status at which hot flashes begin. S. M. McKinlay et al. (1992) report data from the MWHS on the relationship of hot flashes to the menopause transition. Figure 1 summarizes a complex analysis of 1178 women in the cohort who were premenopausal at the first follow-up. At three contact points prior to the inception of perimenopause, the rate of hot flash reporting is 10%. This rate slowly increases as irregularity in menses is observed. Hot flash reporting peaks to about 50% at the contact just prior to when menopause is defined. By the fourth postmenopausal contact (about 4 years after FMP), the rate of hot flash reporting has declined to 20%. These findings contradict the widely held clinical impression that hot flashes begin to increase after last menstrual period. S. M. McKinlay et al. also found that the rate of hot flash reporting is related to the duration of the perimenopause. Women with a perimenopause of less than 6 months (estimated at 10% of women) have much lower rates of symptom reporting.

Some women report never experiencing hot flashes, while others report experiencing hot flashes throughout the day. There are no good population data on the distribution of hot flash frequency across women. Data from the MWHS show that 19% of postmenopausal women report having never experienced a hot flash, and of those who experienced hot flashes, only 19% said they were very bothersome. The most bothersome symptom experienced was menstrual flow problems. Although only 13% of women reported this symptom, 53% of those who did reported this symptom as very bothersome. From the high variability among women of hot flashes experienced, it is clear that factors other than hormonal changes affect this symptom experience (Table I).

Depression and Mood

A long-held notion that continues to persist, despite evidence to the contrary, is that menopausal women are likely to become depressed (Kaufert, Gilbert, & Hassard, 1988; S. M. McKinlay & Jefferys, 1974; Winokur, 1973). This presumption prevails among women in general (Avis & McKinlay, 1991) as well as among clinicians (Cowan, Warren, & Young, 1985; Roberts, 1985). Much of the research that gives rise to this perceived relationship is derived from clinic or patient populations of women who self-select into treatment (J. B. McKinlay et al., 1987a). Some cross-sectional research has shown more frequent depressed mood among peri- or postmenopausal women than among premenopausal women (Ballinger 1975; Bungay,

TABLE I   Symptom Reporting in Postmenopausal Women Anytime during Study

Symptom	Percent reporting experiencing symptom (%)	Percent reporting symptom as very bothersome (%)[a]
Hot flashes	81	19
Night sweats	58	20
Menstrual flow problems	13	53
Vaginal dryness	20	15

Note. Data from Massachusetts Women's Health Study ($n = 1109$).

[a]Of those who reported experiencing symptom.

Vessey, & McPherson, 1980; Hunter, Battersby, & Whitehead, 1986; Jaszmann, van Lith, & Zaat, 1969b), while other studies have not (Kaufert, et al., 1988; Matthews et al., 1990; McKinlay, McKinlay, & Brambilla, 1987b).

In a Canadian study of middle-aged women, Kaufert et al. (1988) looked at the association between menopausal status and a symptom index that included the following three symptoms: irritability, nervous tension, and feeling blue or depressed. Over the six interviews, they found no association between menopausal status and the psychological symptom scores. The Pittsburgh Healthy Women Study compared psychological characteristics and symptoms between pre- and postmenopausal women, controlling for age, and found that natural menopause did not adversely affect anxiety, anger, total symptoms, depression, or perceived stress (Matthews et al., 1990).

Cross-sectional data, however, can neither control for premenopausal depression nor characterize the transition through menopause. Longitudinal data are necessary to study women as they proceed through menopause and to control for premenopausal depression.

Using data from the MWHS, Avis, Brambilla, McKinlay, and Vass (1994), addressed the effect of change in menopause status on depression (as measured by self-reported depressive symptoms), while controlling for prior depression. Depression was measured by the CES-D scale, a well-established scale measuring depressive symptomatology, developed by the Center for Epidemiological Studies (Radloff, 1977) and often used in epidemiological research. The CES-D consists of 20 self-report items concerning depressed mood. Scores range from 0 to 60, with those scoring 16 and above generally classified as at high risk for clinical depression (Myers & Weissmann, 1980). To study change in menopause status, a menopause transition variable was created that took into account a woman's menopausal status at the two time points (27 months apart) at which depression was measured (referred to as T_1 and T_2). Women were classified into five categories: premenopausal at both T_1 and T_2 (pre–pre), premenopausal at T_1 and perimenopausal at T_2 (pre–peri), perimenopausal at both T_1 and T_2 (peri–peri), pre- or perimenopausal at T_1 and postmenopausal at T_2 (pre/peri–post), and postmenopausal at both T_1 and T_2 (post–post).

The rate of depression according to transition pattern and premenopausal depression is graphically shown in Figure 2. This figure clearly shows that across all menopause statuses, those women who were classified as depressed at T_1 had higher rates of depression at T_2. For women who were *not* depressed at T_1 the rate of depression at T_2 increases slightly as women move from pre–pre to pre–peri, and is highest for women who have remained perimenopausal for at least 27 months. The rate of depression begins to decrease as women move from peri- to postmenopause, and is lowest for those women who have been postmenopausal for at least 27 months. Although these results show that depression is moderately associated with the perimenopause status, they also show that this depression is *transitory;* as women become postmenopausal, their rates of depression decline.

In a logistic regression analysis of T_2 depression on premenopausal depression and menopausal transition, the variable most predictive of subsequent depression

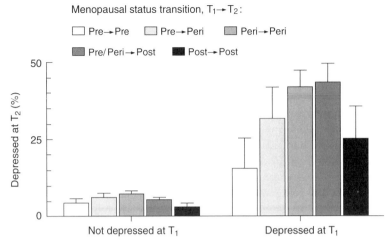

FIGURE 2   Percentage of women classified as depressed at T_2, by depression status at T_1 and menopausal transition. Reprinted by permission of the publisher from: A longitudinal analysis of the association
between menopause and depression: Results from the Massachusetts Women's Health Study, Avis et al.,
Annals of Epidemiology, 4, 214–220. Copyright 1994 by Elsevier Science.

was prior depression. There was also a moderately significant, though much smaller,
effect of menopausal transition. Further analyses revealed that this effect was due to
the peri–peri group, which significantly differed from the pre–pre group. The peri–
peri group also differed significantly from the post–post group when the latter was
used as the comparison group, suggesting that the increased rate of depression is
transitory. These results suggest that the majority of depression during menopause
can be attributed to prior depression, though there is a slight elevation of depression
among women who have been perimenopausal for at least 27 months.

It has been hypothesized that the relation between menopause and depression
can be explained by symptoms. Further analyses of these data examined whether
this increased rate of depression among the peri–peri women could be attributed
to symptoms associated with menopause (i.e., hot flashes, night sweats, menstrual
problems). When menopausal symptoms was added to the regression model, it
became a significant predictor of T_2 depression and menopausal transition was no
longer statistically significant. Over all menopause transition categories, those
women who reported experiencing hot flashes, night sweats, and/or menstrual
problems consistently showed higher rates of depression.

Results from this large, community-based sample of women do not show evidence that onset of menopause is significantly associated with increased risk of
depression. Experiencing a long perimenopausal period (at least 27 months), however, was moderately associated with increased, but transitory, risk of depression.
This increased depression was largely explained by menopausal symptoms.

Sleep

While sleep disturbances are thought to be associated with menopause, it is unclear whether they are directly related to hormonal changes or are secondary to hot flashes. Episodes of wakening and insomnia occur with hot flashes (Erlik, 1981); both are reduced by estrogen replacement therapy, and women with severe vasomotor symptoms are at risk for sleep disturbances. However, a review by Regestein (1994) found that menopause per se explained only a small part of the increase in sleep disturbances at menopause. One study that included asymptomatic women did not find that menopause status was related to sleep quality. However, peri- and postmenopausal women who were experiencing hot flashes tended to spend more time in bed, have a lower mean sleep efficiency index, and have greater rapid eye movement latency than asymptomatic women (Shaver, Giblin, Lentz, & Lee, 1988). In a longitudinal study, Hunter (1992) found that poor health, lack of regular exercise, and difficulty coping with symptoms before menopause may also predict sleep problems.

Memory

Like sleep disturbances, memory complaints have also been thought to be associated with menopause (Hamburger, Liu, & Rebar, 1987; Kopera, 1973; Malleson, 1953). The effect of menopausal hormonal changes on memory, however, has not been well studied. Most studies in this area have looked at the effect of estrogen replacement therapy (ERT) on cognitive functioning. Several mechanisms have been proposed to explain the effect of estrogen replacement on cognitive functioning. Estrogen might influence the concentration of certain neurotransmitters (Luine, Park, Joh, Reis, & McEwen, 1980), induce anatomical changes in the nerve cells in the ventromedial hypothalamus (McEwen, 1991), improve carotid artery blood flow (Gangar et al., 1991), or improve depressed mood (Aylward, 1973). Research on the effect of ERT on cognitive functioning, however, has reported contradictory results, with some studies showing improved memory among women taking ERT (Campbell & Whitehead, 1977; Fedor-Freybergh, 1977; Kimura, 1995; Sherwin, 1988) and other studies showing no effect (Barrett-Connor & Kritz-Silverstein, 1993; Ditkoff, Crary, Cristo, & Lobo, 1991; Rauramo, Langerspetz, Engblom, & Punnonen, 1975; Vanhulle & Demol, 1976). A recent review of this research concluded that while there are plausible biological mechanisms that might account for a beneficial effect of estrogen therapy on cognition, the studies conducted in women have substantial methodologic problems and have produced conflicting results (Yaffe, Sawaya, Lieberburg, & Grady, 1998). Except for Barrett-Connor and Kritz-Silverstein, these studies generally have small sample sizes and limited tests of cognitive function. Further, most studies have been conducted with recently postmenopausal women and have not separated the effect of estrogen on cognitive function from its effect on symptom relief (particularly sleep). There have been no good studies on the effect of naturally occurring hormonal changes during menopause and their relation to memory or on the effect of ERT on cognitive function separate from its effect on dysphoric mood and somatic symptoms (Barrett-Connor & Kritz-Silverstein, 1993).

Summary

Menopause is thought to alter central nervous system function as manifested by hot flashes, mood changes, and memory and sleep disturbances. However, only vasomotor symptoms such as hot flashes and night sweats have been clearly associated with menopause. Furthermore, the interrelationships among these factors and their causal ordering are not understood. It is not known if changes in reproductive hormones are directly responsible for symptoms or if any mood or memory changes are secondary to hot flashes. Moreover, not all women experience menopausal symptoms. The next section reviews factors related to menopause symptomatology.

Although menopausal symptoms are related to depression (Avis et al., 1994), correlational studies of mood and hormone levels have failed to show a relation between depressed mood and estrogen levels (Avis, McKinlay, Vass, Brambilla, & Longcope, 1993; Ballinger, Browning, & Smith, 1987). These results suggest that other factors mediate the relation between hormonal level and depressed mood. These factors are explained in the following section.

PSYCHOSOCIAL AND CULTURAL FACTORS ASSOCIATED WITH MENOPAUSE

Meaning of Menopause at Societal/Cultural and Individual Levels

Societal Level

In the seventeenth and eighteenth centuries in Western societies, a woman had two roles: mother and housewife. Those women who could not have children were called "barren." During these centuries, negative attitudes toward the menopause began to emerge. Because menopausal women were unable to perform one of the two roles society gave them, many believed menopause caused most, if not all, of the illnesses suffered by middle-aged women. Moreover, it wasn't unusual for a physician to tell his patient that her illness resulted from neglecting her husband and children, or even from too much education.

In the nineteenth century, two prominent physicians, Edward Tilt and Andrew Currier published works on menopause. Tilt (1857) attributed over a hundred diseases to the menopause, including tuberculosis and diabetes. Although Tilt regarded the menopausal process as "perilous" he did believe that afterward there is a great improvement in the general health and often in physical looks. Since menopause was thought to be the cause of so many illnesses affecting women, physicians sought to develop some form of treatment for it. By the end of the nineteenth century, menopause was viewed as a deficiency disease directly related to the malfunction of the ovaries. Therapy for this condition included prescribing ovarian juice, powdered ovaries, and powdered ovarian tablets, each of which was obtained from the ovaries of horses. Then, in 1929, Butenandt isolated a hormone from the urine of a pregnant woman. This hormone, later known as estrone, was believed to be the missing ingredient in menopausal women. It was only a matter of time before a synthetic version was developed, and in 1938, estrogen therapy, though controversial, became a form of treatment. And even today, the debate over hormone replacement therapy continues.

Today, women have other roles and we are less inclined to think that menopause is traumatic because a woman can no longer fulfill her reproductive role. Furthermore, for some women, menopause provides freedom from worry about contraception and pregnancy, as well as relief from the annoyance and/or symptoms associated with menstrual periods. However, in our society, which extols youthfulness and sexuality, menopause is feared because it signifies aging, a lack of sexual attractiveness. In the 1960s, experts referred to the menopausal woman's body in a repulsive way: "Her spinal column is 'hump-backed,' her vagina is a 'dry, rigid tube,' and hair grows on her face . . . her breasts are particularly of concern . . . often the 'skin of the breasts coarsens and is covered with scales'" (Wilson, 1966).

Cross-cultural and anthropological studies provide evidence that the meaning of this event varies greatly across cultures. How a society views menopause is influenced by how it views aging and women in general. Menopause is often viewed as a positive event in women's lives in non-Western cultures where menopause removes constraints and prohibitions imposed on menstruating women. In countries where women have low status or are not allowed to show sexuality (such as India), menopause is seen positively as it provides freedom to go out in public and do things usually forbidden to women. Among South Asian women, the end of childbearing and the menstrual cycle are welcomed. While social status is tied to motherhood, it is motherhood that is valued and not biological fertility itself (Vatuk, 1992).

Among both Mayan and Greek women, menopause is seen as a positive event, although for different reasons. Mayan women marry young, do not practice birth control, and spend most of their reproductive years either pregnant or lactating. Pregnancy is viewed as dangerous and stressful, and menopause frees women from restrictions and pregnancy. Although Greek women attempt to curtail family size and often use abortion as a means of birth control, menopause also frees Greek women from taboos and restrictions. A postmenopausal Greek woman is allowed to participate fully in church activities, as she is no longer viewed as a sexual threat to the community. Both Mayan and Greek women report better sexual relationships with their husbands following menopause, as the fear of pregnancy is eliminated (Beyene, 1986). In other cultures, menopause is given little thought. In Papago culture, menopause may be completely ignored to the extent that the language contains no word for menopause (Griffen, 1982; Kearns, 1982). In Japan there is no word to describe hot flashes (Lock, 1986). The lack of a Japanese word to describe hot flashes is remarkable in a language that is infinitely more sensitive than is English in its ability to describe bodily states (e.g., there are over 20 words to describe the state of the stomach).

In Western societies women are valued for sexual attractiveness and do not face restrictions found in other cultures. Aging, especially among women, is not revered, but rather viewed quite negatively. In these societies menopause takes on a very different meaning. However, as shown in the next section, this negative view is found more among society as a whole than among menopausal women themselves.

Individual Level

The general emphasis on loss with respect to menopause has meant that the developmental context and potential for growth at this time has often been ignored (Notman, 1990). In the 1940s, psychoanalytic writers such as Helen Deutsch and Ruth Benedek viewed menopause in terms of reproductive loss. They regarded menopause as a critical event in the life of a middle-aged woman, which threatened her adjustment and self-concept. Deutsch even went so far as to say that the inability to reproduce was a psychological death for all women. Benedek (1950), on the other hand, also believed that menopause provided a release of constructive energy— that menopause desexualizes emotional needs, thus freeing energies. This notion of increased energy following menopause is also seen in Margaret Mead's writings about postmenopausal zest.

Neugarten (1968), one of the first to look at midlife development, described a shift in adulthood with respect to salient issues, where the 50s become an important turning point with an increase in reflection and introspection in both men and women. As one of the first investigators of the psychology of menopause, she concluded that, unlike early childhood, the biological events in adulthood were not necessarily the important events in understanding the psychology of adulthood. More recently, Pollock (1981) viewed aging as a life course process involving development as well as decline. He viewed losses and the process of mourning as potentially liberating. Thus, in adult development, the inevitable losses and declines in function can stimulate new development and new psychological organization.

Most life-span theorists agree that there is continuity with respect to turning points and that the response to menopause is a function of the woman's premenopausal personality and life patterns. Benedek (1950) and Deutsch (1945) also felt that a woman's reactions to menopause are similar to her reactions to puberty. The menopause itself does not turn a healthy functioning woman into an involutional psychotic (Bart & Grossman, 1978). This perspective is also seen in Costa and McCrae's (1980) view that personality remains essentially stable over the life-span.

How a women views menopause might be related to several factors: (1) the value she places on being young and attractive and her views of women and roles in general; (2) how she feels about where she is in her life cycle in terms of family and career; and (3) other physiological changes. If a women is childless, menopause brings a clear end to possibilities. To a childless woman who had hoped for children, menopause signifies the closing off of opportunities. The associated sadness or depression she may experience is not due to loss of femininity or hormonal depletion, but to the real loss of opportunities (Notman, 1990). For other women, not concerned with continued fertility, the end of menses may bring new sexual freedom.

Although the stereotypical view is that women view menopause quite negatively, research on women's attitudes toward the menopause has not found such negativity among middle-aged women (Avis & McKinlay, 1991; Barentson, Foekma, Bezemer, & Stiphout, 1994; Frey, 1982; Krescovich, 1980; Leiblum & Swartzman, 1986; Millette, 1981; Neugarten, Wood, Kraines, & Loomis, 1963). In 1963 Neugarten published a classic paper (Neugarten et al., 1963) that reported that women's attitudes toward menopause were much more positive than the medical community believed. In a study of women's experiences in different phases of the life cycle, Martin (1987) found systematic differences among women according to age. The "vast majority" of older women saw menopause in a positive light. Younger women, however, tended to share the medical view of menopause. A review of the research on women's attitudes toward menopause across a wide range of populations and cultures shows that women consistently feel relief over the cessation of menses and do not agree with statements that they become less sexually attractive following menopause. These studies also find that postmenopausal women generally have a more positive view of menopause than premenopausal women (Avis, 1996).

Avis and McKinlay (1991) reported data from the MWHS showing that women's attitudes become more positive as they experience menopause. At baseline the majority of women reported feeling relief (42.2%), followed by neutral feelings (35.5%). Some women reported mixed feelings (19.6%), but very few women reported feeling regret (2.7%). Feelings toward menopause were significantly related to menopause status, with women who had a surgical menopause most likely to report relief and the premenopausal women least likely to report relief. In general, women who had a surgical menopause were more likely to have negative attitudes regarding the menopause experience. This is consistent with other findings that women who have a surgical menopause are an atypical subgroup (S. M. McKinlay & McKinlay, 1986). Postmenopausal women were generally most likely to report positive or neutral feelings regarding the cessation of menses. The percentage of women reporting relief was very similar to that found by S. M. McKinlay and Jefferys (1974) (over two decades earlier) and just slightly higher than that found by Lock (34%) in a Japanese sample (1986). This finding, therefore, is remarkably stable over different generations and different cultures. The direction of attitude change for women who were premenopausal at the beginning of the study and later became postmenopausal was overwhelmingly toward more positive attitudes. Thus, the experience of menopause led to more positive, rather than negative, attitudes.

Responses to various statements about menopause revealed that a high percentage of women believed that women become depressed or irritable during the menopause, but otherwise believed that menopause has little effect on women. A comparison of responses to these statements with those found by Neugarten et al. (1963) reveal differences between the two studies. More women in the MWHS agreed with the statement that women become depressed or irritable during menopause (70% vs. 57%), while many fewer agreed with the statement that women lose their minds during menopause (21% vs. 51%). One should note that the Neugarten et al. sample consisted of 100 highly educated women aged 45–55, who were not differentiated by menopause status, but excluded women who had a surgical menopause (Table II).

Menopause in Biopsychosocial Context

This chapter emphasizes the variation among cultures and individuals with respect to their response to the physiological event of menopause. The interplay of the biological, psychological, and social aspects of menopause is clearly seen as one examines factors related to menopausal symptoms, both vasomotor and psychological.

TABLE II   Percent Who Agree with the Statements about Menopause by Concurrent Menopausal Status

Statement	Surgical ($n = 78$)	Natural ($n = 261$)	Peri ($n = 1628$)	Pre ($n = 525$)
Transmenopause				
Become depressed or irritable[a]	78	69	73	63
With interests, don't notice	76	79	75	78
Worry about losing mind[c]	32	26	21	19
Postmenopause				
No longer "real" women	19	18	19	22
Does not change women	71	77	73	78
Women feel regret[b]	14	17	16	17

Note. Adapted by permission of the publisher from Avis and McKinlay (1991). A longitudinal analysis of women's attitudes towards menopause: Results from the Massachusetts Women's Health Study. *Maturitas 13*, 65–79. Copyright 1991 by Elsevier Science.

[a]$p < .001$.
[b]$p < .01$.
[c]$p < .05$.

Vasomotor Symptoms

As previously mentioned, considerable individual variation is found among women in the manifestation of menopausal signs and symptoms. Factors thought to be related to symptomatology include sociocultural (Beyene, 1986; Kaufert, 1982; Lock, 1986), psychological (Avis & McKinlay, 1991; Hunter, 1992; Swartzman, Edelberg, & Kemmann, 1990), menstrual/reproductive (Beyene, 1986; Hunter, 1992), dietary (Beyene, 1986), as well as hormonal changes (Kronenberg, 1990).

As early as last century the diversity in the experience of menopause was noted. Currier (1897) described both within and between society variations. Among European women he identified "highly-bred," "civilized" women and "those with many troubles and ills" as the primary sufferers of severe menopausal symptomatology. He also remarked on the apparently very different experiences in Eskimos and American Indians compared to the French and Irish.

Cultural Influences

It is well established that menopause symptomatology differs across cultures. For example, hot flashes are uncommon in Mayan women (Beyene, 1986). Japanese and Indonesian women report far fewer hot flashes than women in Western societies (Agoestina & van Keep, 1984; Lock, 1986). Researchers in North America and Europe have shown that many of the symptoms that women expect, or that have been attributed to menopause in the medical literature, are components of a stereotype of the menopausal woman, rather than a reflection of actual experience in the majority of women. In societies where women acquire social, religious, or political power in postmenopausal years, menopausal symptoms are minimal.

An International Health Foundation study on menopause in seven Asian countries found low levels of vasomotor and psychic complaints among menopausal women (Payer, 1991). Flint's work with the Rajput women in India produced similar findings (Flint, 1975). She reports that Rajput women have very few problems with menopause, other than menstrual cycle changes. South Asian women do not explicitly associate any physical or psychosocial difficulties with the physiological process of menopause (Vatuk, 1992).

It is difficult to determine the extent to which these societal differences are due to genetic, dietary, reproductive, or cultural factors. In addition to different societal views of menopause, countries also differ in the number of children women have, exercise patterns, and diet. In the absence of cross-cultural studies that can control for, or vary, these factors, it is difficult to assess their relative contribution to symptom reporting. Beyene (1986) points out this difficulty in comparing Greek and Mayan women. She reports that although menopause is viewed positively among both Greek and Mayan women, Mayan women do not report experiencing hot flashes, while Greek women do. She points out that there are several differences between these two cultures: diets vary dramatically, as do fertility patterns. Mayan women eat little animal protein and no milk products. They have a high incidence of vitamin deficiency and anemia. Mayan women also spend most of their reproductive years either pregnant or lactating and have very few menstrual cycles. It is unknown to what extent these differences might account for differences in symptoms.

Another example of this complex interaction is seen in a comparative analysis of studies using similar methodology by Avis et al. (1993). These analyses compared the diversity of menopause experience by comparing symptom reporting in three distinct population groups of women in the United States, Canada, and Japan, all aged 45–55 at the time of survey. These three populations represent differences in culture and beliefs as well as in societal and health care system responses. These comparisons are unique because they are based on three distinct studies that employed similar methodology and used identical questions.

The development of items for common use was agreed on among the investigators (Sonja McKinlay, Massachusetts; Patricia Kaufert, Manitoba; and Margaret Lock, Japan). Women were also asked in the same manner about health, symptoms, use of medication, and chronic health problems. Every effort was made to ensure that the questions used in the Japanese survey measured the same underlying concepts as those used in the Canadian and United States surveys. In all three studies, women were asked to respond to a list of 16 core symptoms. For the Japanese sample the symptom list was translated and back-translated from English to Japanese.

Symptom reporting in the Japanese women was generally low. A comparison with the Canadian and United States data showed that Japanese women had lower frequencies on most of the symptoms shared in common among the three studies. Diarrhea/constipation was the only symptom that was highest in the Japanese sample. Although women in all three studies were aged 45–55, the percentage of Japanese women reporting hot flashes or night sweats was considerably lower (14.7%) than it was for the Canadian (36%) or United States women (38%). Table III

TABLE III   The Percentage of Women Reporting Hot Flashes/Sweats and Feeling Blue/Depressed in Each Study by Menopause Status

Menopause status	Hot flashes/sweats			Feeling blue/depressed		
	Japan	Canada	U.S.A.	Japan	Canada	U.S.A.
Surgical menopause	19.8	38.3	44.4	9.9	23.1	39.1
Natural menopause	16.8	45.5	42.6	8.9	23.0	33.8
Perimenopause	19.8	45.2	37.3	9.9	23.2	38.1
Premenopause	9.7	19.3	13.8	12.7	24.1	29.1

Note. Adapted by permission of the publisher from Avis et al. (1993). The evolution of menopausal symptoms. In H. Burger (Ed.), *Bailliere's Clinical Endocrinology and Metabolism, 7(1),* 17–32. Copyright 1993 by Bailliere Tindall.

shows the relationship between symptom reporting and menopause status in the three studies. As seen here, the Japanese rates for combined hot flashes/night sweats are consistently low across all menopause status categories. Thus, although an association between menopausal status and vasomotor symptoms was found in the Japanese sample, as in the North American samples, the prevalence of these symptoms was low.

Whether the low incidence of vasomotor symptoms reflects cultural, psychological, or physiological differences, or some combination of all three, requires further examination. Japanese women may not perceive these heat changes as remarkable and/or they may experience them at a much lower rate, possibly because of the much lower fat content in their diets. Another hypothesis is that the low rate of hot flash reporting among Japanese women may be due to phytoestrogens in their diet (Adlercreutz et al., 1992).

Cross-cultural research thus clearly shows that menopause is not experienced universally among women. This research suggests that possible factors that may influence menopausal symptoms include cultural views of menopause, behavioral factors such as diet and exercise, and reproductive factors.

Psychosocial Influences

There is also evidence that psychological factors influence menopausal symptoms. Laboratory studies have shown increased reporting of hot flashes during stress (Swartzman et al., 1990). Other evidence for a psychological component to hot flashes comes from the results of clinical trials of estrogen replacement therapy (ERT). Studies of ERT's effectiveness that include a placebo control have often found a significant placebo effect on symptom reduction (e.g., Clayden, Bell, & Pollard, 1974; Coope, Thomson, & Poller, 1975; Poller, Thomson, & Coope, 1980). Other studies have shown that premenopausal attitudes toward menopause are predictive of menopausal symptomatology (Avis & McKinlay, 1991; Hunter, 1992; Matthews, 1992). The Healthy Women Study, a longitudinal study of 541 community-based women, found that women who expected to experience vasomotor symptoms during the menopause showed increased depressive symptoms and anger postmenopause (Matthews, 1992). This study also found that women who expected that information and positive expectations during the menopause would facilitate good experiences during the menopause had lower levels of depression and fewer symptoms.

In the MWHS, Avis and McKinlay (1991) also found that negative attitudes toward menopause prior to experiencing menopause were related to symptom reporting during menopause. Those women who held more positive attitudes toward menopause when they were premenopausal were *less* likely to subsequently report hot flashes. For example, as shown in Table IV, only 37% of those who agreed with the statement, "women with other interests don't notice the meno-

TABLE IV   Percent Reporting Hot Flashes and Night Sweats during Menopause according to Prior Attitudes toward Menopause

	Hot flashes		Night sweats	
Attitude prior to menopause	Agree	Disagree	Agree	Disagree
Transmenopause				
Become depressed or irritable	43 (45/105)[a]	37 (15/40)	23 (24/105)	25 (10/40)
With interests, don't notice	37 (52/141)	56 (10/18)	21 (30/141)	22 (4/18)
Worry about losing mind	42 (15/36)	39 (44/114)	33[b] (12/36)	17 (19/114)
Postmenopause				
No longer "real" women	36 (16/45)	39 (46/118)	27 (12/45)	19 (22/118)
Does not change women	37[b] (49/133)	56 (18/32)	19[b] (25/133)	37 (12/32)
Women feel regret	33 (11/33)	42 (56/134)	21 (7/33)	23 (31/134)

Note. Reprinted by permission of the publisher from Avis and McKinlay (1991). A longitudinal analysis of women's attitudes towards menopause: Results from the Massachusetts Women's Health Study. *Maturitas, 13,* 65–79. Copyright 1991 by Elsevier Science.

[a]Ratios in parentheses refer to number of women who reported symptom divided by number who agreed or disagreed with statement.

[b]$p < .05$.

pause" subsequently reported hot flashes, while 56% who disagreed later reported hot flashes. In general, fewer women reported experiencing night sweats than reported hot flashes, but there was also a relationship between prior attitudes and subsequent reporting of night sweats. Only 19% of those who agreed with the statement, "menopause does not change women" reported sweats, while 37% who disagreed reported sweats. These results provide confirmation that expectations regarding menopause can be related to symptom reporting. This finding is consistent with other research on menopausal symptoms (Matthews, 1992), as well as previous research on menstrual symptoms (Brooks-Gunn and Ruble, 1982). There are at least two possible explanations for the role of expectations/attitudes in subsequent symptom reporting. These negative attitudes may become a self-fulfilling prophecy and/or women may base these expectancies on past responses to other physiological changes or events.

Depression and Mood

The relationship between menopause and depression also exemplifies the complex interaction of biological, psychological, and sociocultural factors. Cross-sectional studies of depression and menopause have shown that psychosocial factors account for more of the variation in depressed mood among women at the time of menopause than does menopause itself (Ballinger, 1976; Dennerstein, 1987; Greene & Cooke, 1980; J. B. McKinlay et al., 1987b). Greene and Cooke (1980) conducted a detailed cross-sectional study of postmenopausal women in Glasgow and found that stressful life events involving exits from a woman's social network were associated with reports of psychological symptoms. These events accounted for a greater proportion of the variation in reports of psychological symptoms than did menopause status. Bart (1971) analyzed mental hospital records of 533 women aged 40–59 and found that the lack of meaningful roles and the consequent loss of self-esteem, rather than hormonal changes, seemed to account for menopausal depression. In a survey of women aged 40–55 in the general population, Ballinger (1975) found that the death of a parent and changing patterns of relations with children were related to psychiatric morbidity. In an analysis of the relative contributions of health, social circumstances, and menopause to depression, J. B. McKinlay et al. (1987b) found that the variables most associated with depression were lower education, marital status (widowed, divorced, separated women have higher rates), physical health, and stress from worry about others. Other studies have also shown that socioeconomic status is related to depression (Holte & Mikkelson, 1991; Hunter et al., 1986).

Longitudinal data suggest that prior depression is the primary factor related to depression during menopause. In addition to the previously reported findings of Avis et al. (1994), Hunter (1990) also found that depressed mood during the menopause was most strongly predicted by premenopausal depression. Hunter further found that negative stereotyped beliefs about the menopause, being under stress before the menopause, together with not working outside the home and defining oneself as belonging to the working class were related to depression. Together, these factors accounted for 51% of the variation in depressed mood when these women became peri- or postmenopausal.

Cross-cultural studies show that there is a cultural component to this relationship as well (Avis et al., 1993). In the Avis et al. analysis comparing Massachusetts, Canadian, and Japanese women, the rates of reporting feeling blue and depressed were clearly highest in the United States sample and lowest in the Japanese sample (see Table III). Interestingly, they found a significant interaction among country, status, and feeling blue or depressed, suggesting that the pattern of reporting feeling blue or depressed by status varied across countries. In the Japanese and Canadian samples, the highest rates of feeling blue or depressed were found among the premenopausal women. In the United States sample the highest rates were in the perimenopausal women. Also, in the Canadian sample there are essentially no differences among the statuses. These different patterns across countries clearly argue against a direct link between decline in estrogen and depression. Attempts to associate menopause and depression through cross-cultural comparisons, however, are complicated by variations in the meaning of menopause as well as the presentation of depressive symptoms (Townsend & Carbone, 1980).

Summary

This review shows that menopause is not experienced universally by women across and within cultures. Differences in symptom reporting are related to culture, expectations, and prior experience. The reporting of vasomotor symptoms is related to symptoms prior to menopause as well as expectations about menopause. Some research suggests that women who report more problems associated with menstruation experience more symptoms during menopause (Hunter, 1992). It could be that such women expect a more difficult menopause, or there could be a physiological connection. The research in the area of depression suggests that the majority of depression among middle-aged women is associated with prior depression and/or life circumstances.

Taken as a whole, these findings suggest that the so-called menopausal syndrome may be related more to personal characteristics or past experiences than to menopause per se. Thus, the image of the depressed woman who dreads menopause and feels that afterward she will no longer be a true woman may well come from those women who are depressed to begin with and may bear little relationship to menopause itself. The subgroup of women reporting negative attitudes and health problems may be the same group who also report menstrual symptoms and other problems, thus supporting Neugarten's thesis that for a subgroup of women, negative menopausal experiences are due to problems in the life course and are not merely the effect of the life event itself (Neugarten & Kraines, 1965). Recent data from the MWHS provide further support that general symptom reporting prior to menopause is highly predictive of menopausal symptom reporting (Avis et al., 1994).

It thus appears that a developmental perspective within a cultural context is essential in understanding women's experience of menopause. Clearly, a woman's psychological state, her attitudes toward menopause, and how she generally responds to symptoms are important predictors of how she will experience menopause. It also appears that, for the majority of women, other events in her life and how she views aging and midlife are more important to her than the biological fact of cessation of menses.

LONG-TERM CHANGES FOLLOWING MENOPAUSE

Menopause is the only physiological change in women directly associated with midlife. However, the hormonal changes accompanying menopause are thought to impact on other bodily systems, in particular the musculoskeletal, cardiovascular, and urogenital systems. Changes in these systems are thought to precipitate increases in heart disease, diabetes, hypertension, osteoporosis, urinary incontinence, and autoimmune disease (Bjorntorp, 1988). It is currently unknown, however, to what extent changes in these systems are directly associated with reductions in estrogen, aging, or concurrent behavioral changes.

Musculoskeletal

Osteoporosis, a condition characterized by loss of bone mass resulting in increased porosity, brittleness, and fragility of bone, is one of the leading causes of morbidity and mortality in the elderly (Riggs & Melton, 1986, 1992). Osteoporosis affects over 20 million Americans and leads to approximately 1.3 million osteoporotic fractures in the United States each year (Riggs & Melton, 1992). The vertebral column is one of the most common sites of bone loss, leading to curvature of the spine, loss of height, and pain (Riggs et al., 1986). The most serious consequence of osteoporosis is the increased risk for a bone fracture, especially in the hip. The relationship between osteoporosis and fracture, however, is still debated (U.S. Congress, Office of Technology Assessment, 1992). Bone mass in older women is a function of two major factors: peak amount of bone mass and rate of bone loss (Heaney et al., 1982). Peak bone mass is determined to a large extent by genetic inheritance (Pollitzer & Anderson, 1989) and other factors such as diet and physical activity (Kanders, Dempster, & Lindsay, 1988). Hormonal status exerts it greatest effect on rate of bone loss.

Women lose about 50% of their trabecular bone and 30% of their cortical bone mass over their lifetime, about half of which is lost during the 10 years after menopause (Riggs & Melton, 1986, 1992). Estrogen appears to protect bone and stimulate calcium absorption, while FSH is thought to interfere with parathormone, which prevents loss of calcium in the urine and helps transport calcium. Although there is an acceleration of bone loss with the cessation of menses, it is unclear when menopausal bone loss begins. Further, different bone sites may vary in their rate of bone loss (Sowers & LaPietra, 1995). Data from the MWHS show that bone loss is easily detectable in the late perimenopause and is equally rapid in the 12 months before and after the last menstrual period. This finding is consistent with other studies of late perimenopausal women (Pouilles, Tremollieres, & Ribot, 1993; Sowers, Clark, Hollis, Wallace, & Jannausch, 1992).

It is important to point out that most of the studies in this area have been conducted on white women. Existing data suggest that African-American women are at lower risk for hip and spinal fractures than white women. Some studies suggest that African-American women may not experience the same postmenopausal bone loss as white women (Krolner & Pors Nielson, 1982; Mazess, 1982; Ruegsegger, Dambacher, Ruegsegger, Fischer, & Anliker, 1984). A recent prospective study of African-American and white women found a higher average bone mass in younger

African-American women and a slower rate of bone loss in the early menopausal period in African-American women as compared to white women. The rates of bone loss in women more than 5 years postmenopausal did not differ (Luckey, Wallenstein, Lapinski, & Meier, 1996).

Cardiovascular

In the United States, cardiovascular disease is the leading cause of death for both men and women. It has often been purported that cardiovascular disease in women significantly increases postmenopause. Before age 50, rates of heart disease are higher in men than in women. However, after age 50, the approximate average age of menopause, the risk of heart disease begins to rise more steeply in women than men. The incidence of coronary artery disease in men and women becomes equal around age 75 (NCHS, 1990). This has led to the belief that estrogen deficiency plays a major role in the acceleration of cardiovascular disease in women (Eaker et al., 1993). However, women do not show an obvious "bump" in heart disease around the time of menopause. This narrowing of the "gender gap" appears to be a function of changing rates in both men and women (McKinlay et al., 1994).

Further, mortality from heart disease does not substantially increase for women following menopause. In fact, the actual rate of increase from age 40 onward is fairly consistent (Bush, 1990). Tracey (1966) demonstrated that when mortality rates for CHD in women are plotted on a log scale, the rate of increase at different ages is completely smooth. The reduced sex difference in mortality appears to be more a result of a leveling of male mortality than an increase in female mortality.

While data do not show an obvious increase in cardiovascular morbidity or mortality following menopause, menopause may still have an impact on cardiovascular risk. Researchers have explored various links between cardiovascular disease risk factors and estrogen levels. The strongest link appears to be with lipids and lipoproteins. Natural menopause has been found to be associated with an unfavorable decrease in HDL cholesterol and an increase in LDL cholesterol (Brown et al., 1993; Matthews et al., 1989). However, only about 25 and 50 percent of estrogen's apparent cardioprotective effect can be attributed to its effect on lipids and lipoproteins.

Some evidence suggests that estrogen also has direct effects on the cardiovascular system including the possible ability to increase coronary artery vascular reactivity, prevent acetylcholine-induced coronary vasoconstriction, increase vasodilation, improve cardiac output, and lower systemic vascular resistance. There are only limited or inconsistent data regarding other possible effects of estrogen on cardiovascular risk factors such as glucose and insulin levels, clotting and coagulation, and weight and body composition.

This is an area of active investigation in which researchers are attempting to sort out the relative impact of age, hormonal changes, and lifestyle factors that may impact changes in cardiovascular risk factors at mid-life.

Body Composition

It has been well documented that body composition changes with age in both men and women. Cross-sectional and longitudinal studies alike have shown that weight (or fatness) increases in adulthood and throughout middle-age, then begins to decline after the sixth decade of life (Kuczmarski et al., 1994; Garn & Clark, 1976). More important, the ratio of lean body mass to fat mass decreases with age. Increase in weight (or fatness), excessive weight change, and the placement of fat (waist/hip ratio, WHR) have all been linked to morbidity in adulthood. Obesity is a major risk factor for several chronic diseases (e.g., coronary artery disease, diabetes, hypertension, and certain types of cancers), and changes in body composition are considered potential risk factors for coronary artery disease, hyperlipidemia, and osteoporosis (Bjorntorp, 1988).

Changes in weight among middle-aged women have not been directly linked to menopause status (Wing, Matthews, Kuller, Meilahn, & Plantinga, 1991). However, menopause may be associated with accelerated loss of lean body mass and an increase in fat mass (Aloia, McGowan, Vaswani, Ross, & Cohn, 1991; Ley, Lees, & Stevenson, 1992). Ley et al. (1992) found that postmenopausal women had a significantly greater prevalence of an android fat distribution than did premenopausal women. Premenopausally, female sex steroid hormones regulate the accumulation of fat in the gluteal-femoral region by activating lipoprotein lipase. Fat mobilization to the hip area is hormonally regulated to accommodate pregnancy (Rebuffe-Scrive, 1988). After menopause, the regulation of fat placement is more equally distributed and it is speculated that these same hormones regulate the mobilization of fat in the abdominal region (Rebuffe-Scrive, 1988), thus increasing the WHR.

The question remains as to what direct effect (if any) menopause status has on these events. Weight gain (and its inherent risk factors) is common throughout adulthood as well as at the time of menopause. Therefore, there is great difficulty in distinguishing the effects of aging from the effects of menopause. Changes in body composition could be attributed to neuroendocrine function, energy balance, lifestyle factors (e.g., alcohol, smoking, exercise), genetic factors, or psychosocial factors. Although these changes begin to appear around the time of menopause, the extent to which they are due to menopause, aging, or lifestyle changes is unclear.

Urogenital

Urinary Incontinence

Urinary symptoms, including incontinence, have often been thought to be part of the menopausal syndrome. The belief is that because bladder and urethral tissue are estrogen sensitive, there is a causal relationship between estrogen deficiency and incontinence. However, it is difficult to determine whether urinary changes are a direct result of estrogen deficiency or are part of the general aging process (Versi, 1990). In a study of 600 working women aged 35–60 years of age, Osborne (1976) did not find an increase in stress incontinence at menopause. In a study of 10,000 women, Thomas, Plymat, Blannin, and Meade (1980) did not find an increase in prevalence of urinary incontinence in women aged 45–60. Neither Hording et al. (1986) nor Hagstad and Jansen (1986) found an increase in incontinence between age-matched pre- and postmenopausal women.

Studies of the effect of ERT on urinary incontinence have yielded mixed results (Versi, 1990). Although uncontrolled trials have shown subjective improvement (Versi & Cardozo, 1988), results of placebo controlled trials are not as favorable. Neither Fantl, Wyman, Anderson, Matt, and Bump (1988) nor Versi et al. (1990) found significant effects of ERT in postmenopausal women with stress incontinence.

Sexuality

It is generally thought that sexual activity declines with age (Dennerstein & Burrows, 1982; Kinsey, Pomeroy, Martin, & Gebhard, 1953; Pfeiffer, Verwoerdt, & Davis, 1972). For women, however, there is some controversy over the relative contribution of menopause to this decline. It is difficult to determine whether this age-associated decline in sexual activity is due to menopause and declining estrogen levels, age, or other age-related circumstances, such as male partner sexual problems. Furthermore, it is not clear whether frequency alone declines, or whether sexual interest and dissatisfaction decline also. Kinsey et al. (1953) and Masters and Johnson (1966) argued that changes in sexual activity for women were largely explained by the decline in sexual functioning in their male partners. More recent researchers attribute changes in women's sexual activity to declining estrogen levels (Davidson, Gray, & Smith, 1983; Hallstrom, 1977). Declines in estrogen reduce the elasticity of vaginal musculature, and lubrication diminishes, often causing dyspareunia. It is unclear, however, which (if any) aspects of sexual activity are affected by lowered estrogen levels and whether these changes are inevitable. Conclusions in this area have been hampered by numerous methodological limitations of the research. The research is often cross-sectional (Bachmann et al., 1985; Hallstrom, 1977; Hunter et al., 1986) and/or based on patient populations. Often only a few aspects of sexuality are studied, few other variables are included, and/or the sample sizes are quite small (McCoy & Davidson, 1985). Several recent studies using large community-based samples are now addressing these issues. A recent study of 2000 middle-aged women in Australia did not find any association between menopause status and libido or frequency of sexual activity (Dennerstein, Dudley, Hopper, & Burger, 1997). Findings from the Massachusetts Women's Health Study II also show no relation between menopause status and frequency of sexual activity, although results from the MWHS did find an age-related decline in frequency (Avis, Stellato, Crawford, & Johannes, 1995). Satisfaction with sexual relationships has not been found to be related to menopause status or age (Avis et al., 1995). Additional longitudinal research is needed to examine the complex interplay of age, hormones, health, psychosocial characteristics, and partner characteristics on different aspects of sexual functioning (frequency of various activities, interest, desire, satisfaction) for women at midlife.

Breast Cancer

Breast cancer is clearly a hormonally mediated disease (Howe & Rohan, 1993). Risk is modified by markers of hormonal status such as age of menarche, pregnancy, and age of menopause (Howe & Rohan, 1993). Menopause is important for breast cancer in that late age of natural menopause consistently has been shown to elevate breast cancer risk (Brinton, 1990; Howe & Rohan, 1993). Early menopause, particularly if it involves surgical removal of both ovaries, greatly reduces risk (Trichopoulos, MacMahon, & Cole, 1972). Because of the well-recognized role of hormonal factors in breast cancer, there is considerable concern over the effect of exogenous hormone use in increasing a woman's risk for breast cancer.

Although all of the aforementioned conditions or diseases are thought to increase following menopause, the actual *rate* of increase in breast cancer decreases postmenopause. Although incidence rates increase with age, the increase is less steep after about age 45–50 than in reproductive years (Kelsey & Horn-Ross, 1993). This strongly suggests the involvement of reproductive hormones in breast cancer etiology.

Hormone Replacement Therapy

Hormone replacement therapy is currently touted as an antidote to these long-term consequences of menopause/aging. In evaluating the effectiveness of hormone therapy in preventing disease and disability, it is necessary to consider the two primary types of hormone therapy: estrogen alone (ERT) or estrogen combined with a progestin (combined therapy or HRT). Estrogen alone gained widespread use in the mid-1960s when it was promoted aggressively by pharmaceutical companies and by books such as Wilson's *Feminine Forever*. In the mid-1970s, however, three studies showed that estrogen considerably increased a woman's risk for endometrial cancer (Mack et al., 1976; Smith et al., 1975; Ziel & Finkle, 1975). Based on these findings, unopposed estrogen is generally not recommended for women who still have a uterus. In response to these studies, the pharmaceutical companies began searching for a way to counter this effect of estrogen. The combination of estrogen and a progestin prevents an excess of estrogen from building up in the endometrium and reduces a woman's risk of endometrial cancer.

The strongest evidence for a preventive effect of HRT is found for preventing bone loss (Ettinger, Genant, & Cann, 1985; Genant, Baylink, & Gallagher, 1989; Lindsay & Cosman, 1990; Lindsay et al., 1980). However, while research suggests that estrogen use can retard bone loss, once estrogen replacement stops, the bone loss resumes (Lindsay et al., 1978). Further, more recent evidence suggests that estrogen use even up to 10 years postmenopause provides little benefit for women 75 years and older, who have the highest risk of fracture (Felson et al., 1993). Studies have also shown that beginning hormone therapy later in life may provide almost as much protection against osteoporotic fracture as lifelong therapy started at menopause (Ettinger & Grady, 1994; Schneider Barrett-Connor & Morton, 1997).

Hormone replacement therapy is often cited as providing a protective effect for cardiovascular disease. However, there are a number of limitations regarding our current knowledge of the effect of estrogen on CHD. The primary limitation is that to date the majority of data on HRT use and CHD are derived from observational studies of women who take HRT compared to those who do not. Although these studies show that estrogen users are less likely to develop CHD, it is crucial to consider that there are several potential biases in observational studies. First, selection bias is widely recognized as a problem in observational studies. Comparisons of HRT users versus non-users have found that hormone users, prior to the use of HRT, have a better cardiovascular risk factor profile than non-estrogen users. HRT users, in general, have higher levels of HDL cholesterol and leisure physical activity, as well as lower levels of apolipoprotein B, blood pressure, weight, and fasting insulin (Derby et al., 1993; Johannes et al., 1994). Second, hormone users are more likely than non-users to interact with the health care system and to engage in a variety of prevention-related behaviors, such as mammograms, pap smears, and cholesterol checks. Third, hormone users have been shown to be generally more compliant with respect to medication taking (Petitti, 1994). These biases are likely to lead to overstating the cardioprotective effect of exogonous estrogen.

To further complicate the question of whether estrogen is cardioprotective, the existing long-term data are primarily on the effect of estrogen alone. The data on the cardioprotective effect of adding a progestin are limited and inconsistent (Barrett-Connor, 1996). While there has been some clinical trial evidence that estrogen can have a favorable impact on cardiovascular risk (The Postmenopausal Estrogen/Progestin Interventions (PEPI) Trial Investigators, 1995), how this translates into cardiovascular disease is still unknown. This is one of the major research questions being addressed by the Women's Health Initiative.

One of the primary potential risks associated with long-term use of HRT is breast cancer. As previously mentioned, there is considerable evidence that breast cancer is hormonally mediated. However, whether exogenous estrogen increases a woman's risk for breast cancer remains controversial. As Barrett-Connor (1994) recently pointed out, of four recent meta-analyses on the relation between estrogen use and increased breast cancer, two of these analyses concluded that there was no risk (Armstrong, 1988; Dupont & Page, 1991), while the other two concluded that there was a small increased risk (Sillero-Arenas et al., 1992; Steinberg et al., 1991). The studies reported in these meta-analyses are limited, however, in that most of the women studied had used estrogen for less than 10 years, earlier studies that showed no association had poor study design, and dosages have changed over time. Barrett-Connor further points out that such observational studies have inherent biases such as the fact that estrogen users have more physician contact. Further, most of the studies to date look at the effect of estrogen alone. Combined therapy has not been in use long enough to determine the potential impact of the addition of a progestin, which may increase risk. The most recent and comprehensive meta analysis concluded that the risk of breast cancer increases in relation to the increasing duration of use in current or recent users of HRT but not in past users: the effects of HRT are more adverse in thinner than heavier women, the breast cancers diagnosed in women who use HRT are less advanced clinically than those diagnosed in never users, and progestins do not reduce increased risk associated with estrogens (Collaborative Group on Hormonal Factors in Breast Cancer in Oxford, England, 1997).

Estrogen and progesterone are potent hormones and the effects of regular usage for 20–30 years are essentially unknown. Our only available information comes from continuing research on oral contraceptives, which include different pharmaceuticals at different doses. Women who choose to take exogenous hormones for the rest of their postmenopausal lives or for many years may be at risk for a variety of as yet unknown effects. Some of these long-term effects are currently being studied as part of the Women's Health Initiative. As potential alternatives to estrogen replacement therapy, a new class of compounds called selective estrogen receptor modulators (SERMS) are being developed. SERMS may be thought of as "designer estrogens," compounds that are tailored to possess estrogen agonist-like actions on bone tissues and serum lipids while displaying estrogen antagonist properties in the breast and uterus. Tamoxifen, the first SERM in clinical use, seems to block estrogenic effects in breast tissue, but evidence is accumulating that it may stimulate uterine tissue, increasing the risk of hyperplasia and endometrial cancer. Raloxifene, a newer SERM, is thought to have favorable effects on bone density and blood lipids while blocking estrogen receptors in the breast as well as the uterus. Recent data, however, suggest that although raloxifene has some effect on lipids, this is less than estrogens and that raloxifene also increases hot flashes (Walsh, Kuller, Wild, Paul, Farmer, Lawrence, Shah, & Anderson, 1998). SERMS are very new therapies at this time. Their actual impact on lipids and long-term cardioprotective effects are unknown (Rifkind & Rossouw, 1998).

Despite the risks of HRT, many women are clearly drawn to the benefits of hormone therapy. Many of these benefits, however, can be achieved through other much safer means. While epidemiologists continue to study the risks and benefits of ERT, it is important to also study its alternatives. Lifestyle changes such as smoking cessation, weight reduction, and exercise are effective alternatives to ERT for reducing risk of coronary heart disease (Manson et al., 1992) and may be beneficial in preventing osteoporosis (Dalsky, 1987; Sinaki, 1989), although systematic evidence is lacking on this issue.

CONCLUSIONS

This chapter provides a review of women's health at midlife with a primary focus on menopause and the long-term changes following menopause. It is apparent from this review that the physiological and hormonal changes associated with menopause do not affect all women the same and that women differ in how they respond to this physiological event. Factors that influence a woman's response appear to be cultural, behavioral, psychosocial, as well as physiological. There is also evidence that women who experience a more difficult time during menstruation have a more difficult menopause. This may reflect a consistent pattern of responding to physiological changes and/or symptoms or reflect an underlying physiological mechanism related to both experiences. Although Western societies often hold negative views of menopause, menopausal and postmenopausal women often have more positive views than society as a whole. In fact, following menopause, many women experience a new period of developmental growth and increased energy. How an individual woman responds to menopause is a complex interaction of physiology, her current life circumstances, attitudes/concerns about fertility, the culture in which she lives, and her history of responding to physiological changes/symptoms.

There is still a great deal we do not know about menopause. We know little about the factors that influence the perception of and response to perimenopausal symptoms and the effect of the perimenopause transition on the musculoskeletal, cardiovascular, urogenital, and other biological systems. Further, our current knowledge of the menopausal transition is primarily limited to white women. We know very little about the range of experiences in women of other racial/ethnic backgrounds. Future research needs to study this life transition among women of diverse racial/ethnic groups, determine long-term health changes that are directly attributable to menopause versus those due to aging, and better understand the risks and benefits of hormone replacement therapy and its alternatives.

REFERENCES

Adena, M. A., & Gallagher, H. G. (1982). Cigarette smoking and age at menopause. *Annals of Human Biology, 9*, 121–130.

Adlercreutz, H., Hamalaiven, O., Gorbach, S., & Grodin, B. (1992). Dietary phytoestrogens and the menopause in Japan. *Lancet, 339*, 12333.

Agoestina, T., & van Keep, P. A. (1984). The climacteric in Bandung, West Java Province, Indonesia. A survey of 1025 women between 40 and 55 years of age. *Maturitas, 6*, 327–33.

Aloia, J. F., McGowan, D. M., Vaswani, A. N., Ross, P., & Cohn, S. H. (1991). Relationship of menopause to skeletal and muscle mass. *American Journal of Clinical Nutrition, 53*, 1378–1383.

Anderson, E., Hamburger, S., Liu, J. H., & Rebar, R. W. (1987). Characteristics of menopausal women seeking assistance. *American Journal of Obstetrics and Gynecology, 156*, 428–433.

Armstrong, B. K. (1988). Estrogen therapy after the menopause—Boom or bane? *Medical Journal of Australia, 18*, 213–214.

Avis, N. E. (1996). Women's perceptions of the menopause. *European Menopause Journal, 3,* 80–84.

Avis, N. E., Brambilla, D. J., McKinlay, S. M., & Vass, K. (1994). A longitudinal analysis of the association between menopause and depression: Results from the Massachusetts Women's Health Study. *Annals of Epidemiology, 4,* 214–220.

Avis, N. E., Crawford, S. L., & McKinlay, S. M. (1997). Psychosocial, behavioral, and health factors related to menopause symptomatology. *Women's Health: Research on Gender, Behavior, and Policy, 3,* 103–120.

Avis, N. E., Kaufert, P. A., Lock, M., McKinlay, S. M., & Vass, K. (1993). The evolution of menopausal symptoms. In H. Burger (Ed.), *Bailliere's clinical endocrinology and metabolism* (Vol. 7(1), pp. 17–32). London: Bailliere Tindall.

Avis, N. E., & McKinlay, S. M. (1991). A longitudinal analysis of women's attitudes towards the menopause: Results from the Massachusetts Women's Health Study. *Maturitas, 13,* 65–79.

Avis, N. E., & McKinlay, S. M. (1995). The Massachusetts Women's Health Study: An epidemiologic investigation of the menopause. *Journal of the American Medical Women's Association, 50,* 45–63.

Avis, N. E., McKinlay, S. M., Vass, K., Brambilla, D., & Longcope, J. (1993, June). *Hormone levels, symptoms, and the relation between menopause and depression.* Paper presented at the 7th International Congress on the Menopause, Stockholm, Sweden.

Avis, N. E., Stellato, R., Crawford, S., & Johannes, C. (1995). How does menopause impact sexual activity? *Menopause, 2,* 245 (abstract).

Aylward, M. (1973). Plasma tryptophan levels and mental depression in postmenopausal subjects: Effects of oral piperazine-oestrone sulphate. *International Research Communications Systems Medical Science, 1,* 30–34.

Bachmann, G. A., Leiblum, S. R., Sandler, B., Ainsley, W., Narcessian, R., Shelden, R., & Hymans, H. N. (1985). Correlates of sexual desire in post-menopausal women. *Maturitas, 7,* 211–216.

Ballinger, C. B. (1975). Psychiatric morbidity and the menopause screening of general population sample. *British Medical Journal, 3,* 344–346.

Ballinger, C. B. (1976). Psychiatric morbidity and the menopause: Clinical features. *British Medical Journal, 1,* 1183–1185.

Ballinger, C. B., Browning, M. C. K., & Smith, A. H. W. (1987). Hormone profiles and psychological symptoms in perimenopausal women. *Maturitas, 9,* 235–251.

Barentsen, R., Foekema, H. A., Bezemer, W., & van Stiphout, F. L. M. (1994). The view of women aged 45–65 and their partners on aspects of the climacteric phase of life. *European Journal of Obstetrics, Gynecology, and Reproductive Biology, 57,* 95–101.

Barnett, R. C., & Baruch, G. K. (1978). Women in the middle years: A critique of research and theory. *Psychology of Women Quarterly, 3,* 187–197.

Barrett-Connor, E. (1994). Postmenopausal estrogen and the risk of breast cancer. *Annals of Epidemiology, 4,* 177–180.

Barrett-Connor, E. (1996). The menopause, hormone replacement, and cardiovascular disease: The epidemiologic evidence. *Maturitas, 23,* 227–234.

Barrett-Connor, E., & Kritz-Silverstein, D. (1993). Estrogen replacement therapy and cognitive function in older women. *Journal of the American Medical Association, 20,* 2637–2641.

Bart, P. B. (1971). Depression in middle-aged women. In V. Gornick & B. K. Moran (Eds.), *Women in sexist society and studies in power and powerlessness.* New York: Basic Books.

Bart, P. B., & Grossman, M. (1978). Menopause. In M. T. Notman & C. C. Nadelson (Eds.), *The woman patient* (Vol. 1). New York: Plenum Press.

Bean, J. A., Leeper, J. D., Wallace, R. B., Sherman, B. M., & Jagger, H. (1979). Variations in the reporting of menstrual histories. *American Journal of Epidemiology, 109,* 181–185.

Bell, S. E. (1990). Sociological perspectives on the medicalization of menopause. *Annals of the New York Academy of Sciences, 592,* 173–178.

Benedek, T. (1950). Climacterium: A developmental phase. *Psychoanalytic Quarterly, 19(1),* 1–27.

Beyene, Y. (1986). Cultural significance and physiological manifestations of menopause: A biocultural analysis. *Culture, Medicine and Psychiatry, 10,* 47–71.

Bjorntorp, V. A. (1988). The associations between obesity, adipose tissue. Distribution and disease. *Acta Medica Scandinavica, 723(Suppl),* 121–134.

Brambilla, D. J., & McKinlay, S. M. (1989). A prospective study of factors affecting age at menopause. *Journal of Clinical Epidemiology, 42,* 1031–1039.

Brambilla, D. J., McKinlay, S. M., & Johannes, C. B. (1994). Defining the perimenopause for application in epidemiologic investigations. *American Journal of Epidemiology, 140,* 1091–1095.

Brinton, L. A. (1990). Menopause and the risk of breast cancer. *Annals of the New York Academy of Sciences, 592,* 357–362.

Brooks-Gunn, J., & Ruble, D. N. (1982). The development of menstrual-related beliefs and behaviors during early adolescence. *Child Development, 53,* 1567–1577.

Brown, J. R. W. C., & Brown, M. E. A. (1976). Psychiatric disorders associated with the menopause. In R. J. Beard (Ed.), *The menopause: A guide to current research and practice.* Baltimore, MD: University Park Press.

Brown, S. A., Hutchinson, R., Morrisett, J., Boerwinkle, E., Davis, C. E., & Gotto, A. M. (1993). Plasma lipid, lipoprotein cholesterol and apopprotein distributions in selected US communities. *Arteriosclerosis and Thrombosis, 13,* 1139–1158.

Bungay, G. T., Vessey, M. P., & McPherson, C. K. (1980). Study of symptoms in middle life with special reference to menopause. *British Medical Journal, ii,* 181–183.

Bush, T. L. (1990). The epidemiology of cardiovascular disease in postmenopausal women. *Annals of the New York Academy of Sciences, 592,* 263–271.

Bush, T. L., Barrett-Connor, E., Cowan, L. D., Criqui, M. H., Wallace, R. B., & Suchindran, C. M. (1987). Cardiovascular mortality and noncontraceptive use of estrogen in women: Results from the Lipid Research Clinics Program Follow-Up Study. *Circulation, 75,* 1102–1109.

Campbell, S., & Whitehead, M. (1977). Oestrogen therapy and the menopausal syndrome. *Clinical Obstetrics and Gynaecology, 4,* 31–47.

Chapman, S. (1979). Advertising and psychotropic drugs: The place of myth in ideological production. *Social Science and Medicine, 13A,* 751–764.

Clayden, J. R., Bell, J. W., & Pollard, P. (1974). Menopausal flushing: Double-blind trial of a non-hormonal medication. *British Medical Journal, 1,* 409–412.

Collaborative Group on Hormonal Factors in Breast Cancer. (1997). Breast Cancer and hormone replacement therapy: Collaborative reanalysis of data from 51 epidemiologic studies of 52,705 women with breast cancer and 108,411 women without breast cancer. *Lancet, 350,* 1047–1059.

Coope, J., Thomson, J. M., & Poller, L. (1975). Effects of "natural oestrogen" replacement therapy on menopausal symptoms and blood clotting. *British Medical Journal, 4,* 139–143.

Costa, P. T., & McCrae, R. R. (1980). Still stable after all these years: Personality as a key to some issues in aging. In P. B. Baltes & O. G. Brim, Jr. (Eds.), *Life-span development and behavior* (Vol. 3, pp. 65–102). New York: Academic Press.

Cowan, G., Warren, L. W., & Young, J. L. (1985). Medical perceptions of menopausal symptoms. *Psychology of Women Quarterly, 9(1),* 3–14.

Currier, A. F. (1897). *The menopause.* New York: Appleton.

Dalsky, G. J. (1987). Exercise: Its effects on bone mineral content. *Clinical Obstetrics and Gynecology, 30,* 820–832.

Davidson, J. M., Gray, G. S., & Smith, E. R. (1983). The sexual psychoendocrinology of aging. In J. Meites (Ed.), *Neuroendocrinology of aging* (pp. 221–258). New York: Plenum Press.

Dennerstein, L. (1987). Depression in the menopause. *Obstetrics and Gynecology Clinics of North America, 4(1),* 33–48.

Dennerstein, L., & Burrows, G. D. (1982). Hormone replacement therapy and sexuality in women. *Clinical Endocrinology and Metabolism, 11,* 661–670.

Dennerstein, L., Dudley, E., Hopper, J., & Burger, H. (1997). Sexuality, hormones and the menopausal transition. *Maturitas, 26,* 83–93.

Derby, C. A., Hume, A. L., Barbour, M. M., McPhillips, J. B., Lasater, T., & Carleton, R. A. (1993). Correlates of postmenopausal estrogen use and trends through the 1980s in two southeastern New England communities. *American Journal of Epidemiology, 137,* 1125–1135.

Deutsch, H. (1945). *The psychology of women: A psychoanalytic interpretation.* New York: Grune and Stratton.

Ditkoff, E. C., Crary, W. G., Cristo, M., & Lobo, R. A. (1991). Estrogen improves psychological function in asymptomatic postmenopausal women. *Obstetrics and Gynecology, 78,* 991–995.

Dupont, W. D., & Page, D. L. (1991). Menopausal estrogen replacement therapy and breast cancer. *Archives of Internal Medicine, 151,* 67–72.

Eaker, E. D., Chesbro, J. H., Sacks, F. M., Wenger, N. K., Whisnant, J. P., & Winston, M. (1993). Cardiovascular disease in women. *Circulation, 88,* 1999–2009.

Erikson, E. H. (1950). *Childhood and society.* New York: Norton.

Erlik, Y., Tataryn, I. V., Meldrum, D. R., Lomax, P., Bajorek, J. G., & Judd, H. L. (1981). Association of waking episodes with menopausal hot flushes. *Journal of the American Medical Association, 245*(17), 1741–1744.

Ettinger, B., Genant, H. K., & Cann, C. E. (1985). Long-term estrogen replacement therapy prevents bone loss and fractures. *Annals of Internal Medicine, 102*(3), 319–324.

Ettinger, B., & Grady, D. (1994). Maximizing the benefit of estrogen therapy for prevention of osteoporosis. *Menopause, 1,* 19–24.

Fantl, J. A., Wyman, J. F., Anderson, R. L., Matt, D. W., & Bump, D. C. (1988). Postmenopausal urinary incontinence: Comparison between non-estrogen supplemented and estrogen-supplemented women. *Obstetrics and Gynecology, 71,* 823.

Fedor-Freybergh, P. (1977). The influence of oestrogen on the well-being and mental performance in climacteric and postmenopausal women. *Acta Obstetrics Gynecology Scandinavia, 64,* 5–69.

Felson, D. T., Zhang, Y., Hannan, M. T., Kiel, D. P., Wilson, P. W., & Anderson, J. J. (1993). The effect of postmenopausal estrogen therapy on bone density in elderly women. *The New England Journal of Medicine, 329* (16), 1141–1146.

Flint, M. (1975). The menopause: Reward or punishment? *Psychosomatics, 15,* 161–163.

Frey, K. (1982). Middle-aged women's experience and perceptions of menopause. *Women and Health, 6,* 25–36.

Gangar, K. F., Vyas, S., Whitehead, M., Crook, D., Meire, H., & Campbell, S. (1991). Pulsatility index in internal carotid artery in relation to transdermal oestradiol and time since menopause. *The Lancet, 338,* 839–842.

Garn, S. M., & Clark, D. C. (1976). Trends in fatness and origins of obesity. *Pediatrics, 57,* 443–456.

Genant, H. K., Baylink, D. J., & Gallagher, J. C. (1989). Estrogens in the prevention of osteoporosis in postmenopausal women. *American Journal of Obstetrics and Gynecology, 161* (6, Pt. 2), 1842–1846.

Gilligan, C. (1979). Woman's place in man's life cycle. *Harvard Educational Review, 49,* 431–446.

Gilligan, C. (1982). *In a different voice: Psychological theory and women's development.* Cambridge, MA: Harvard University Press.

Grady, D., Rubin, S. M., Petitti, D. B., Fox, C. S., Black, D., & Ettinger, B. (1992). Hormone therapy to prevent disease and prolong life in postmenopausal women. *Annals of Internal Medicine, 117,* 1016–1037.

Greene, J. G., & Cooke, D. J. (1976). A factor analytic study of climacteric symptoms. *Journal of Psychosomatic Research, 40,* 425–430.

Greene, J. G., & Cooke, D. J. (1980). Life stress and symptoms at the climacterium. *British Journal of Psychiatry, 136,* 486–491.

Griffen, J. (1982). Cultural models for coping with menopause. In A. M. Voda, M. Dinnerstein, & S. R. O'Donnell (Eds.), *Changing perspectives on menopause.* Austin, TX: University of Texas Press.

Groeneveld, F. P. M., Bareman, F. P., Barensten, R., & Dokter, H. (1993). Relations between attitude toward menopause, well-being, and medical attention among women aged 45 to 60 years. *Maturitas, 17,* 77–88.

Hagstad, A. (1986). The epidemiology of climacteric symptoms. *Acta Obstetricia et Gynecologica Scandanavica, 134S,* 59–65.

Hallstrom, T. (1977). Sexuality in the climacteric. *Clinics in Obstetrics and Gynecology, 4,* 277–239.

Heaney, R. P., Gallagher, J. C., Johnston, C. C., Neer, R., Parfitt, A. M., & Whedon, G. D. (1982). Calcium nutrition and bone health in the elderly. *American Journal of Clinical Nutrition, 36,* 986–1013.

Holte, A., & Mikkelsen, A. (1991). Psychosocial determinants of climacteric complaints. *Maturitas, 13,* 205–215.

Hording, U., Pedersen, K. H., Sidenius, K., & Hedegaard, L. (1986). Urinary incontinence in 45-year-old women. An epidemiologic survey. *Scandanavian Journal of Urology and Nephrology, 20,* 183–186.

Howe, G. R., & Rohan, T. E. (1993). The epidemiology of breast cancer in women. In J. Lorrain (Ed.), *Comprehensive management of menopause.* New York: Springer Verlag.

Howell, M. C. (1974). What medical schools teach about women. *The New England Journal of Medicine, 291,* 304–307.

Hunter, M. S. (1990). Somatic experience of the menopause: A prospective study. *Psychosomatic Medicine, 52,* 357–367.

Hunter, M. (1992). The South-East England longitudinal study of the climacteric and postmenopause. *Maturitas, 14,* 117–126.

Hunter, M. S., Battersby, R., & Whitehead, M. (1986). Relationships between psychological symptoms, somatic complaints and menopausal status. *Maturitas, 8,* 217–228.

Jaszmann, L., van Lith, N. D., & Zaat, J. C. A. (1969a). The age at menopause in the Netherlands. *International Journal of Fertility, 14,* 106–117.

Jaszmann, L., van Lith, N. D., & Zaat, J. C. A. (1969b). The perimenopausal symptoms: The statistical analysis of a survey—Part A. *Medical Gynaecology and Sociology, 4,* 268–277.

Jick, H., & Porter, J. (1977). Relation between smoking and age of natural menopause. *Lancet, 1,* 1354–1355.

Johannes, C. B., Crawford, S. L., Posner, J. G., & McKinlay, S. M. (1994). Longitudinal patterns and correlates of HRT use in middle-aged women. *American Journal of Epidemiology, 140,* 439–452.

Kanders, B., Dempster, D. W., & Lindsay, R. (1988). Interaction of calcium nutrition and physical activity on bone mass in young women. *Journal of Bone Mineral Research, 3*(2), 145–149.

Kaufert, P. A. (1982). Anthropology and the menopause: The development of a theoretical framework. *Maturitas, 4,* 181–193.

Kaufert, P. A., Gilbert, P., & Hassard, T. (1988). Researching the symptoms of menopause: An exercise in methodology. *Maturitas, 10,* 117–131.

Kaufert, P., Lock, M., McKinlay, S., Beyene, Y., Coope, J., Davis, D., Eliasson, M., Gognalons-Nicolet, M., Goodman, M., & Holte, A. (1986). Menopause research: The Korpilampi Workshop. *Social Science and Medicine, 22*(11), 1285–1289.

Kaufert, P. A., & McKinlay, S. M. (1985). Estrogen replacement therapy: The production of medical knowledge and the emergence of policy. In E. Lewin & V. Olesen (Eds.), *Women, health and healing: Toward a new perspective.* New York: Tavistock.

Kaufman, D. W., Sloane, D., Rosenberg, L., Miettinen, O. S., & Shapiro, S. (1980). Cigarette smoking and age at natural menopause. *American Journal of Public Health, 70,* 420–422.

Kaufman, D. W., Slone, D., Rosenberg, L., Miettinen, O. S., & Shapiro, S. (1980). Cigarette smoking and age at natural menopause. *American Journal of Public Health, 70,* 420–422.

Kearns, B. J. R. (1982). Perceptions of menopause by Papago women. In A. M. Voda, M. Dinnerstein, & S. R. O'Donnell (Eds.), *Changing perspectives on menopause.* Austin, TX: University of Texas Press.

Kelsey, J. L., & Horn-Ross, P. L. (1993). Breast cancer: Magnitude of the problem and descriptive epidemiology. *Epidemiologic Reviews, 15*(1), 7–16.

Kimura, D. (1995). Estrogen replacement therapy may protect against intellectual decline in postmenopausal women. *Hormones and Behavior, 29,* 312–321.

Kinsey, A. C., Pomeroy, W. B., Martin, C. E., & Gebhard, P. H. (1953). *Sexual behavior in the human female.* Philadelphia: W. B. Saunders.

Kopera, H. (1973). Estrogens and psychic functions. *Frontiers Hormone Research, 2,* 118–133.

Krailo, M. D., & Pike, M. C. (1983). Estimation of the distribution of age at natural menopause. *American Journal of Epidemiology, 117,* 356–61.

Krescovich, E. A. S. (1980). A comparison of attitudes toward menopause held by women during the three phases of the climacterium. *Issues of Mental Health in Nursing, 2*(3), 59–69.

Krolner, B., & Pors, N. S. (1982). Bone and mineral content of the lumbar spine in normal and osteoporotic women: Cross-sectional and longitudinal studies. *Clinical Science, 62,* 329–336.

Kronenberg, F. (1990). Hot flashes: Epidemiology and physiology. *Annals of the New York Academy of Sciences, 592,* 52–86.

Kuczmarski, R. J., Flegal, K. M., Campbell, S. M., & Johnson, C. L. (1994). Increasing prevalence of overweight among U.S. adults. *Journal of the American Medical Association, 272,* 205–211.

Leiblum, S. R., & Swartzman, L. C. (1986). Women's attitudes toward the menopause: An update. *Maturitas, 8,* 47–56.

Levinson, D. (1978). *The seasons of a man's life.* New York: Ballantine Books.

Ley, C. J., Lees, B., & Stevenson, J. C. (1992). Sex- and menopause-associated changes in body-fat distribution. *American Journal of Clinical Nutrition, 55,* 950–954.

Lindsay, R., & Cosman, F. (1990). Estrogen in prevention and treatment of osteoporosis. *Annals of the New York Academy of Sciences, 592,* 326–333.

Lindsay, R., Hart, D. M., Maclean, A., Clark, A. C., Kraszewski, A., & Garwood, J. (1978). Bone response to termination of estrogen treatment. *The Lancet, i,* 1325–1327.

Lindsay, R., Hart, D. M., Forrest, C., & Baird, C. (1980). Prevention of spinal osteoporosis in oophorectomized women. *The Lancet, 2,* 1151–1154.

Lock, M. (1985). Models and practice in medicine: Menopause as syndrome or life transition. In R. A. Hahn & A. D. Gaines (Eds.), *Physicians of western medicine.* Boston: Reidel.

Lock, M. (1986). Ambiguities of aging: Japanese experience and perceptions of menopause. *Culture, Medicine and Psychiatry, 10,* 23–46.

Luckey, M. M., Wallenstein, S., Lapinski, R., & Meier, D. E. (1996). A prospective study of bone loss in African-American and white women—a clinical research center study. *Journal of Clinical Endocrinology and Metabolism, 81,* 2948–2956.

Luine, V. N., Park, D., Joh, T., Reis, D., & McEwen, B. (1980). Immuno-chemical demonstration of increased choline acetyltransferase concentration in rat preoptic area after estradiol administration. *Brain Research, 191,* 273–277.

Mack, T. M., Pike, M. C., Henderson, M. E., Pfeffer, R. I., Gerkins, V. R., Arthur, M., & Brown, S. E. (1976). Estrogens and endometrial cancer in a retirement community. *The New England Journal of Medicine, 294,* 1262–1267.

Magursky, V., Mesko, M., & Sokolik, L. (1975). Age at menopause and onset of the climacteric in women of Martin District. *International Journal of Fertility, 20,* 17–23.

Malleson, J. (1953). An endocrine factor in certain affective disorders. *The Lancet, 2,* 158–164.

Manson, J., Tosteson, H., Satterfield, S., Hebert, P., O'Connor, G. T., Baring, J. E., & Hennekens, C. H. (1992). The primary prevention of myocardial infarction. *New England Journal of Medicine, 326,* 1406–1416.

Martin, E. (1987). *The woman in the body.* Boston: Beacon Press.

Masters, W. H., & Johnson, V. E. (1966). *Human sexual response.* Boston: Little, Brown.

Matthews, K. (1992). Myths and realities of the menopause. *Psychosomatic Medicine, 54,* 1–9.

Matthews, K. A., Meilhan, E., Kuller, L. H., Kelsey, S. F., Caggiula, A. W., & Wing, R. R. (1989). Menopause and risk factors for coronary heart disease. *The New England Journal of Medicine, 321,* 641–646.

Matthews, K. A., Wing, R. R., Kuller, L. H., Meilahn, E. N., Kelsey, S. F., Costello, J. E., & Caggiula, A. (1990). Influences of natural menopause on psychological characteristics and symptoms of middle-aged healthy women. *Journal of Consulting and Clinical Psychology, 58,* 345–351.

Mazess, R. B. 91982). On aging bone mass. *Clinical Orthopedics and Related Research, 165,* 239–252.

McCrea, F. (1983). The politics of menopause: The discovery of a deficiency disease. *Social Problems, 31,* 111–123.

McEwen, B. S. (1991). Steroid hormones are multifunctional messengers to the brain. *Trends in Endocrinology Metabolism, 2,* 62–67.

McKinlay, J. B., Crawford, S., McKinlay, S. M., & Sellers, D. E. (1994). On the reported gender difference in coronary heart disease: An illustration of the social construction of epidemiologic rates. In S. M. Czajkowski, D. R. Hill, & T. B. Clarkson (eds.), *Women, behavior, and cardiovascular disease* (pp. 223–252). National Institutes of Health Publication No. 94-339.

McKinlay, J. B., McKinlay, S. M., & Brambilla, D. J. (1987a). Health status and utilization behavior associated with menopause. *American Journal of Epidemiology, 125,* 110–121.

McKinlay, J. B., McKinlay, S. M., & Brambilla, D. J. (1987b). The relative contributions of endocrine changes and social circumstances to depression in mid-aged women. *Journal of Health and Social Behavior, 28,* 345–363.

McKinlay, S. M., Bifano, N. L., & McKinlay, J. B. (1985). Smoking and age at menopause in women. *Annals of Internal Medicine, 103,* 350–356.

McKinlay, S. M., Brambilla, D. J., Avis, N. E., & McKinlay, J. B. (1991). Women's experience of the menopause. *Current Obstetrics and Gynecology, 1,* 3–7.

McKinlay, S. M., Brambilla, D. J., & Posner, J. G. (1992). The normal menopause transition. *Journal of Human Biology, 4,* 37–46.

McKinlay, S. M., & Jefferys, M. (1974). The menopausal syndrome. *British Journal of Preventive Social Medicine, 28,* 108–115.

McKinlay, S. M., Jefferys, M., & Thompson, B. (1972). An investigation of the age at onset of menopause. *Journal of Biosocial Science, 4,* 161–173.

McKinlay, S. M., & McKinlay, J. B. (1973). Selected studies of the menopause—A methodological critique. *Journal of Biosocial Science, 5,* 533–554.

McKinlay, S. M., & McKinlay, J. B. (1986). Health status and health care utilization by menopausal women. In M. Notelovitz & D. van Keep (Eds.), *The Climacteric Perspective.* Lancaster: MTP Press Limited.

Millette, B. M. (1981). Menopause: A survey of attitudes and knowledge. *Issues of Health Care for Women, 3,* 263–276.

Morse, C., Smith, A., Dennerstein, L., Green, A., Hopper, J., & Burger, H. (1994). The treatment-seeking women at menopause. *Maturitas, 18,* 61–173.

Myers, J. K., & Weissmann, M. (1980). Use of a self-report symptom scale to detect depression in a community sample. *American Journal of Psychiatry, 137,* 1081–1084.

National Center for Health Statistics (NCHS). (1990). *Vital statistics of the United States, Vol. II, Morality, Pt. B* (DHHS Public Health Service Pub. No. (PHS) 90-1102). Washington DC: U.S. Government Printing Office.

Neugarten, B. L. (1968). Adult personality: Toward a psychology of the life cycle. In *Middle age and aging* (pp. 137–147). Chicago: University of Chicago Press.

Neugarten, B. L., & Kraines, R. J. (1965). "Menopausal symptoms" in women of various ages. *Psychosomatic Medicine, 27(3),* 266–273.

Neugarten, B. L., Wood, V., Kraines, R. J., & Loomis, B. (1963). Women's attitudes toward the menopause. *Vitae Human, 6,* 140–151.

Notman, M. (1978). Women and mid-life: A different perspective. *Psychiatric Opinion, 15(9),* 15–25.

Notman, M. (1979). Midlife concerns of women: Implications of the menopause. *American Journal of Psychiatry, 136,* 1270–1274.

Notman, M. (1990). Menopause and adult development. *Annals of the New York Academy of Sciences, 592,* 149–155.

Osborne, J. L. (1976). Postmenopausal changes in micturition habits and in urine flow and urethral pressure studies. In S. Campbell (Ed.), *The management of the menopause and postmenopausal years.* Boston: MTP Publications.

Paganini-Hill, A., & Henderson, V. W. (1996). The effects of hormone replacement therapy, lipoprotein cholesterol levels, and other factors on a clock drawing task in older women. *Journal of the American Geriatrics Society, 44,* 818–822.

Paganini-Hill, A., Krailo, M. D., & Pike, M. C. (1984). Age at natural menopause and breast cancer risk: The effect of errors in recall. *American Journal of Epidemiology, 119,* 81–85.

Parlee, M. B. (1974). Stereotypic beliefs about menstruation: A methodological note on the Moos Menstrual Distress Questionnaire. *Psychosomatic Medicine, 36,* 229.

Payer, L. (1991). The menopause in various cultures. In H. Burger & M. Boulet (Eds.), *A portrait of the menopause.* Park Ridge, New Jersey: Parthenon.

Petitti, D. (1994). Coronary heart disease and estrogen replacement therapy: Can compliance bias explain the results of observational studies? *Annals of Epidemiology, 4,* 115–118.

Pfeiffer, E., Verwoerdt, A., & Davis, G. (1972). Sexual behavior in middle life. *American Journal of Psychiatry, 128,* 1262–1267.

Poller, L., Thomson, J. M., & Coope, J. (1980). A double-blind cross-over study of piperazine oestrone sulphate and placebo with coagulation studies. *British Journal of Obstetrics and Gynaecology, 87,* 718–725.

Pollitzer, W. S., & Anderson, J. J. B. (1989). Ethnic and genetic differences in bone mass: A review with a hereditary v. environmental perspective. *American Journal of Clinical Nutrition, 50*(6), 1244–1259.

Pollock, G. (1981). Aging and aged: Development on pathology. In *The course of life: Psychoanalytic contributions toward understanding personality development* (Vol. 3, pp. 549–585). Washington, DC: U.S. Government Printing Office.

Postmenopausal Estrogen/Progestin Intervention Writing Group. (1995). Effects of estrogen or estrogen/progestin regimens on heart disease risk factors in postmenopausal women: The Postmenopausal Estrogen/Progestin Intervention. *Journal of the American Medical Association, 273,* 199–208.

Pouilles, J. M., Tremollieres, F., & Ribot, C. (1993). The effects of menopause on longitudinal bone loss from the spine. *Calcified Tissue International, 52,* 340–343.

Prather, J., & Fidell, L. (1975). Sex differences in the content and style of medical advertisements. *Social Science and Medicine, 9,* 23–26.

Radloff, L. (1977). The CES-D scale: A self-reported depression scale for research in the general population. *Applied Psychology Measurements, 137,* 385–401.

Rauramo, L., Langerspetz, K., Engblom, P., & Punnonen, R. (1975). The effect of castration and peroral estrogen therapy on some psychological functions. *Frontiers in Hormone Research, 8,* 133–151.

Rebuffe-Scrive, M. (1988). Metabolic difference in fat depots. In C. Bouchard and F. E. Johnson (Eds.), *Fat distribution during growth and later health outcomes* (pp. 163–174). New York: Alan Liss.

Regestein, Q. R. (1994). Menopausal aspects of sleep disturbance. In J. Lorrain (Ed.), *Comprehensive management of menopause.* New York: Springer Verlag.

Reuben, D. (1969). *Everything you always wanted to know about sex, but were afraid to ask.* New York: David McKay.

Rifkind, B. M., & Rossouw, J. E. (1998). Of designer drugs, magic bullets, and gold standards. *Journal of the American Medical Association, 279,* 1483–1451.

Riggs, B. L., & Melton, L. J. (1986). Involutional osteoporosis. *The New England Journal of Medicine, 314,* 1676–1686.

Riggs, B. L., & Melton, L. J. (1992). The prevention and treatment of osteoporosis. *The New England Journal of Medicine, 327,* 620–627.

Riggs, B. L., Wahner, H. W., Melton, L. J., Richelson, L. S., Judd, H. L., & Offord, K. P. (1986). Rates of bone loss in the appendicular and axial skeletons of women. Evidence of substantial vertebral bone loss before menopause. *Journal of Clinical Investigation, 77,* 1487–1491.

Roberts, H. (1985). *The patient patients: Women and their doctors.* London: Pandora Press.

Rose, L. (1977). What is menopause? In L. Rose (Ed.), *The menopause book* (pp. 1–17). New York: Hawthorn Books.

Ruegsegger, P., Dambacher, M. A., Ruegsegger, E., Fischer, J. A., & Anliker, M. (1984). Bone loss in premenopausal women. *Journal of Bone and Joint Surgery, 66a,* 1015–1023.

Schneider, D., Barrett-Connor, E., & Morton, D. (1997). Timing of postmenopausal estrogen for optimal bone mineral density. The Rancho Bernardo Study. *Journal of the American Medical Association, 277,* 543–547.

Scully, D., & Bart, P. (1973). A funny thing happened on the way to the orifice: Women in gynecology textbooks. *American Journal of Sociology, 73,* 1045–1051.

Shaver, J., Giblin, E., Lentz, M., & Lee, K. (1988). Sleep patterns and stability in perimenopausal women. *Sleep, 11,* 556–561.

Sherwin, B. B. (1988). Estrogen and/or androgen replacement therapy and cognitive functioning in surgically menopausal women. *Psychoneuroendocrinology, 13,* 345–357.

Sillero-Arenas, M., Delgado-Rodriguez, M., Rodigues-Canteras, R., Bueno-Cavanillas, A., & Galvez-Vargas, R. (1992). Menopausal hormone replacement therapy and breast cancer: A meta-analysis. *Obestetrics and Gynecology, 79,* 286–294.

Sinaki, M. (1989). Exercise and osteoporosis. *Archives of Physical and Medical Rehabilitation, 70,* 220–229.

Smith, D. C., Prentice, R., Thompson, D. J., & Hermann, W. L. (1975). Association of extrogenous estrogen and endometrial carcinoma. *The New England Journal of Medicine, 293(23),* 1164–1167.

Smith-Rosenberg, C. (1973). Puberty to menopause: The cycle of femininity in nineteenth-century America. *Feminist Studies, 1,* 58–72.

Sowers, M. R., Clark, M. K., Hollis, B., Wallace, R. B., & Jannausch, M. (1992). Radial bone mineral density in pre- and post-perimenopausal women: A prospective study of rates and risk factors for loss. *Journal of Bone Mineral Research, 7,* 647–657.

Sowers, M. R., & La Pietra, M. T. (1995). Menopause: Its epidemiology and potential association with chronic diseases. *Epidemiologic Reviews, 17,* 287–302.

Stampfer, M. J., Colditz, G. A., Willet, W. C., Manson, J. E., Rosner, B., & Speizer, F. E. (1991). Postmenopausal estrogen therapy and cardiovascular disease. *The New England Journal of Medicine, 325,* 756–762.

Stearns, P. (1975, October). Interpreting the medical literature on aging. In *Newberry Library, Family and Community History Colloquia: The physician and social history,* Chicago.

Steinberg, K. K., Thacker, S. B., Smith, S. J., Stroup, D. F., Zack, M. M., Flanders, W. D., & Berkelman, R. L. (1991). A meta-analysis of the effect of estrogen replacement therapy on the risk of breast cancer. *Journal of the American Medical Association, 265,* 1985–1989.

Stellato, R. K., Crawford, S. L., McKinlay, S. M., & Longcope, C. (1998). Can follicle-stimulating hormone be used to define menopausal status? *Endocrine Practice, 4,* 137–141.

Swartzman, L. C., Edelberg, R., & Kemmann, E. (1990). The menopausal hot flush: Symptom reports and concomitant physiological changes. *Journal of Behavioral Medicine, 13*(1), 15–31.

Thomas, T. M., Plymat, K. R., Blannin, J., & Meade, T. W. (1980). Prevalence of urinary incontinence. *British Medical Journal, 281,* 1243.

Tilt, E. J. (1857). *The change in life in health.* London: Churchill.

Townsend, J. M., & Carbone, C. L. (1980). Menopausal syndrome: Illness or social role—a transcultural analysis. *Culture, Medicine and Psychiatry, 4,* 229–248.

Tracey, R. E. (1966). Sex difference in coronary disease: Two opposing views. *Journal of Chronic Diseases, 19,* 1245–1251.

Treloar, A. E. (1974). Menarche, menopause and intervening fecundability. *Human Biology, 46,* 89–107.

Trichopoulos, D., MacMahon, B., & Cole, P. (1972). Menopause breast cancer risk. *Journal of the National Cancer Institute, 48,* 605–613.

U.S. Congress & Office of Technology Assessment. (1992). *Policy issues in the prevention and treatment of osteoporosis.* Washington, DC: U.S. Government Printing Office.

Vanhulle, G., & Demol, R. (1976). A double-blind study into the influence of estriol on a number of psychological tests in post-menopausal women. In P. A. van Keep, R. B. Greenblatt, & M. Albeux-Fernet (Eds.), *Consensus on menopausal research* (pp. 94–99). Lancaster, England: MTP Press Ltd.

Vatuk, S. (1992). Sexuality and the middle-aged woman in South Asia. In V. Kerns & J. K. Brown (Eds.), *In her prime: New views of middle-aged women.* Urbana: University of Illinois Press.

Versi, E. (1990). Incontinence in the climacteric. *Clinical Obstetrics and Gynecology, 33*(2), 392.

Versi, E., & Cardozo, L. D. (1988). Oestrogens and lower urinary tract function. In J. W. W. Studd & M. I. Whitehead (eds.), *The menopause.* Oxford: Blackwell Scientific Publications.

Versi, E., Cardozo, L. D., Tapp, A., Cooper, D. J., Brincat, M., & Studd, J. W. W. (1990). The long-term effect of hormone implant therapy on the lower urinary tract. *International Urogynecology Journal, 1,* 87–90.

Walsh, B. W., Kuller, L. H., Wild, R. A., Paul, S., Farmer, M., Lawrence, J. B., Shah, A. S., & Anderson, P. W. (1998). Effects of raloxifene on serum lipids and coagulation factors in healthy postmenopausal women. *Journal of the American Medical Association, 279,* 1445–1451.

Weideger, P. (1977). *Menstruation and menopause.* New York: Delta.

Whelan, E. A., Sandler, D. P., McConnaughey, D. R., & Weinberg, C. R. (1990). Menstrual and reproductive characteristics and age at natural menopause. *American Journal of Epidemiology, 131*(4), 625.

Willett, W., Stampfer, M. J., Bain, C., Lipnick, R., Speizer, F. E., Rosner, B., Cramer, D., & Hennekens, C. (1983). Cigarette smoking, relative weight, and menopause. *American Journal of Epidemiology, 117,* 651–658.

Wilson, R. A. (1966). *Feminine forever.* New York: M. Evans.

Wing, R. R., Matthews, K. A., Kuller, L. H., Meilahn, E. N., & Plantinga, P. L. (1991). Weight gain at the time of menopause. *Archives of Internal Medicine, 151,* 97–102.

Winokur, G. (1973). Depression in the menopause. *American Journal of Psychiatry, 130,* 92–93.

World Health Organization Scientific Group. (1996). Research on the Menopause in the 1990s. World Health Organization Technical Services Report Series No. 886. Geneva: World Health Organization.

Yaffe, K., Sawaya, G., Lieberburg, I., & Grady, D. (1998). Estrogen therapy in postmenopausal women: Effects on cognitive function and dementia. *Journal of the American Medical Association, 279,* 688–695.

Ziel, H. K., & Finkle, W. D. (1975). Increased risk of endometrial carcinoma among users of conjugated estrogens. *The New England Journal of Medicine, 293*(23), 1167–1170.

Cardiovascular Health: A Challenge for Midlife

Ilene C. Siegler

Department of Psychiatry and Behavioral Sciences, Duke University Medical Center, Durham, North Carolina; and School of Public Health, University of North Carolina, Durham, North Carolina

Berton H. Kaplan

Department of Epidemiology, School of Public Health, University of North Carolina, Durham, North Carolina

Dean D. Von Dras

Department of Psychology, Washington University, St. Louis, Missouri

Daniel B. Mark

Department of Medicine, Duke University Medical Center, Durham, North Carolina

In this chapter the focus is on psychosocial factors and cardiovascular disease, primarily coronary heart disease (CHD) and hypertension, about which there is a large literature on psychophysiology and behavioral epidemiology (see Blaskovich & Katkin, 1993; Ostfeld & Eaker, 1983; Siegman & Smith, 1994). In the introduction to this volume Willis and Reid use ages 45–64 as middle-aged and talk about the projected baby-boomer boom as the 1946–1964 cohorts move into, through, and out of middle-age. Indeed, the popular press has made an industry of speculating on the future cultural changes (Gerber, Wolff, Klores, & Brown, 1989). How these cohorts deal with cardiovascular disease and its associated risk factors will have a lot to do with their quality of life when they are elderly in the near future. The societal impact of these cohorts will continue to influence those who will become middle-aged after them. Adding an understanding of cardiovascular health to the psychology of adult development and aging, particularly the study of middle age, has the opportunity to advance our understanding of the causes and consequences of cardiovascular disease during the middle and later years. This chapter will cover three areas: (1) A brief review of past and current age-related prevalence of heart disease; (2) A discussion of the role of personality and risk behavior in midlife as a way to increase prevention of CHD; and (3) an examination of the impact of CHD on quality of life for middle-aged persons with heart disease. This chapter is a small subset of the literature on developmental health psychology (Siegler, 1989). Relevant data has been reviewed in chapters in *Handbook of the Psychology of Aging* by Eisdorfer and Wilkie (1977), Siegler and Costa (1985). Elias, Elias, and Elias (1990), and Contrada, Leventhal, and O'Leary (1990).

UNDERSTANDING HEART DISEASE

A useful brief introduction to the understanding of heart disease is provided by Sullivan (1987). He notes that major problems can include circulation in the coronary arteries that supply blood directly to the heart, the heart muscle itself, the heart valves, or maintenance of the rhythm of the heartbeat. Thus, heart disease is one of the disorders of the cardiovascular system, which includes the heart and the blood vessels. Other diseases of the cardiovascular system also become increasingly common with advancing age. Prominent among these are hypertension (or high blood pressure) and cerebrovascular accidents (stroke). An excellent chapter detailing the consequences of hypertension on cognitive functioning over the life cycle is that by Elias et al. (1995). Smith and Leon (1992) have written an excellent primer on CHD for the behavioral scientist.

> Wenger et al. (1995) put the amount of heart disease in the population into perspective. Cardiovascular disease is the leading cause of morbidity and mortality in the United States, accounting for almost 50% of all deaths. Coronary heart disease (CHD) with its manifestations of stable angina pectoris (chest pain), unstable angina, acute myocardial infarction (heart attack) and sudden death affects 13.5 million Americans. Nearly 1.5 million Americans sustain myocardial infarction each year of which almost 500,000 episodes are fatal. Myocardial infarctions can occur at young age: 5 percent occur in people younger than age 40, and 45 percent occur in people under age 65.
>
> The almost 1 million survivors of myocardial infarction each year and the more than 7 million patients with stable angina pectoris are candidates for cardiac rehabilitation, as are patients following revascularization with coronary artery bypass graft surgery (CABG) (309,000 patients in 1993, 45 percent under age 65) or percutaneous transluminal coronary angioplasty (PTCA) and other trans-catheter interventional procedures (362,000 in 1993, 54 percent under age 65). (Wenger et al., 1995, p. 1)

A brochure from the National Heart, Lung, and Blood Institute (1992) gives understandable definitions of disease:

> What is coronary heart disease? Like any muscle, the heart needs a constant supply of oxygen and nutrients that are carried to it by the blood in the coronary arteries. When the coronary arteries become narrowed or clogged and cannot supply enough blood to the heart, the result is CHD. If not enough oxygen-carrying blood reaches the heart, the heart may respond with a pain called angina. The pain is usually felt in the chest or

sometimes in the left arm and shoulder. (However, the same inadequate blood supply may cause no symptoms, a condition called silent angina.)

When the blood supply is cut off completely, the result is a heart attack. The part of the heart that does not receive oxygen begins to die and some of the heart muscle may be permanently damaged.

What causes CHD? CHD is caused by a thickening of the inside walls of the coronary arteries. This thickening, called atherosclerosis, narrows the space through which blood can flow, decreasing and sometimes completely cutting off the supply of oxygen and nutrients to the heart.

Atherosclerosis usually occurs when a person has high levels of cholesterol, a fat-like substance, in the blood. Cholesterol and fat, circulating in the blood, build up on the walls of the arteries. This buildup narrows the arteries and can slow or block the flow of blood. When the level of cholesterol in the blood is high, there is a greater chance that it will be deposited onto the artery walls. This process begins in most people during childhood and the teenage years, and worsens as they get older.

CHANGING RATES OF DISEASE

Because of declining rates of coronary disease in the United States, cardiovascular disease is increasingly a disease of later life. The ""first heart attack" was the archetypal sign of middle age. Perhaps the result of this shift in the timing of heart disease will be to lengthen the period we call middle age. Recent mortality figures suggest that progress has been made in reducing mortality from cardiovascular disease during the middle years. We know that risk factors are related to disease prevalence in the middle and later years, and it is suggested that the decline in rates of CHD is due to risk factor modification (USDHHS, 1994). Data from the most recent health statistics show that this is true. In 1980, for persons aged 25–44, the leading causes of death were (1) injuries, (2) cancers, and (3) heart disease. By 1991, HIV had replaced heart disease as the third cause of death. At ages 45–64 in 1980 the causes of death were (1) heart, (2) cancer, (3) cerebrovascular, and (4) injuries, but in 1991 cancer and heart disease had changed positions (USDHS, 1994). Because more older people die than younger people do, age-adjusted mortality still shows heart disease as the nation's number one killer.

Kannel and Thom (1994) have reviewed the epidemiology of cardiovascular diseases. Although rates of disease have declined considerably in the past 25 years, it is still a major health problem. Most of the data on age-related incidence (new cases) of disease come from the 36-year follow-up of persons aged 35–94 who participated in the Framingham Study. Average annual rates for first major cardiovascular events rose from 5 per 1000 men at ages 35–44 to 59 per 1000 men at ages 85–95; the comparable rates for women were 2 per 1000 and 66 per 1000. For women, the comparable rates are achieved about 10 years later than men (p. 186). As Kannel and Thom state, ""Whether attributable more to changes in disease-promoting lifestyle or to better medical care of those already afflicted, it is clear that cardiovascular disease is not an inevitable burden of aging or genetic make-up" (p. 187–188).

Advice to reduce risky behaviors and increase protective behaviors are now found in the popular press as well as in the physician's office. Two questions are important for this chapter: (1) Is midlife a good time to try to make those behavioral changes? and (2) Do we know anything about the psychological factors underlying risky behaviors that will help to understand them? The major risky behaviors have to do with smoking, sedentary lifestyle, overweight, eating and drinking recommended amounts of foods, and controlling hypertension and controlling cholesterol. Major protective factors appear to relate to social support and, for women, taking estrogen replacement.

MIDLIFE AS A TIME FOR BEHAVIOR CHANGE

From a public health perspective behavior change may be enhanced during the middle years as individuals start to experience health problems, the deaths of parents and friends, and, as Elliot Jaques (1965) noted many years ago in defining middle age, individuals may actually feel mortal for the first time and thus motivated to change their behavior. For women, the menopause provides an interesting opportunity to reduce coronary risk with estrogen replacement therapy (Matthews, 1992). Current data (see Adami & Persson, 1995; Colditz et al., 1995) find that the benefits in reduction of CHD for women tends to balance the increased risk for breast cancer. Whether this is because of healthier women choosing to take estrogens or other factors is not known (see Matthews, Kuller, Wing, Meilahn, & Planinga, 1996a,b). Furthermore, taking estrogens at the time of menopause can reduce the risk of fracture 30 years later. This is a consequential decision that each woman should make individually with consultation from her own physician. Thus, the middle years are important for consequences that are not apparent until many years later.

UNDERSTANDING RISKY BEHAVIOR

One way to understand risk factor behavior is to conceptualize risk behaviors as characteristic ways of coping with stress and to see if personality as a characteristic way of dealing with the environment is associated with risky behavior in middle and later life. Evidence from our ongoing work suggests that this is so. The UNC Alumni Heart Study is a longitudinal study of members of the "baby boom" cohort who are now starting to turn 50 years old (see Lipkus, Barefoot, Williams, & Siegler, 1994; Siegler et al., 1990; Siegler, Peterson, Barefoot, Harvin, et al., 1992; Siegler, Peterson, Barefoot, & Williams, 1992).

Individuals in the UNC Alumni Heart Study were asked to report on the extent to which they handled stress by engaging in various risky behaviors. Individuals were first asked whether their habits were affected by stress. In order of frequency,

78.2% reported changes in sleep patterns, 64% in eating, 53% in exercising, 51% in smoking, 37% in caffeine, 28% in alcohol use, and 16% in use of prescription drugs. Individuals then indicated the direction of the change, which was for most people eating more, sleeping less, drinking more caffeine and alcohol, smoking more, using more drugs, with an even split on exercise. These preliminary data show that all of the risk factors are nominated as coping behaviors and that except for smoking and using prescription drugs, which increased only under stress, all of the other risk factors both increase and decrease as a function of stress. Thus, part of the association between habits and the development of coronary heart disease may be due to the individual's characteristic ways of coping with stress.

Thus, it is reasonable to ask if there are significant correlations between adult personality functioning and risky behaviors. The answer is yes, as seen in data shown in Table I from the UNC Alumni Heart Study (UNCAHS). The NEO Personality Inventory (Costa & McCrae, 1992/1985) was completed by members of the UNCAHS as part of the second adult follow-up in 1988. All measures of risk behaviors were reported at the first adult enrollment period in 1987 except for social support, which was measured at the third adult follow-up in 1989. The five-factor model of personality is well represented in the domains of the NEO-PI (John, 1990), as is known to be reasonably stable during the ages from 40 to 43, when all of the risk and protective and personality indices were measured (Costa & McCrae, 1994). All five personality domains are related to health behaviors; but clearly neuroticism is the most prevalent domain. Individuals who rated themselves high in neuroticism were more likely to be practicing health-damaging behaviors and thus were more hostile, have a higher body mass index, drink more alcohol, and be a current smoker. In terms of health-protective factors of social support and exercise, those lower in neuroticism were higher on social support and exercised more. Extraversion had different relationships. Hostility was related to introversion, while social support, exercise, as well as body mass index and alcohol were associated with

TABLE I   NEO Personality Factors and Risk Behaviors in the UNC Alumni Heart Study

Measure	Neuroticism	Extraversion	Openness	Agreeableness	Conscientiousness
Hostility	.49	−.16	−.08	−.50	−.05
Body mass Index	.08	.05	−.03	−.05	−.07
Alcohol amount	.07	.06	.06	−.10	—
Current smoker	.05	—	.05	—	—
Social support	−.19	.25	.16	.20	.09
Exercise	−.05	.12	−.07	—	—

Note. All coefficients are statistically significant at $p < .001$.

extraversion. Openness is associated with increases in exercise, social support, smoking and drinking, and a lower body mass index. Agreeableness was associated with higher social support, and antagonism with hostility, body mass index, and alcohol use. Conscientiousness was opposite to neuroticism with highly conscientious persons more likely to have high social support and to exercise more, while having lower hostility and body mass index.

Similar patterns of correlation were found on the NEO and risk factors and participants in the Baltimore Longitudinal Study of Aging (Siegler & Costa, 1993). Replication in the two study populations are important because they suggest associations across the full adult age-span in very different populations. Furthermore, it is interesting that there are personality associations with both positive and negative health behaviors. Social support is one of the few protective factors, and as such suggests that midlife is also an opportunity to better understand other behaviors that are health promoting. For example, Kaplan (1992) argued that it is equally important to study the components of behavior that are not coronary prone or Type B behaviors in order to understand how potentially protective mechanisms might work. Modifying risky behaviors in order to prevent disease is primary prevention. Activities to prevent disease recurrence or progression is called secondary prevention. Wenger et al. (1995) note that only 11–20% of persons with CHD have participated in cardiac rehabilitation programs. These programs are designed to improve exercise tolerance and habits, lipid profiles, body weight, glucose and blood pressure levels, and cessation of smoking, along with reductions in stress, anxiety, and depression (p. 1–2).

MIDDLE AGE WITH HEART DISEASE

A final question of theoretical interest to students of aging is very hard to study in real life, that is, what role does age play in our understanding of CHD? This is hard to answer for a number of reasons: (1) Disease prevalence is age related; (2) Diseases are still rare events. In studies of normal populations, we do not find high rates of CHD in middle age, and so must turn to clinical populations; (3) In studies of persons with CHD the research questions are generally not attempting to find the role of age, but rather to understand how, controlling for age, we can understand disease prognosis.

Kannel and Thom (1994) report estimates from the National Health Interview Survey that show that 2.9% of the population has coronary heart disease. The prevalence for men is 85.9 per 1000 population aged 45–64 and 168.9 at ages 65 and over. For women, the prevalences are 25.6 per 1000 women aged 45–64 and 113 per 1000 women at age 65 and over (p. 188).

Relatively few studies have assessed the impact of heart disease on personality functioning. One paper from the Western Electric Study (Lebovits, Shekelle, Ostfeld, & Paul, 1967) assessed the impact of coronary heart disease and angina pectoris on personality change as measured with the MMPI (at age 48 as baseline) as a function of surviving a CHD diagnosis 5 years later. Personality changes for survivors of CHD were found for hypochondriasis, depression, and hysteria, all indicating increases in these traits, which may reflect an increase in awareness of bodily symptoms that was reported by the respondents.

Our discussion here will focus on findings from our work on patients undergoing diagnostic coronary angiography at Duke Medical Center who have been shown to have established coronary disease (Califf et al., 1989). Mark et al. (1992) reported that age was related to return to work in the first year following a diagnosis of heart disease for white but not for black patients. Individuals who returned to work had a mean age of 54 (48–58 is 25th–75th percentile), while those who did not had a mean age of 58 (52–61 is 25th–75th percentile). Our previous work with this population has shown that socioeconomic factors and social support are related to mortality in those with disease, in a population with a mean age of 52 (48–58 is the 25th–75th percentile) evaluated for heart disease from 1974 to 1980 (Williams et al., 1992). We were able to show that, controlling for disease severity, persons with high social support, indexed by being married or having a confident and higher income, demonstrated extended survival postdiagnosis. The Mediators of Social Support (MOSS) Study is designed to understand why social support is protective (Mark et al., 1995). The MOSS study started enrolling patients in 1992. They are followed for 3 years and the initial cohort has just completed the study. The current mean age is 62 years old. As part of the baseline MOSS protocol we have been measuring the impact of illness on functioning using the short form health survey (SF-36); this measures patients' perceptions of medical outcomes, which has been interpreted as a component of quality of life. Understanding quality of life has become increasingly important in evaluating aging and health concerns (see Abeles, Gift, & Ory, 1994). As mortality from CHD decreases, more people live longer with the disease.

Quality of life was measured with the SF-36 (Ware & Sherbourne, 1992; Ware & Associates, 1993). This 36-item index uses some fairly standard measures of functional and self-rated health including the pain and disability components of physical and mental illnesses. Furthermore, it has been widely used and there are norms available for the population by age and gender as well as from specialized studies of persons with specific chronic diseases. Thus, as a general quick and comparative scan, it has much to recommend it. The scores range from 0 to 100 and can be interpreted as the percentage with excellent quality of life.

We can compare data from persons in the MOSS study at age 45–54 who were all being evaluated for coronary disease. Their mean scores ranging from 43.07 to 66.87 are compared to those reported by Spiro et al. (1994) from the Normative Aging Study. Men initially screened for health but measured at age 50–54 had scores ranging from 64 to 90. National data provided by Ware & Associates (1993) for the general population at age 45–54 ranged from 61.79 to 84.61. Thus, variations in quality of life do vary in middle age as a function of the health status of the middle-aged sample being studied. Although heart disease is not very frequent in middle age, when middle-aged persons do get heart disease it has serious consequences for their perceptions of health.

Can we not look at age versus health in middle age? We can begin to model this by looking at age, sex, and group designations as an index of disease severity within the MOSS sample. Because the MOSS protocol studies almost everyone referred for diagnostic cardiac catheterization at Duke University Medical Center, we can compare individuals' quality of life at the time of diagnosis. This includes 963 persons who did not have significant coronary artery disease upon examination, 1366 persons who were treated surgically, and two groups of medically treated patients, 202 who were considered high risk and 243 considered low risk on the basis of their hazard scores (at the time the subjects rated their quality of life they did not have the results of their catheterization). Thus, at this point in the study the baseline quality of life scores reflect the impact of the symptoms and disease severity that led to the diagnosis.

Analysis of the components of Quality of Life in the MOSS patients suggests that quality of life varies by age, gender, and disease group. A series of three-way analysis of variances were calculated for eight of the quality of life indices that are composed of multi-items scales. There were gender effects for all indices of quality of life, with the men consistently higher than the women. Men are 62% of the total population, 70% of persons treated surgically, 71% of low-risk medically treated persons, 54% of high-risk medically treated persons, and 54% of those without significant CHD. In general, the women in each group are on average 4 years older than the men, and tend to be concentrated in the two extreme groups. This may also reflect the willingness of women to report symptoms at higher rates than men. The significant age effects are shown in the data in Table II.

As can be seen from Table II, the PF physical functioning (which is a 10-item activities-of-daily-living scale) and the RP role physical (the extent that physical health impairs work or other activities) fall linearly with age. The SF social func-

TABLE II   Aging and the Quality of Life in MOSS Patients

Mean age, SD	38.61, 5.13	49.48, 2.89	59.56, 2.92	69.37, 2.87	78.44, 3.08
Range, N	< 44, 279	44–54, 613	55–64, 759	65–74, 774	> 75, 304
PF	67.26	62.49	56.93	49.97	38.25
RP	48.55	43.34	39.15	30.88	21.44
SF	69.77	69.97	68.57	65.42	59.07
MH	63.72	66.85	69.56	72.87	70.86

Note. PF, physical functioning, 10-item ADL; RP, role physical, extent that health interferes with ADL; SF, social functioning, extent that health interferes with social activities; MH, mental health, happy, not depressed, 5 items.

tioning disrupted by health does not appear to drop until age 75, and in the MH mental health scale of reports of being happy and not depressed, the means rise slightly with age.

Thus, these interesting findings from the MOSS study suggest that the impact of age on quality of life for persons with established heart disease varies as a function of the index of quality of life. For areas of psychological functioning, MH in particular, those who were the oldest had the least impact on their quality of life due to having heart disease, whereas the impact on the role that physical health plays in activities of daily living is severe.

CONCLUSION

Middle age is an important time for risk factor modification, whether it is primary or secondary prevention. Understanding the psychology of adult development during midlife should help to prevent the onset of CHD and reduce the impact in those affected.

ACKNOWLEDGMENTS

Preparation of this chapter has been supported by the following research and training grants from the National Institutes of Health, R01-HL36587, R01 HL45702 and R01 HL55356 from the National Heart, Lung, and Blood Institute; T32 MH19109 from the National Institute of Mental Health; and R01 AG12458 from the National Institute on Aging.

REFERENCES

Abeles, R. P., Gift, H. C., & Ory, M. G. (Eds.). (1994). *Aging and quality of life.* New York: Springer.

Adami, H-O., & Persson, I. (1995). Hormone replacement and breast cancer: A remaining controversy? Editorial. *Journal of the American Medical Association 274(2),* 178–179.

Blascovich, J., & Katkin, E. S. (Eds.). (1993). *Cardiovascular reactivity to psychological stress and disease.* Washington, DC: American Psychological Association.

Califf, R. M., Harrell, F. E., Lee, K. L., Rankin, J. S., Hlatky, M. A., Mark, D. B., Jones, R. H., Muhlbaier, L. H., Oldham, N. H., & Pryor, D. B. (1989). The evolution of a medical and surgical therapy for coronary artery disease: A 15 year perspective. *Journal of the American Medical Association, 261*(14), 2077–2086.

Colditz, G. A., Hankinson, S. E., Hunter, D. J., Willett, W. C., Manson, J. E., Stampfer, M. J., Henne-kens, C., Rosner, B., & Speitzer, F. E. (1995). The use of estrogens and progestins and the risk of breast cancer in postmenopausal women. *New England Journal of Medicine, 332*(24), 1589–1593.

Contrada, R. J. (1994). Personality and anger in cardiovascular disease: Toward a psychological model. In A. W. Siegman & T. W. Smith (Eds.), *Anger, hostility and the heart* (pp. 149–171). Hillsdale, NJ: Erlbaum.

Contrada, R. J., Leventhal, H., & O'Leary, A. (1990). Personality and health. In L. A. Pervin (Ed.), *Handbook of personality* (pp. 638–669). New York: Guilford Press.

Costa, P. T., & McCrae, R. R. (1992/1985). NEO-PIR Professional Manual. Odessa, FL: Psychological Assessment Resources.

Costa, P. T., & McCrae, R. R. (1994). Set like plaster? Evidence for the stability of adult personality. In T. F. Heatherton & J. L. Weinberger (Eds.), *Can personality change?* (pp. 21–40). Washington, DC: American Psychological Association.

Dawber, T. R. (1990). *The Framingham Study: The epidemiology of atherosclerotic disease.* Cambridge, MA: Harvard University Press.

Eisdorfer, C., & Wilkie, F. (1977). Stress, disease, aging and behavior. In J. E. Birren & K. W. Schaie (Eds.), *Handbook of the psychology of aging* (pp. 251–275). New York: Van Nostrand Reinhold.

Elias, M. F., Elias, P. K., Cobb, J., D'Agostino, R., White, L. R., & Wolf, P. A. (1995). Blood pressure affects cognitive functioning: The Framingham Studies revisited (pp. 121–143). In J. E. Dimsdale & A. Braum (Eds.), *Quality of life in behavioral medicine research.* Hillsdale, NJ: Erlbaum.

Elias, M. F., Elias, P. K., & Elias, J. W. (1990). Biological and health influences. In J. E. Birren & K. W. Schaie (Eds.), *Handbook of the psychology of aging* (3rd ed., pp. 79–102). New York: Academic Press.

Gerber, J., Wolff, J., Klores, W., & Brown, G. (1989). *Life-trends: Your future for the next 30 years.* New York: Avon Books.

Jaques, E. (1965). Death and the mid-life crisis. *International Journal of Psychoanalysis, 46,* 502–514.

John, O. P. (1990). The ""Big five" factor taxonomy: Dimensions of personality in the natural language and in questionnaires. In L. A. Pervin (Ed.), *Handbook of personality* (pp. 66–100). New York: Guilford Press.

Kannel, W. B., & Thom, T. J. (1994). Incidence, prevalence and mortality of cardiovascular diseases. In R. C. Schalant & R. W. Alexander (Eds.), *The heart, arteries and veins* (8th ed.). New York: McGraw Hill.

Kaplan, B. H. (1992). Social health and the forgiving heart: The type B story. *Journal of Behavioral Medicine, 15*(1), 3–14.

Lebovits, B. Z., Shekelle, R. B., Ostfeld, A. M., & Paul, O. (1967). Prospective and retrospective psychological studies of coronary heart disease. *Psychosomatic Medicine, 29,* 265–272.

Lipkus, I. M., Barefoot, J. C., Williams, R. B., & Siegler, I. C. (1994). Personality measures as predictors of smoking initiation and cessation. *Health Psychology, 13*(2), 149–155.

Mark, D. B., Clapp-Channing, N. E., Barefoot, J. C., Gorkin, L., Siegler, I. C., & Williams, R. B. (1994, April). *Women with coronary heart disease are at higher risk for low social support and depression than men: Results from the MOSS Study.* Paper presented at the Society of Behavioral Medicine, Boston, MA.

Mark, D. B., Clapp-Channing, N. E., Lam, L. C., Barefoot, J. C., Siegler, I. C., & Williams, R. B. (1995, November). *Medical care: Access, utilization, and cost.* Paper presented at the Conference on Socio-economic Status and Cardiovascular Health and Disease. Bethesda, MD.

Mark, D. B., Lam, L. C., Lee, K., Clapp-Channing, N. E., Williams, R. B., Pryor, D. B., Califf, R. M., & Hlatky, M. A. (1992). Identification of patients with coronary disease at high risk for loss of employment. *Circulation, 86,* 1485–1494.

Mark, D. B., Lam, L. C., Lee, K. L., Jones, R. H., Pryor, D. B., Stack, R. S., Williams, R. B., Clapp-Channing, N. E., Califf, R. M., & Hlatky, M. A. (1994). Effects of coronary angioplasty, coronary by-pass surgery, and medical therapy on employment in patients with coronary artery disease. *Annals of Internal Medicine, 120,* 111–117.

Matthews, K. A. (1988). CHD and Type A behaviors: Update on and alternative to the Booth-Kewley and Friedman quantitative review. *Psychological Bulletin, 104,* 373–380.

Matthews, K. A. (1992). Myths and realities of the menopause. *Psychosomatic Medicine, 54,* 1–9.

Matthews, K. A., Kuller, L. H., Wing, R. R., Meilahn, E. N., & Plantinga, P. (1996a). Prior to use of estrogen replacement therapy, are users healthier than nonusers? *American Journal of Epidemiology, 143,* 971–982.

Matthews, K. A., Kuller, L. H., Wing, R. R., Meilahn, E. N., & Plantinga, P. (1996b). Health prior to hormone use: Matthews et al. reply to Grodstein. *American Journal of Epidemiology, 143,* 983–995.

McCrae, R. R., & Costa, P. T. (1990). *Personality in adulthood.* New York: Guilford Press.

National Heart, Lung, and Blood Institute. (1992). *Facts about coronary heart disease* (NIH Pub No. 92-2265). Bethesda, MD: NHLBI Information Center.

Ostfeld, A. M., & Eaker, E. D. (Eds.). (1983). *Measuring psychosocial variables in epidemiologic studies of cardiovascular disease* (NIH Pub. No. 85-2270). Proceedings of a workshop December 11–14; USDHS.

Siegler, I. C. (1989). Developmental health psychology. In M. Storandt & G. R. VandenBos (Eds.), *The adult years: Continuity and change* (pp. 119–142). Washington, DC: American Psychological Association.

Siegler, I. C. (1995, March). Social support in established coronary heart disease: Report of ongoing findings from the MOSS Study. In T. E. Seeman and I. C. Siegler (Cochairs), *Social support.* Society of Behavioral Medicine, San Diego, CA.

Siegler, I. C., & Costa, P. T. (1985). Health behavior relationships. In J. E. Birren & K. W. Schaie (Eds.), *Handbook of the psychology of aging* (2nd ed., pp. 144–166). New York: Van Nostrand Reinhold.

Siegler, I. C., & Costa, P. T. (1993, July). Health and personality in longitudinal studies: Findings from the UNCAHS and the BLSA. In E. Olbrich (Chair), *Longitudinal studies of aging: Medical and psychosocial aspects.* Symposium conducted at the XVth International Congress of Gerontology, Budapest, Hungary.

Siegler, I. C., Peterson, B. L., Barefoot, J. C., Harvin, S. H., Dahlstrom, W. G., Kaplan, B. H., Costa, P. T., & Williams, R. B. (1992). Using college alumni populations in epidemiologic research: The UNC Alumni Heart Study. *Journal of Clinical Epidemiology, 45*(11), 1243–1250.

Siegler, I. C., Peterson, B. L., Barefoot, J. C., & Williams, R. B. (1992). Hostility during late adolescence predicts coronary risk factors at mid-life. *American Journal of Epidemiology, 136*(2), 146–154.

Siegler, I. C., Zonderman, A. B., Barefoot, J. C., Williams, R. B., Jr., Costa, P. T., Jr., & McCrae, R. R. (1990). Predicting personality from college MMPI scores: Implications for follow-up studies in psychosomatic medicine. *Psychosomatic Medicine, 52,* 644–652.

Siegman, A. W., & Smith, T. W. (Eds.). (1994). *Anger, hostility and the heart.* Hillsdale, NJ: Erlbaum.

Smith T. W., & Leon, A. S. (1992). *Coronary heart disease: A behavioral perspective.* Chicago, IL: Research Press.

Spiro, A., Miller, D., Clark, J., Kressin, N., Bosse, R., & Kazis, L. (1994, August). *Quality of life in adulthood: Effects of age and illness.* Paper presented at the American Psychological Association, Los Angeles, CA.

Sullivan, R. J. (1987). Cardiovascular system. In G. L. Maddox, R. C. Atchley, L. W. Poon, R. S. Roth, I. C. Siegler, & R. M. Steinberg (Eds.), *The encyclopedia of aging* (pp. 84–89). New York: Springer.

U.S. Department of Health and Human Services (USDHHS). (1994). *Health, United States, 1993* (DHHS Pub. No. 94-1232). Hyattsville, MD: PHS, CDC, NCHS.

Ware, J. E., & Associates. (1993). *SF-36 Health Survey: Manual and interpretation guide.* Boston, MA: The Health Institute, New England Medical Center.

Ware, J. E., & Sherbourne, C. D. (1992). The MOS 36-item short-form health survey (SF-36) I. Conceptual framework and item selection. *Medical Care, 30*(6), 473–483.

Wenger, N. K., Froelicher, E. S., Smith, L. K., Ades, P. A., Berra, K., Blumenthal, J. A., Certo, C. M. E., Dattilo, A. M., Davis, D., DeBusk, R. F., et al. (1995). *Cardiac rehabilitation as secondary prevention. Clinical Practise Guideline for Clinicians, No 17* (AHCPR Pub. No. 96-0673). Rockville, MD: U.S. Department of Health and Human Services, Public Health Service, Agency for Health Care Policy and Research, and National Heart, Lung, and Blood Institute.

Williams, R. B., Barefoot, J. C., Califf, R. M., Haney, T. L., Saunders, W. B., Pryor, D. B., Hlatky, M. A., Siegler, I. C., & Mark, D. B. (1992). Prognostic importance of social and economic resources among medically treated patients with angiographically documented coronary artery disease. *Journal of the American Medical Association, 267,* 520–524.

PART III

Psychosocial Functioning at Midlife

Psychosocial issues during middle age are reviewed in the third part of the text. Chapters are presented that focus on psychological and social functioning and include the contribution of Corey Lee M. Keyes and Carol D. Ryff on current thinking about psychological well-being in middle age in their chapter, "Psychological Well-Being in Midlife." Next, Margaret Clark-Plaskie and Margie E. Lachman review the importance of autonomy in their chapter on "The Sense of Control in Midlife." The important concerns of "Gender Roles and Gender Identity in Midlife" are discussed in the chapter by Margaret Hellie Huyck. Current thinking on intellectual development is discussed by Sherry L. Willis and K. Warner Schaie in their chapter "Intellectual Development in Midlife." Occupational functioning at midlife is addressed by Bruce J. Avolio and John J. Sosik in this chapter, "A Life-Span Framework for Assessing the Impact of Work on White-Collar Workers." James D. Reid and Sherry L. Willis finish the volume with their chapter, "Middle Age: New Thoughts, New Directions."

CHAPTER 7

Psychological Well-Being
in Midlife

Corey Lee M. Keyes

*Department of Sociology, Emory University, Atlanta, Georgia; and Department of Behavioral Sciences and Health
Education, The Rollins School of Public Health, Atlanta, Georgia*

Carol D. Ryff

*Department of Psychology, The Institute on Aging and Adult Life, University of Wisconsin
Madison, Wisconsin*

INTRODUCTION

Psychological well-being at midlife has not been an explicit target of prior scientific inquiry. There are, rather, domains of study in which psychological functioning in middle adulthood is addressed via other endeavors. Three areas of research illustrate this indirect expression of interest in well-being at midlife. First, studies of successful aging (e.g., Baltes & Baltes, 1990; Ryff, 1982) frequently include midlife in theoretical and empirical formulations as a prelude or precursor to old age. These formulations draw attention to developmental aspects of psychological well-being, such as how different life periods might involve distinct psychological challenges and gains (or losses). A second literature on subjective well-being, involving large survey studies, has frequently questioned the relationship between age (one of several sociodemographic factors of interest) and reports of happiness and life satisfaction (e.g., Diener, 1984; Herzog, Rodgers, & Woodworth, 1982). This work typically treats age in continuous, linear fashion, which means specific periods of adult life are not fully illuminated. Finally, another category of literature, guided by a diverse array of substantive questions, provides knowledge of midlife well-being vis-à-vis particular life domains, such as work (e.g., Baruch, 1984; Coleman & Antonucci, 1983), parenthood (e.g., McLanahan & Adams, 1987), or multiple roles across domains (e.g., Thoits, 1983). Thus, the focus in this realm is specific areas of life experience and their effects on psychological functioning.

Across these domains of inquiry, the task of articulating the essential meaning of psychological well-being has never been center stage. Thus, dependent measures are typically selected from among well used standards, with the greater conceptual effort going to formulate independent variables or intervening variables (see Ryff & Essex, 1992a). We argue that this approach has perpetuated impoverished conceptions and measures of well-being. Our chapter begins therefore with an examination of theory relevant to defining positive psychological functioning. We propose a multidimensional formulation of well-being derived from the synthesis of prior theories. We then review empirical studies that have addressed how men and women of different ages (typically young, middle-aged, and old-aged adults) evaluate themselves on different dimensions of well-being, the extent to which they see progress or decline in their own well-being over time, and whether individual self-evaluations of well-being vary across cultures. We then discuss an explanatory framework that emphasizes adults' life experiences as factors influencing well-being. A key feature of the guiding framework is the focus on how experience is interpreted via social psychological processes (e.g., social comparisons). We illustrate this approach with findings on the experience of parenting in middle adulthood. Finally, we conclude with suggestions for new directions in the study of social well-being in midlife.

A THEORY-DRIVEN PERSPECTIVE ON PSYCHOLOGICAL WELL-BEING

Our approach to the conceptualization of well-being is theoretical and holistic (Ryff, 1985, 1989a, 1989b). Not only do we start with theory, but we try to capture a wide range of meanings. We attempt to cover positive and negative, as well as psychological and social aspects of functioning. Theorists from various domains examined psychological functioning and crafted exemplars of health and well-being. From personality and clinical psychology, we draw upon Maslow's (1968) conception of self actualization, Roger's (1961) description of the fully functioning person; Jung's (1933; Von Franz, 1964) formulation of individuation, and Allport's (1961) depiction of maturity (see Ryff, 1985, for a detailed review). A theme in psychological portrayals of healthy functioning is *eudaimonia*. To Aristotle, a life characterized as full and healthy entails recognizing and working to realize inner talents and potential (Waterman, 1984). Theorists of adult development, too, delineate the challenges people encounter, and the fruits of surmounting each task, throughout life. Notably, there is Erikson's (1959) psychosocial stages and tasks,

Buhler's (1935; Buhler & Massarik, 1968) basic life tendencies, moving toward life fulfillment, and Neugarten's (1968, 1973) depiction of personality changes in adulthood and old age (see Ryff, 1982, 1984, for detailed reviews). In the area of mental health, Jahoda (1958) enumerates several criteria of positive mental health, counteracting the tendency to equate well-being with the absence of illness.

The various conceptions of positive functioning converge on several themes. These points of convergence in early conceptual writings (Ryff, 1985, 1989a, 1989b) provided core definitions for different aspects of well-being. What follows is a brief description of each dimension (see Ryff, 1989a, for detailed descriptions). Table I contains core definitions for each end of the continuum for each dimension.

TABLE I   Definitions of Theory-Guided Dimensions of Well-Being

Self-Acceptance
  High scorer: possesses a positive attitude toward the self; acknowledges and accepts multiple aspects of self including good and bad qualities; feels positive about past life.
  Low scorer: feels dissatisfied with self; is disappointed with what has occurred in past life; is troubled about certain personal qualities; wishes to be different than what he or she is.
Positive Relations with Others
  High scorer: has warm, satisfying, trusting relationships with others; is concerned about the welfare of others; capable of strong empathy, affection, and intimacy; understands give and take of human relationships.
  Low scorer: has few close, trusting relationships with others; finds it difficult to be warm, open, and concerned about others; is isolated and frustrated in interpersonal relationships; not willing to make compromises to sustain important ties with others.
Autonomy
  High scorer: is self-determining and independent; able to resist social pressures to think and act in certain ways; regulates behavior from within; evaluates self by personal standards.
  Low scorer: is concerned about the expectations and evaluations of others; relies on judgments of others to make important decisions; conforms to social pressures to think and act in certain ways.
Environmental Mastery
  High scorer: has a sense of mastery and competence in managing the environment; controls complex array of external activities; makes effective use of surrounding opportunities; able to choose or create contexts suitable to personal needs and values.
  Low scorer: has difficulty managing everyday affairs; feels unable to change or improve surrounding context; is unaware of surrounding opportunities; lacks sense of control over external world.
Purpose in Life
  High scorer: has goals in life and a sense of directedness; feels there is meaning to present and past life; holds beliefs that give life purpose; has aims and objectives for living.
  Low scorer: lacks a sense of meaning in life; has few goals or aims, lacks sense of direction; does not see purpose in past life; has no outlooks or beliefs that give life meaning.
Personal Growth
  High scorer: has a feeling of continued development; sees self as growing and expanding; is open to new experiences; has sense of realizing his or her potential; sees improvement in self and behavior over time; is changing in ways that reflect more self-knowledge and effectiveness.
  Low scorer: has a sense of personal stagnation; lacks sense of improvement or expansion over time; feels bored and uninterested with life; feels unable to develop new attitudes or behaviors.

Self-Acceptance is a ubiquitous criterion of wellness. Healthy people hold positive attitudes toward themselves. In addition to being the embodiment of mental health (Jahoda), accepting oneself is in the thoughts and actions of self-actualizers (Maslow), optimally functioning people (Rogers), and the mature person (Allport). Throughout life, too, positive regard for oneself is integral to adapting to life's challenges and enabling oneself to accomplish goals (Erikson).

Positive Relation with Others is the interpersonal counterpart to self-acceptance. Positive regard for others, as well as oneself, earmarks the healthy individual. Developing and maintaining warm and trusting interpersonal relationships pervades depictions of positive functioning. The ability to love (Jahoda), to feel empathy and affection for all human beings (Maslow), to develop warm relations with others (Rogers, Erikson) characterizes a healthy individual. Others note the challenge to feel and act on a sense of responsibility to others (Erikson). In all, interpersonal warmth delineates a happy and healthy person.

Two related though distinct dimensions emphasize the ability to engage the social milieu. **Autonomy** is the counterpart to submissiveness and blind obedience to other people and society. Healthy people are capable of, and comfortable with, making decisions independently and regulating their behavior from internal standards. In the case of **Environmental Mastery,** people engage and shape their milieus to reflect their needs and personality. That is, healthy people can choose or create environments compatible with their physical and psychological needs.

Autonomy and mastery imply that one is cognizant of personal standards and needs. Paraphrasing an old religious supplication, a healthy person *has the courage to change what can and should be changed, the serenity to accept what cannot be changed, and the wisdom to know the difference.* Theoretically, self actualizing (Maslow), optimally functioning (Rogers), and individuated (Jung) people gain approval from internal standards rather than other people and society. Throughout life, people experience a burgeoning sense of psychological freedom, turning inward and reflecting on themselves, their lives, and what they live for each day (Erikson, Jung, Neugarten). Beyond the internal reflection, healthy and mature (Allport) people participate in important social activities, thereby engaging their surroundings. Moreover, during midlife, people orchestrate complex environments (Buhler, Neugarten) and shape society by nurturing youth and young adults (Erikson).

Purpose in Life incorporates the criterion that healthy people possess goals, intentions, and a sense of direction, from which they feel that their lives are meaningful. Mature persons (Allport) feel a purpose to their lives, and they believe they can live out their plan. Generically, life-span theories (Buhler, Erikson, Jung) depict the stages and trajectories of life as goals or tasks such as industriousness (youth), intimacy (young adulthood), socially active (middle adulthood), and psychologically integrated (later adulthood).

Personal Growth, the final criterion of psychological well-being, entails feelings of, and striving toward, exploration and development. The desire and attempt to grow characterize self-actualizers (Maslow). Openness to new experiences and opportunities, a predecessor to growth, exemplifies the fully functioning person (Rogers). A central feature in life-span theories (Buhler, Erikson, Jung, Neugarten) is the individual's drive to grow, building on past achievements and milestones.

In sum, prior theories point to the multifaceted nature of psychological well-being. It includes fundamental aspects of self-evaluation (i.e., self-acceptance), the quality of ties to others (i.e., positive relations with others), the capacity to be self-determining (i.e., autonomy) and to manage one's surroundings (i.e., environmental mastery), investment in living (i.e., purpose in life), and continued self-realization (i.e., personal growth). The following section summarizes the translation of the theoretical constructs to the empirical level.

EMPIRICAL STUDIES

The Measurement of Well-Being

The preceding six dimensions of well-being were operationalized with structured, self-report scales. Based on the theoretical definitions, items were written to describe individuals who possessed or did not possess the various qualities of well-being (as outlined in Table I). The items pools for all dimensions were subjected to various refinement procedures (see Ryff, 1989b), such as the requirement that each item had to correlate more highly with its own scale than with any other scale. The 20-item parent scales demonstrated high internal reliability (alpha coefficients ranged from .86 to .93) and temporal reliability (test–retest coefficients ranged from .81 to .88). The scales correlated modestly and positively with existing measures of positive functioning (i.e., life satisfaction, affect balance, self-esteem, and internal control) and correlated modestly and negatively with extant measures of negative functioning (i.e., depression, powerful other control, chance control) (see Ryff, 1989b, for details).

Recently, data were obtained from a national probability sample of English-speaking adults, aged 25 or older (Ryff & Keyes, 1995). Respondents completed telephone interviews that included a dramatically reduced version of the six well-being scales.[1] We examined whether and how well the multidimensional structure of well-being manifests in a representative cross-section of adults. Results of confirmatory factor analyses bolster the underlying theory and specification of the multidimensional model of well-being. Confirmatory procedures require *a priori* specification of factorial models to compare how well the data (i.e., correlations or covariances) coincide with each model. We compared the fit of the

[1]The shortened scales include 3 of the original 20 items. Items were selected to maximize representation of the conceptual diversity within each construct. Exploratory factor analyses revealed that each dimension as measured with the 20-item parent scales consisted of 3 facets that correspond to theory. One item was selected from each of the 3 facets within each dimension.

multidimensional (i.e., six-factor) model with a unidimensional, a superfactor, and an artifact model. In the superfactor model, the six latent constructs are effects of a higher order latent construct called "Psychological Well-Being." The unidimensional model purports that the items measure a single dimension of wellness. Two versions of an artifact model suggest that respondents answer items to portray a positive image to the interviewer.

Compared with the unidimensional and the two artifact models, the multidimensional model is the best fitting model. Theory suggests, and data confirm, that well-being is a multifaceted phenomenon. Artifacts of measurement do not appear to wield much, if any, influence on the manifestation of well-being. More convincingly, the superfactor model fits the data better than the multidimensional model, suggesting that the six factors belong to a single conceptual domain of psychological well-being.

In sum, the six scales consisting of 20 items display internal consistency, stability over time, and convergent and discriminant validity. Using reduced scales (i.e., three items per scale) over the telephone with a representative sample of adults, the multidimensional model provides the best explanation for the data. The six, though smaller, scales fit into an even better, "superfactor," model. In short, six factors fit the data *and* measure a single latent construct called psychological well-being. Parsimony exists, but at a higher order. A hierarchical structure exists in which general well-being manifests through six distinct domains of functioning specified *a priori* by guiding psychological theory.

Well-Being in Midlife: Age-Difference Analyses

Next, we review several studies that take various "snapshots" of the functioning and well-being of midlife adults. Emphasizing snapshots of midlife, the following studies utilize cross-sectional data and involve discussion of age differences. We characterize midlife by comparing the functioning of midlife with younger and older adults. Of interest is how profiles of well-being in midlife compare with profiles of functioning in younger and later periods. Such comparisons offer clues regarding possible life course changes, as well as cohort differences.

Ironically, the rich array of theories guiding creation of the six new scales of well-being generates few unambiguous hypotheses about the manifestation of well-being over the life course. Moreover, each of the six scales of well-being and their respective dimensions are amalgams of developmental and personality theories and concepts. We therefore approach the life course patterning of well-being as a more inductive than deductive (i.e., hypotheses testing) enterprise. The question of interest is whether, in its contours of wellness, midlife looks noticeably different from younger and older adulthood. Throughout, young adulthood encompasses ages 18–29, midlife includes ages 30–64, and older adulthood involves ages 65 years and older.

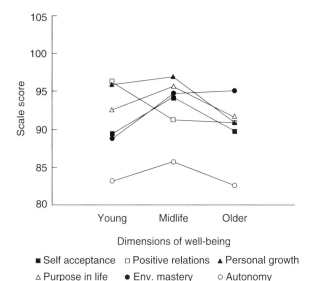

FIGURE 1   Age differences on the six 20-item measures of well-being, Study 1.

Mean-level comparisons between young, middle-aged, and older adults in Study 1 (Ryff, 1989b) reveal differential age profiles on most of the 20-item scales (see Figure 1). Subjects are a nonrandom sample of adults from Wisconsin. The young adults' (n = 133) ages averaged around 20 (SD = 1.6), midlife adults' (n = 108) ages averaged close to 50 (SD = 9.4), and the older adults' (n = 80) ages averaged around 75 (SD = 7.1). We find incremental age profiles for environmental mastery and autonomy. Midlife and older adults possess more environmental mastery, and midlife adults feel more autonomy than younger adults. Midlife adults also report higher levels of purpose in life and personal growth compared to older adults. On the other hand, adults in each age group report nearly identical levels of self-acceptance and positive relationships with others. We observe a statistically signifi-cant main effect of gender for only one criterion of wellness, and none of the psychological well-being age profiles depends on the gender of the adults. In partic-ular, women at all stages of life say they have more positive and warm interpersonal relationships than men.

Using the same 20-item scales, we find many of the same age profiles in Study 2 (Ryff, 1991a) (see Figure 2). As in Study 1, subjects are a nonrandom sample of adults from Wisconsin. The young adults' (n = 123) ages averaged around 19 (SD = 1.5), midlife adults' (n = 95) ages averaged close to 46 (SD = 8.3), and older adults' (n = 90) ages averaged around 73 (SD = 5.6). Once again, current ratings of environmental mastery and autonomy increase, while personal growth decreases, with age. Midlife adults feel more autonomy and environmental mastery than

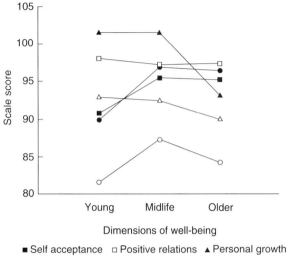

FIGURE 2   Age differences on the six 20-item measures of well-being, Study 2.

younger adults, and they report more personal growth than older adults. Adults at each life stage exhibit nearly identical levels of positive relationships with others. However, compared with Study 1, self acceptance shows increments with age, whereas purpose in life does not vary with age. Again, gender has a main effect only on well-being. Women say they have more positive relations than men.

Using the dramatically smaller scales, analyses of age differences in the nationally representative sample replicates many of the previous findings (Ryff & Keyes, 1998) (see Figure 3). In this study, the young adults' ($n = 133$) ages averaged around 27 ($SD = 1.5$), midlife adults' ($n = 805$) ages averaged close to 44 ($SD = 9.9$), and the older adults' ($n = 160$) ages averaged around 72 ($SD = 5.3$). Compared with the adults in Study 1 and Study 2, the young adults in the national study are slightly older, while the midlife and older adults are about the same ages on average across the three studies. Purpose in life and personal growth continue to show decremental age profiles. Environmental mastery continues to show age increments. As in Study 1, self-acceptance shows no age differences. Unlike in Study 1 and Study 2, we do not observe age differences in autonomy, and we find a statistically significant increment in positive relations with others. Older adults, in particular, express more positive interpersonal relations than younger adults. Gender continues to display main effects only on well-being and only for the criterion of positive relations with others. Regardless of their stage in life, women have more positive and warm interpersonal relationships than men.

In sum, across three sets of data having wide variation in depth of measurement (i.e., from 20 to 3 item scales), using different modes of administration (i.e., self-administered and telephone interviews), and with different sampling techniques (i.e., purposive and random national samples), we observe replicable age profiles. In all three studies, feelings of personal growth and purpose in life decline, while a sense of environmental mastery increases, with age. In two of the three studies, self-acceptance and positive relationships with others tend to be the same among the various age groups. Moreover, in two of the three studies, feelings of autonomy tend to increase with age, especially from younger to midlife adulthood.

Taken together, these findings suggest that midlife is a time when people function particularly well relative to those who are younger or older. The capacity to be self-determining (i.e., autonomy) and to manage one's surroundings (i.e., environmental mastery) show marked improvement in midlife, compared with young adulthood. Investment in living (i.e., purpose in life), and the desire for continued self-realization (i.e., personal growth) remains consistently high from young adulthood into midlife, but they drop sharply during older adulthood. Interestingly, self-evaluation (i.e., self-acceptance), on one hand, and other-evaluation (i.e., positive relations with others), on the other hand, display similar profiles over the life course. Perhaps aspects of wellness that involve assessments of oneself or the relationship of the "self" and other people remain salient throughout life.

Assuming that the observed mean-level difference reflects, in part, true developmental changes, we might conjecture that well-being is not a unitary phenomenon that is completely stable over time. Well-being manifests over the life course in

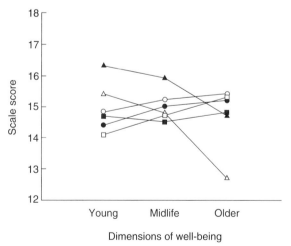

FIGURE 3   Age differences on the six 3-item measures of well-being, Study 3.

many ways, suggesting a multidirectionality to profiles of positive functioning. Compared with youth, midlife is a time of gains in all areas of wellness. From midlife through older adulthood, some aspects of well-being remain constant, while others tend to decline.

Theoretically, the results suggest that the subjective organization of the life course (see Ryff, 1984) might play a part in how people assess their functioning. Whereas everyone has an outlook situated in the present, the amount of past or future one has depends, in part, on age (see also Carstensen, 1995). Young adulthood is temporally *prospective,* that is, a time when people have more of a future than a past. Older adulthood, in contrast, is *retrospective,* a time when people have more of a past than a future. Midlife is temporally *balanced* between the past and future.

There is also an implicit temporality to the actual dimensions of well-being. Positive relations with others, autonomy, and environmental mastery are, for example, anchored predominantly in the present, emphasizing how people see themselves functioning at the current time. How people construe their futures is, however, salient in the dimensions of personal growth and purpose in life. Both scales emphasize personal goals, aspirations, a sense of direction, and the belief in continual development, all of which consist of some projection of the self into the future. In contrast, self-acceptance contains some reference to functioning in the past—accepting oneself involves evaluation of accomplishments and one's "lived" life.

Putting these temporal observations together, it appears that there is some degree of fit between one's placement in the life course with the past versus present versus future orientation of particular dimensions of well-being. For example, older adults, whose outlooks are largely retrospective, consistently exhibited lower levels of purpose in life and personal growth (dimensions rooted partly in one's future) than younger and midlife adults. Younger adults, whose outlooks are largely prospective, showed trends of scores lower on self-acceptance (a dimension rooted partly in one's past) than midlife and older adults, but none of the differences were statistically significant. Consistent with the temporal balancing of past and future, midlife adults tended to exhibit the highest overall profiles of well-being.

Temporal Assessments: Perceptions of Progress and Decline in Well-Being

Continuing the theme of time and functioning, Study 2 reported earlier (Ryff, 1991a) included examination of temporal aspects of functioning via the correspondence of past, current, future, and ideal well-being over the life course. To assess ideal well-being, subjects responded to items of well-being with regard to how they would most like to function. To assess past well-being, subjects answered items in terms of how they functioned in the past. For young adults, the past refers to their adolescence. The past for middle-aged adults is young adulthood (20–25 years of age). For older adults, the past involves their midlife (40–50 years of age). To obtain future ratings, subjects answered items in terms of how they believe they might function during their subsequent stage in life. Young adults projected themselves into their midlife (40–50 years of age). The middle-aged adults predicted their well-being during old age (65–70 years of age). The older adults projected their well-being into the 10 to 15 years from their current age.

Figure 4 depicts the profile of functioning on the four temporal dimensions for each group of adults. Because the configuration of the temporal profiles are nearly identical for the six dimensions of well-being, Figure 4 contains the average well-being (i.e., over the six scales) for ideal, future, present, and past well-being for each group of adults (see Ryff, 1991a, for more detailed analyses).

Ideal ratings of all aspects of well-being decline over the span of life. With age, people appear to lower their standards of functioning, perhaps adapting to expected decrements during later life. Older adults envision markedly lower ideal levels of well-being than midlife and younger adults. Interestingly, the discrepancy between how people would like to be and how they currently function diminishes with age. Younger adults expect to function better in the future than they do now. Midlife adults believe they will function about the same in the future as now. Older adults predict a decrement in well-being in the future. Past assessments of well-being indicate less of a discrepancy between past and present functioning for older, unlike midlife and younger, adults.

In short, midlife appears to be the temporal bench-mark for well-being throughout the life course. Younger and older adults construe midlife as the time in their lives when they function best. Focusing on midlife, younger adults expect to do

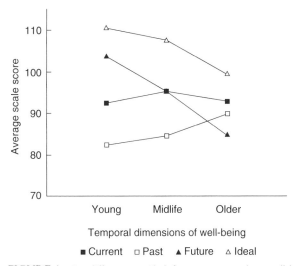

FIGURE 4   Age differences on ideal, future, present, and past well-being.

better in the future, and older adults believe they did better in the past. As we discussed earlier, midlife adults tend to function better in the present than older adults (and sometimes younger adults) on most facets of well-being. From all angles, midlife is thus the peak of well-being. It is instructive to note, however, that all adults reveal that they never expect in the future to function at, or beyond, their ideal. Such a finding suggests, on one hand, that adults at all periods of life view their future somewhat pessimistically. People never live up to their ideal levels of functioning. On the other hand, the discrepancy of ideal and future functioning could indicate that all adults view their future motivationally. That is, adults construe life as a process during which there is continual room for growth and challenge, regardless of their predominant temporal outlook (i.e., prospective, balanced, or retrospective).

Cultural Analyses: East/West Differences in Well-Being

Cultures consist of predominant values and practices that reflect either individualistic and independent or collectivistic and interdependent orientations (Markus & Kitayama, 1991; Triandis, 1989). Individualistic societies like that in the United States emphasize individual achievement and personal identity over the achievement and identity of groups. Collectivistic societies promote group achievement and identification with social groups. Insofar as cultures emphasize and support development and functioning consistent with their ideals, we hypothesize cultural differences for criteria of well-being that coincide with broad cultural ideals. The theme of individualism in the United States suggests that aspects of well-being that focus on the self over others (e.g., autonomy and self-acceptance) are encouraged and supported. The theme of collectivism suggests that aspects of well-being that focus on other people over oneself (viz., positive relations with others) are encouraged and supported.

Data from probability samples of midlife adults in South Korea and the United States were compared (Ryff, Lee, & Na, 1993). Both samples come from capital cities that are centers of higher education and political administration, surrounded by rural and agricultural areas. The Korean sample includes 220 adults whose ages average around 54.5 (SD = 4.7). The U.S. sample consists of 215 adults whose ages average around 53.7 years (SD = 6.8). The response rate was exceptionally high (i.e., 92 percent) in South Korea, while the rate of response was typical (i.e., 70%) in the United States. The gender composition (divided about equally between men and women) and educational attainment in each sample are comparable. In addition to the six scales of well-being, open-ended questions inquired into cultural construals of well-being. Through open questions, respondents indicate what aspects of life are important, what facets of life make them unhappy, and what qualities comprise a mature and fulfilled person.

On all six measures, Korean adults display vastly lower levels of well-being, and they exhibit less variation in their responses to each item, compared to the adults from the United States. The vast differences in functioning reflect what appear to be marked cultural differences in the use of six-point response scales. Koreans, for example, are much less likely to give a strongly affirmative answer to a positively phrased item. That is, Korean adults, unlike U.S. adults, do not strongly endorse honorific statements about themselves. The tendency to be self-effacing among Koreans likely reflects different socialization practices and sanctions against self-aggrandizement (see Markus & Kitayama, 1991). On the other hand, for the dimensions of well-being that may be uniquely Western and individualistic (e.g., personal growth, self-acceptance, autonomy), the scores of Korean and U.S. adults could also reflect meaningful differences in which Eastern adults rate themselves lower on aspects of functioning not endorsed by their own culture.

Examination of mean-levels within cultures and comparison of responses to the open-ended questions provide support for the cultural hypothesis. Korean adults display the highest level of well-being for positive relations with others and the lowest level on self-acceptance. Adults in the United States exhibit the highest level of well-being on personal growth, followed closely, however, by positive relations with others. It is also interesting to note similarities in the well-being for men and women in both cultures. Women in Korea and the United States have more positive relations with others and perceive more personal growth than men in Korea and the United States.

The open-ended responses indicate that Korean adults conceive of well-being, maturity, and personal fulfillment through their family rather than through their personal accomplishments and qualities. Midlife Koreans view well-being, for example, as a reflection of the success of their children. Moreover, Koreans define a mature person as one with interdependent qualities like being honest and conscientious, modest and respectful of others, and faithful and responsible. Ryff et al. (1993) asked the same set of open-ended questions of midlife adults in the United States. Surprisingly, the data reveal a prominent theme of interdependence among adults. As in Korea, the U.S. adults conceive of well-being and fulfillment through their family, as well as their marital relationship. Moreover, adults in the United States describe a well-adjusted and mature person as a caring person who is connected with other people. But, harkening to a theme of independence, the U.S. midlife adults, unlike those in Korea, depict a healthy, happy, and fulfilled person as confident, assertive, continually growing, and enjoying life. Moreover, U.S. adults see personal fulfillment as personal accomplishments, rather than children's accomplishments. Still, the theme of interdependence is evident among U.S. midlife adults. Where does this supposed cultural discrepancy originate?

One explanation, originating in a comparison of the homogeneity of cultures, suggests that the stereotype of U.S. adults as individualistic might be overstated. Culture appears to be more diverse in the United States than in South Korea (cf. Triandis, 1989). The ethnic and racial makeup, for instance, of the United States is more heterogeneous than the makeup of Korean society. Korean culture, unlike the culture of the United States, is more uniform, a reflection of which might be found in the consistent theme of interdependence of well-being. There is likely to be much more variation in how people in the United States construe themselves, some seeing the world more interdependently, while others see themselves and their milieu more independently (see also Markus & Kitayama, 1991).

Another explanation implicates the frame of reference people use to answer questions. When defining functioning as the "ideal person," Korean midlife adults suggest most frequently that someone who does "one's best" is the ideal. Describing the ideal person as "an achiever" is somewhat discrepant with the otherwise inter-dependent construal of well-being among Koreans. On the other hand, the U.S. midlife adults define the ideal person as caring and having deep friendships. Each in their own way, Korean and U.S. adults define the ideal person with adjectives that are somewhat discrepant with their cultural modes and values. Such an irony suggests that people might define their ideal mode of functioning with traits that reflect the obverse of their cultural values and practices. The ideal person in an independent culture is caring rather than someone who does "one's best." In an interdependent culture, the ideal person is an achiever, rather than a "caring and friendly" person. The ideal person, in each culture, blends disparate aspects of life, being at once part of his or her culture and beyond his or her culture.

TOWARD EXPLANATIONS OF WELL-BEING

Life Experience as Antecedent

Our efforts to understand human variation in psychological well-being have looked to the experiential substance of people's lives for explanatory influences. Among the kinds of experiences studied are the having and raising of children (Ryff, Lee, Essex, & Schmutte, 1994; Schmutte & Ryff, 1994), growing up with an alcoholic parent (Tweed & Ryff, 1991), educational and occupational achievements in midlife (Hauser et al., 1992), health problems in later life (Heidrich & Ryff, 1993a, 1993b), community relocation among aging women (Ryff & Essex, 1992b), and the social stratification of well-being as adults age (Keyes & Ryff, 1998). Across these experiences and events, the objective has been to link what people are actually dealing with in daily life to evaluations of their own well-being. We emphasize, however, that it is how people construe their experiences, not just experience per se, that matters (see, e.g., Keyes & Ryff, 1998).

Interpretive Mechanisms

We draw on diverse aspects of social psychological theory to elaborate how people give meaning to their life experiences. Rosenberg's (1979) self-concept theory, which incorporates numerous social-psychological perspectives to explicate the mechanisms whereby people derive meaning from their experiences, provided initial conceptual guidance. The theory articulates four mechanisms of self-assessment reflecting distinct ways that people construe events. For each mechanism, the motive for self-esteem often drives how people assess themselves and their experiences. That is, the meaning people attach to some events reflects a concern for maintaining a favorable image. People who maintain favorable self-images should exhibit better adjustment and functioning throughout life (cf. Markus & Herzog, 1991).

The first mechanism, **social comparison,** states that people understand experiences and evaluate themselves by comparing themselves with others. Depending on the people to which someone compares him- or herself, events and experiences lead to negative, neutral, or positive self-assessments. How people compare themselves to others undergoing similar experiences determines how events throughout life affect individuals. The second mechanism, **reflected appraisals,** indicates that people understand themselves by imagining how they look to others. We view ourselves and evaluate aspects of our self-image from what we presume are other peoples' attitudes and evaluations of us. In short, over one's span of life, significant interpersonal relationships (e.g., marriage, parenting) and social networks and contexts (e.g., occupational, religious) affect the social construction of our self-assessments and outlooks.

The **self-perception** mechanism indicates that proposes that, under some conditions, people attribute to themselves attitudes and beliefs from observing their overt behavior. When, in particular, people are uncertain about how they feel toward an issue or about somebody, they observe what they have done to make conclusions about their current attitudes and feelings. Thus, changes in behavior and conditions that can create uncertainty about oneself over the life course can accompany variation in self-observation and ascription of personal attributes. The fourth mechanism, **psychological centrality,** suggests that only certain aspects of our self-image and attributes influence how we feel. A self-image consists of numerous traits and pieces. The components are arranged hierarchically, with some pieces being more important than others. Central components of the self are pieces that are more important for how we define ourselves. Over the life course, what people define as central aspects of their self-images might vary. Moreover, life course events are more likely to affect people when the event challenges a central part of the self-image.

The Sample Case of Midlife Parenting

A study about midlife parenting (Ryff et al., 1994; Schmutte & Ryff, 1994) was conceived within the above interpretive framework. We targeted that period of parental experience when one's children are becoming adults in their own right, and parents are gaining a sense of how their children have "turned out." Grown children thus provide parents with a kind of *fait accompli,* which, in turn, may have important implications for how parents evaluate themselves and their own lives in middle adulthood. We hypothesized that parents' assessments of their grown children's adjustment and attainment would be strongly linked with diverse aspects of their own well-being (e.g., self-acceptance, environmental mastery, purpose in life). Moreover, consistent with our interpretive framework, we expected that the link between children's lives and parental well-being could be explained, in part, by social comparison processes, reflected appraisals, behavioral self-evaluations, and even attributional processes (the extent to which parents take credit or responsibility for how children have turned out). The summary provided below will address only one of these mechanisms, social comparison processes.

The study involved 114 midlife mothers and 101 midlife fathers from separate families who were interviewed regarding their children's accomplishments and adjustment, the interpretive processes, and their own well-being. Each parent judged each of his or her children's level of personal adjustment (e.g., confidence, happiness), social adjustment (e.g., liked by other people), and educational and occupational attainment. Each parent also completed the multidimensional scale of psychological well-being. Two types of social comparisons were obtained. First, parents compared each aspect of their child's functioning—that is, adjustment (social and personal) and attainment (educational and occupational)—with similar aspects of functioning among the children of their siblings and friends. Second, thinking about how they functioned when they were young, the parents compared themselves with their children.

Using regression models and controlling for differences in parental and familial backgrounds, the perception of better adjusted (socially and personally) and successful (educationally and occupationally) children positively predicted all aspects of parental well-being, except for feelings of autonomy. The amount of variance for ratings of children's adjustment was higher than that for children's attainment. Results were the same for mothers and fathers. Adding the social comparison variables into the regression model produced mixed results. Parents' comparisons of their children's adjustment and attainment with other people's children did not explain additional variance in any index of well-being. However, parents' comparisons of themselves with their children, particularly in the domain of adjustment, explained additional variation in parental well-being. The direction of these effects was negative—mothers and fathers who perceived themselves as less adjusted in early adulthood compared with their own young adult children had lower levels of well-being.[2]

---

[2]Further analyses showed complex interactions. The impact of social comparisons of one's child and other children's attainment on some aspects of well-being depends on the parent's role/gender (i.e., mothers vs. fathers). Moreover, for mothers, the impact of social comparisons of one's child and other children's attainment on some aspects of well-being depends on the mother's level of educational attainment. The interested reader is referred to Ryff et al. (1994).

Parenthood in midlife tends to be equated with the syndrome of the "empty nest." Undoubtedly, the migration of children out of the home and into the community disrupts parental lifestyles and stimulates many feelings. But, for as many parents who feel depressed, as many others feel a sense of accomplishment and relief. Rather than focus on the physical absence of children, our research on midlife parenting focuses on the psychological presence of children. Midlife is a time when parents assess the quality of their parenting. Parents who believe their children are adjusted and successful feel healthier vis-à-vis nearly all aspects of well-being. In turn, some features of parents' assessment of their parenting also appear to influence their well-being through social comparison processes. Interestingly, parental comparison of themselves with their children suggests complex dynamics. Parents' views of themselves might be threatened as well as enhanced by the accomplishments and adjustment of their offspring.

FUTURE DIRECTIONS: THE STUDY OF SOCIAL WELL-BEING

Our current work involves scrutiny of the extant multidimensional model of well-being, which we have come to see as possibly lacking in more sociological aspects of well-being. Human wellness may include a social side, which psychological theories may not fully articulate. For instance, Ryff's six dimensions, like many assessments of well-being, capture individuals' assessments of their lives via their accomplishments, ability to formulate and strive toward her goals, or to manipulate the world to satisfy their needs. Abstractly, well-being entails examination of oneself in relation to oneself. Absent from current assessments of functioning are aspects of well-being linked explicitly to other people, community, society, and the world.[3] We have proposed and collected data to evaluate a social model of well-being (Keyes, 1998). Grounded in classical sociological theory (e.g., Durkheim's "Anomie" and Marx's "Alienation" and "Class Consciousness"), the dimensions include (1) Social Coherence, (2) Social Integration, (3) Social Actualization, (4) Social Contribution, and (5) Social Acceptance. In general, socially healthy people find the world around them coherent and interesting; they feel they belong to their community and have something they can contribute to the world; and they think society and other people can improve.

The fundamental nature of the self-concept justifies the exploration of the social dimensions of well-being. Theorists from psychology (James, 1890; Markus & Wurf, 1987) and sociology (Cooley, 1902; Mead, 1934) proffer formulations of the self as both private and social. The self-concept plays an integral part in the feeling,

[3]Exceptions are global life satisfaction with one's neighbors or city, and Ryff's (1989b) "positive relations with others." Still, relationships to other people and society are portrayed as unidirectional (i.e., what one gets therefrom) or as filial (i.e., immediate, interpersonal relations).

perception, and articulation of how individuals function and how they think about their functioning (see also Markus & Herzog, 1991). Recognizing the multidimensional and social nature of well-being provides a more comprehensive and realistic account of the fact that people live out their lives as social creatures.

ACKNOWLEDGMENTS

We greatly appreciate and acknowledge the support and the intellectual stimulation provided by our colleagues in the John D. and Catherine T. MacArthur Research Network on Successful Midlife Development (Dr. Orville Gilbert Brim, Director). Portions of work reported in this chapter are also supported by a grant from the National Institute on Aging (1R01AG08979). Special thanks to Marilyn Essex, Sue Heidrich, Young Hyun Lee, Pamela Schmutte, and Marsha Seltzer for their contributions to the work reviewed here.

REFERENCES

Allport, G. W. (1961). *Pattern and growth in personality.* New York: Holt, Rinehart & Winston.
Baltes, P. B., & Baltes, M. M. (1990). *Successful aging: Perspectives from the behavioral sciences.* New York: Cambridge University Press.
Baruch, G. K. (1984). The psychological well-being of women in the middle years. In G. Baruch & J. Brooks-Gunn (Eds.), *Women in midlife* (pp. 161–180). New York: Plenum.
Buhler, C. (1935). The curve of life as studied in biographies. *Journal of Applied Psychology, 19,* 405–409.
Buhler, C., & Massarik, F. (Eds.). (1968). *The course of human life.* New York: Springer.
Cartensen, L. L. (1995). Evidence for a life-span theory of socioemotional selectivity. *Current Directions in Psychological Science, 4*(5), 151–156.
Coleman, L. M., & Antonucci, T. C. (1983). Impact of work on women at midlife. *Developmental Psychology, 19,* 290–294.
Cooley, C. H. (1902). *Human nature and the social order.* New York: Charles Scribner.
Diener, E. (1984). Subjective well-being. *Psychological Bulletin, 95,* 542–575.
Erikson, E. (1959). Identity and the life cycle. *Psychological Issues, 1,* 18–164.
Hauser, R. M., Sewell, W. H., Logan, J. A., Hauser, T. S., Ryff, C., Caspi, A., & MacDonald, M. (1992). The Wisconsin Longitudinal Study: Adults as parents and children at age 50. *IASSIST Quarterly, 16,* 23–38.
Heidrich, S. M., & Ryff, C. D. (1993a). Physical and mental health in later life: The self-system as mediator. *Psychology and Aging, 8*(3), 327–338.
Heidrich, S. M., & Ryff, C. D. (1993b). The role of social comparison processes in the psychological adaptation of elderly adults. *Journal of Gerontology, 48,* P127–P136.
Herzog, A. R., Rodgers, W. L., & Woodworth, J. (1982). *Subjective well-being among different age groups.* Ann Arbor: University of Michigan, Institute for Social Research, Survey Research Center.
Jahoda, M. (1958). *Current concepts of positive mental health.* New York: Basic Books.
James, W. (1890). *Principles of psychology.* New York: Holt.
Jung, C. G. (1933). *Modern man in search of a soul* (W. S. Dell & C. F. Baynes, Trans.). New York: Harcourt, Brace, & World.
Keyes, C. L. M. (1998). Social well-being. *Social Psychology Quarterly, 61*(2), 121–140.
Keyes, C. L. M., & Ryff, C. D. (1998). Generativity in adult lives: Social structural contours and quality of life consequences. In D. P. McAdams & E. de St. Aubin (Eds.), *Generativity and adult development:*

How and why we care for the next generation (pp. 227–263). Washington, D.C.: American Psychological Association.

Markus, H. R., & Herzog, A. R. (1991). The role of the self-concept in aging. In Schaie, K. W., & Lawton, M. P. (Eds.), *Annual review of gerontology and geriatrics* (pp. 110–135). New York: Springer.

Markus, H. R., & Kitayama, S. (1991). Culture and the self: Implications for cognition, emotion, and motivation. *Psychological Review, 98*(2), 224–253.

Markus, H. R., & Wurf, E. (1987). The dynamic self-concept: A social psychological perspective. *Annual Review of Psychology, 38,* 299–337.

Maslow, A. H. (1968). *Toward a psychology of being* (2nd ed.). New York: Van Nostrand.

McLanahan, S., & Adams, J. (1987). Parenthood and psychological well-being. *Annual Review of Sociology, 13,* 237–257.

Mead, G. H. (1934). *Mind, self, and society.* Chicago, IL: Chicago University Press.

Neugarten, B. L. (1968). The awareness of middle age. In B. L. Neugarten (Ed.), *Middle age and aging* (pp. 93–98). Chicago, IL: University of Chicago Press.

Neugarten, B. L. (1973). Personality change in late life: A developmental perspective. In C. Eisdorfer & M. P. Lawton (Eds.), *The psychology of adult development and aging* (pp. 311–335). Washington, DC: American Psychological Association.

Rogers. C. R. (1961). *On becoming a person.* Boston, MA: Houghton Mifflin.

Rosenberg. M. (1979). *Conceiving the self.* New York: Basic Books.

Ryff, C. D. (1982). Successful aging: A developmental approach. *Gerontologist, 22,* 209–214.

Ryff, C. D. (1984). Personality development from the inside: The subjective experience of change in adulthood and aging. In P. B. Baltes & O. G. Brim (Eds.), *Life-span development and behavior* (Vol. 6, pp. 244–281). New York: Academic Press.

Ryff, C. D. (1985). Adult personality development and the motivation for personal growth. In D. Kleiber & M. Maehr (Eds.), *Advances in motivation and achievement: Motivation and adulthood* (Vol. 4, pp. 55–92). Greenwich, CT: JAI Press.

Ryff, C. D. (1989a). Beyond Ponce de Leon and life satisfaction: New directions in quest of successful aging. *International Journal of Behavioral Development, 12,* 35–55.

Ryff, C. D. (1989b). Happiness is everything, or is it? Explorations on the meaning of psychological well-being. *Journal of Personality and Social Psychology, 57,* 1069–1081.

Ryff, C. D. (1991a). Possible selves in adulthood and old age: A tale of shifting horizons. *Psychology and Aging, 6,* 286–295.

Ryff, C. D. (1991b, November). *Mechanisms of self-evaluation in middle and later adulthood.* Paper presented at the Gerontological Society of America Meetings, San Francisco, CA.

Ryff, C. D. (1995). Psychological well-being in adult life. *Current Directions in Psychological Science, 4,* 99–104.

Ryff, C. D., & Essex, M. J. (1992a). Psychological well-being in middle and later adulthood: Descriptive markers and explanatory processes. In K. W. Schaie & M. P. Lawton (Eds.), *Annual review of gerontology and geriatrics* (Vol. 11, pp. 144–171). New York: Springer.

Ryff, C. D., & Essex, M. J. (1992b). The interpretation of life experience and well-being: The sample case of relocation. *Psychology and Aging, 7,* 507–517.

Ryff, C. D., & Keyes, C. L. M. (1995). The structure of psychological well-being revisited. *Journal of Personality and Social Psychology, 69,* 719–727.

Ryff, C. D., Lee, Y. H., Essex, M. J., & Schmutte, P. S. (1994). My children and me: Midlife evaluations of grown children and self. *Psychology and Aging, 9,* 195–205.

Ryff, C. D., Lee, Y. H., & Na, K. C. (1993, November). *Through the lens of culture: Psychological well-being at midlife.* Paper presented at the Gerontological Society of America Meetings, New Orleans, LA.

Schmutte, P. S., & Ryff, C. D. (1994). Success, social comparison, and self-assessment: Parents' midlife evaluations of sons, daughters, and selves. *Journal of Adult Development, 1,* 109–126.

Thoits, P. A. (1983). Multiple identities and psychological well-being: A reformulation and test of the social isolation hypothesis. *American Sociological Review, 48,* 174–187.

Triandis, H. C. (1989). The self and social behavior in differing cultural contexts. *Psychological Review, 96,* 506–520.

Tweed, S. H., & Ryff, C. D. (1991). Adult children of alcoholics: Profiles of wellness amidst distress. *Journal of Studies on Alcohol, 52,* 133–141.

Von Franz, M. L. (1964). The process of individuation. In C. G. Jung (Ed.), *Man and his symbols* (pp. 158–229). New York: Doubleday.

Waterman, A. S. (1984). *The psychology of individualism.* New York: Praeger.

CHAPTER 8

The Sense of Control in Midlife

Margaret Clark-Plaskie

Empire State College—The State University of New York, Corning, New York

Margie E. Lachman

Department of Psychology, Brandeis University, Waltham, Massachusetts

> Middle-aged men and women, while they by no means regard themselves as being in command of all they survey, nevertheless recognize that they constitute the powerful age-group vis a vis other age groups; that they are the norm-bearers and the decision-makers; and they live in a society which, while it may be oriented towards youth, is controlled by the middle-aged. (Neugarten, 1968, p. 93)

So wrote midlife researcher Bernice Neugarten in response to a *Time* magazine reference to "the command generation" (those between the ages of 40 and 60) in the late 1960s. Is it still the case today that midlife is a time of increased power, influence, and control? If midlife is indeed a period of relatively high actual control in society (e.g., in terms of leadership roles and increased responsibilities), then do middle-aged persons perceive themselves as being more in control and efficacious than do individuals of other ages? What about the generation of "baby-boomers" (those who were born roughly between 1946 and 1964) who are now moving through midlife? To what extent does this cohort have perceptions of control in midlife that differ from those of previous cohorts because of their unique generational experiences? Such questions are addressed in the present chapter, as we examine the sense of control in midlife for individuals and groups within the context of the whole life-span, as well as within societal and historical context.

In this chapter, we first present an overview of theoretical orientations to the study of control and definitions of control constructs. Second, the sense of control across the life-span is examined; this includes a discussion of the important methodological issues in this research, followed by a review of the main results of studies of control in childhood, adolescence, middle adulthood, and later adulthood. The section on middle adulthood highlights aspects of control experiences important in this period of life, such as increased goals and roles and the particularly salient domain of work. Third, individual differences in sense of control in midlife are examined, including the effects of gender, socioeconomic status, culture, and cohort. Within the section on cohort effects, the baby-boomer cohort is discussed in terms of its unique experiences and sense of control in midlife. Finally, we present some concluding remarks, along with a "prescription" for "successful" control in middle age.

WHAT IS THE "SENSE OF CONTROL?"

As noted by Baltes and Baltes (1986), "The meaning of psychological control is not universally shared by researchers on the topic. Psychological control refers to a field of study rather than a singular theoretical construct" (p. xviii). Studies in this field have examined individuals' various beliefs about personal control, correlates of different control beliefs, individuals' subsequent behaviors, and the opportunities for actual control in the environment. According to some theorists, such as White (1959), the need to effectively exert control over outcomes is a basic human drive. Whether it is construed as a motivation or as a belief, sense of control is deemed an important contributor to quality of life (Abeles, 1991).

Locus of Control

One of the constructs that has dominated this field of study for decades is that of perceived locus of control. Rotter (1966) hypothesized that individuals' reactions to reinforcing events are partly determined by their beliefs about the relationships between their actions and the events. Individuals may believe that events are contingent upon their actions (internal locus of control) or that events are contingent upon other people or some outside force such as luck, fate, or chance (external locus of control). Rotter's (1966) general, forced-choice Internal–External Locus of Control Scale has been widely used in psychological control research (see Lefcourt, 1981; Strickland, 1989).

However, concerns have been raised about the effectiveness of solely using a unidimensional and global measure of control, such as Rotter's scale. That is, individuals could believe that their own personal control, luck, chance, fate, and powerful others all contribute to outcomes to varying degrees. But this possibility is hidden when individuals are forced to choose between these different beliefs and are given scores on a single dimension (internal vs. external locus of control). Therefore, some researchers have developed multidimensional measures of control (e.g., Levenson, 1981). Levenson's scale investigates individuals' internal control beliefs, beliefs in chance, and beliefs in powerful others, providing separate scores for each type of belief.

Another important issue in control research is that of global versus domain-specific measurements. Rotter's (1966) scale examines global or general control beliefs, and does not allow for the possibility of different control beliefs in different areas of life. For example, an individual might have high internal control beliefs for social relationships, but not in terms of health. Also, some domains of life may be more highly valued by individuals than others; so if the individual in the above example values relationships more highly than health issues, the relatively lower health internal control beliefs may not be so important. In an effort to study such domain-specific control beliefs, researchers have developed a variety of measures, such as the Health Locus of Control Scale (Wallston & Wallston, 1981) or the PIC Intellectual Control Scales (Lachman, 1986).

Self-Efficacy

Two related constructs are perceived self-efficacy and outcome expectations (Bandura, 1977). These constructs are similarly concerned with individuals' perceptions rather than objective reality. According to Bandura, efficacy expectations refer to individuals' perceptions that they can successfully execute the behaviors required to produce certain outcomes; perceived competence. Outcome expectations, on the other hand, refer to individuals' perceptions that given behaviors will lead to particular outcomes; perceived contingency.

Taken together, perceptions of self-efficacy and outcome expectations may be seen as constituting one's basic sense of control, and research on these constructs has provided much of the initial picture of perceived control from childhood to later adulthood. Both constructs originate from social learning perspectives and thereby acknowledge the role of the environment, especially the social environment, in the development of control perceptions. Studies of locus of control (or outcome expectancies) and self-efficacy beliefs might, then, help us to understand how individuals' sense of control develops as environments and experiences (as well as capabilities) vary with age.

Assimilative and Accommodative Control

Another theory that is particularly useful in understanding the development of control perceptions in adulthood is the dual-process model of primary and secondary control (Heckhausen & Schulz, 1993). According to this model, adults may use primary control or assimilative control strategies (changing circumstances in accordance with personal preferences) and/or secondary control or accommodative control strategies (adjusting personal preferences to situational constraints), and the use of these different strategies may vary with age (Brandtstadter & Renner, 1990).

SENSE OF CONTROL ACROSS THE LIFE-SPAN

Personal control is often believed to increase early in life, remain stable during most of middle age, and slowly but steadily decline after age 55 or so (Brim, 1974). Although some research findings may support this pattern, other findings reveal different, even conflicting, patterns of change and/or stability with age. These mixed results may be at least partly due to the research designs and measurement instruments used in most studies of perceived control (Lachman, 1986; Skinner & Connell, 1986).

Methodological Issues

Given that we are interested in the development of sense of control across the life-span, we would ideally like to investigate how individuals' control beliefs change as they get older. However, the majority of the studies of control are *cross-sectional* in nature; they compare the control beliefs of different individuals, who are different ages, at one point in time. Thus, information is gained about *age differences,* but not necessarily *age changes.* In cross-sectional studies, age changes are confounded with *cohort effects.* Any differences in control beliefs found between individuals of different ages could be due either to their ages or to the unique experiences that have affected them as members of different birth cohorts, or generations. In order to know if the beliefs of particular individuals actually change with age, those individuals would have to be followed and tested over time, as in *longitudinal research.*

Since much of the research is based on cross-sectional data, we should be aware of the possible effects of cohorts, as well as the effects of the types of measurements used (unidimensional vs. multidimensional and global vs. domain-specific), as mentioned earlier, when interpreting findings about sense of control across the life-span.

Childhood

Cross-Sectional Research

As noted by Rodin (1987), cross-sectional studies with children and adolescents show an increase in internality with age, but not a linear increase, as there are both increases and decreases from Grade 1 to 12, and differences by gender. Skinner and Connell (1986) have also observed that numerous cross-sectional studies of the general, bipolar construct of locus of control in children have resulted in inconsistent findings. The one reliable finding, according to Skinner and Connell, is that relative internality increases from about age 5 or 6 to approximately age 7 or 8 (after entering school).

Multidimensional and Domain-Specific Measures

Studies of multiple dimensions and specific domains have revealed more information about children's perceptions of control. For instance, in terms of multiple sources of control, Skinner, Chapman, and Baltes (1982) found that with children aged 6–12, there is an increase in the mean level of perceived effectiveness of effort, and a decrease in the role of luck. They also found that internal and external causes are distinguished more and they become less related to each other with age. Connell (1985) found that among children aged 8–14, there is a decrease in attributions to unknown sources of control for cognitive, social, physical, and general outcomes; a decrease in internal attributions only for physical outcomes; and a linear decrease in attributions to powerful others for cognitive, social, physical, and general outcomes with age. In addition, some researchers have measured beliefs about success and failure outcomes separately. According to Skinner and Connell (1986), the consistent developmental trends in childhood involve increases in perceived internal responsibility for failure outcomes as well as for social events.

In sum, during childhood, there is an increase in relative internality (especially in early childhood), an increased recognition of effort rather than luck, an increased understanding of the sources of control (fewer attributions to "unknown" sources), a decrease in the perceptions of others as the locus of control, and an increase in perceptions of internal responsibility for failures and social outcomes.

Adolescence and Young Adulthood

As Rodin (1990) noted:

> Issues of control and self-determination loom large in adolescence and a sense of one's own efficacy can make the transition to adulthood more successful. (p. 11)

Thus, individuals' sense of control in adolescence depends in part on their earlier perceptions and experiences and may, in turn, affect their subsequent sense of control in midlife. According to Rodin (1990), there is the potential for decreases in sense of control during this transition period. Social comparisons may diminish perceived self-efficacy and physiological changes and social transitions may threaten perceived control and predictability (Hamburg, 1980). However, as Heckhausen (1992) explained, there may be the opportunity for increases in sense of control during this time as well. As in childhood, there are developments in physical and cognitive abilities in adolescence that might positively affect individuals' perceived competence. In addition, there are added age-graded social roles that expand adolescents' opportunities to exert control and experience autonomy.

What does research reveal about the pattern of control perceptions in adolescence? There are few studies that target this particular age group. In some cases, adolescents are included in studies of childhood. In many other instances, the control beliefs of late adolescents, and particularly young college students, are compared to those of older adults (and middle-aged adults, to a lesser extent).

Cross-Sectional Research

Some cross-sectional studies seem to indicate that the general, relative increases in internal control beliefs found in childhood do continue through adolescence and young adulthood, even into midlife. It has been found that young adults have higher internal control beliefs than do children/teens (Ryckman & Malikiosi, 1975; Staats, 1974) and that adults in their thirties have higher internal control beliefs than do young adults (Lao, 1974).

Longitudinal Research

Longitudinal data is helpful in disentangling age and cohort effects. Gatz and Karel (1993) conducted a 20-year longitudinal study of four generations of families. They reported that the overall increases in mean levels of internal control over time were most likely reflective of contextual factors in the culture. However, by comparing their cross-sectional and longitudinal data, they also concluded that there is a *developmental change* toward greater internality as young adults move into early middle adulthood.

Domain-Specific Measures

Although the view that internal control continues to increase throughout young adulthood seems to be supported, the picture may actually be more complicated than indicated in these studies, which use general measures of control. For instance, Bradley and Webb (1976) examined domain-specific control beliefs of individuals aged 13–18, 19–25, 35–50, and 60–90. They found that internal control was lowest for the oldest group in the physical domain, lowest for the youngest and oldest groups in the social domain, and stable across the age groups in the intellectual domain. Thus, there may be different patterns of development across adulthood for control beliefs in different domains.

Middle Adulthood

Cross-Sectional Research

Some cross-sectional studies reveal no differences in the internal control beliefs of young adults and middle-aged adults (Andrisani, 1977; Gatz & Siegler, 1981, Study 3). However, other cross-sectional studies report higher internal control beliefs in middle-aged adults than in young adults (e.g., Staats, 1974). One reason for the seemingly inconsistent findings may be the varied age compositions of the samples being compared (a concern noted by Lachman, 1986). Another reason may again be the confound of age and cohort effects inherent in cross-sectional studies.

Longitudinal Research

Even with longitudinal data, though, several patterns of change and/or stability in locus of control beliefs are found. For instance, in one study, no changes in the level of internal control beliefs were found for individuals aged 46–69 over a 2-year period (Gatz & Siegler 1981, Study 1). However, in another study of individuals aged 46–69, Siegler and Gatz (1985) reported a decrease in internal control beliefs over a 6-year period. In a cross-sequential study of adults aged 35–69, Lachman (1985) found that elderly adults had more internal control beliefs than did middle-aged adults and this did not change over 4 years. The fact that the difference did not change over time might be indicative of a cohort effect, rather than a developmental change. In this vein, although Gatz and Karel (1993) found cross-sectional differences in the control beliefs of middle-aged and older adults (with middle-aged adults having greater internality), their combined longitudinal, cross-sectional, and sequential comparisons revealed that these were actually more likely to be effects of time of measurement, and not developmental changes.

Mulitdimensional and Domain-Specific Measures

The types of control measures used in these studies may also have contributed to the diverse findings. As previously mentioned, Ryckman and Malikiosi (1975) found that internal control beliefs were stable among adults in their 30s to 70s, beliefs in powerful others were stable, except in the 50s when they were lower, and beliefs in chance were highest among adults in their 30s and 40s. In a study of adults aged 21–88, Saltz and Magruder-Habib (1982) found no age differences in internal or powerful others beliefs, but older adults tended to have stronger beliefs in chance.

Control beliefs may vary within specific domains, as well. As discussed earlier, Bradley and Webb (1976) found some similarities and some differences between young, middle-aged, and older adults in locus of control beliefs, depending on the domain. In a study of adults aged 20–89, Lachman (1991) also found differential age patterns in control beliefs, depending on the specific domains, as well as the control measures. In particular, all age groups had similar interpersonal and political control beliefs, and young and middle-aged adults also had similar general, health, and intellectual control beliefs. However, older adults had lower internal beliefs and higher external beliefs in general and for health and intellectual functioning than did young and middle-aged adults. (See Figure 1 for a depiction of the age-group differences in general and domain-specific control beliefs.) Within the intellectual domain, Cornelius and Caspi (1986) also found that self-efficacy remained constant during midlife, but that it declined in later life, when concern about intellectual aging increased.

According to Brandtstadter and Rothermund (1994), though, the effect of domain-specific control perceptions on an individual's overall sense of control depends on the personal importance of the particular domains. Shifts in the subjective importance of goal domains were found in their 8-year longitudinal study of adults aged 30–59, and stability in control perceptions was also found; that is, perceived losses of control within certain domains had little effect on general control beliefs if the importance of the domains had declined during that time period.

The Domain of Work

The importance of the work domain typically continues or even increases in midlife, particularly for professionals and white-collar workers who are "climbing the corporate ladder" (Howard & Bray, 1988). In one study, when asked what was most important in their lives, middle-aged adults emphasized jobs or careers (Ryff, 1989). In another study, Clark and Lachman (1994) categorized middle-aged and older adults' current and future goals by life domain. It was found that a greater percentage of middle-aged adults' current and future goals were in the work domain than in any other life domain. (See Figure 2 for the percentages of middle-aged adults' current goals by domain.)

There seems to be an important, close relationship between this salient domain of work and perceptions of control in midlife. For instance, Clark and Lachman (1994) found that middle-aged adults' perceived internal control was higher for goals in the work domain than for goals in the family, health, leisure, and financial domains, based on rank order. The relationship between work experiences and perceived control in midlife appears to be a reciprocal one. In some studies, types of job and work experiences predict internal control beliefs among middle-aged adults (e.g., Huyck, 1991; Kivett, Watson, & Busch, 1977). Also, Andrisani and Nestel (1976) examined cross-sectional and longitudinal data from nearly 3000 middle-aged men and found that internal control had a systematic influence on work success, and success at work also enhanced expectancies of internal control. In this way, middle-aged adults who believe that they are in control tend to have more successful experiences at work, which, in turn, increases their feelings and expectations of being in control. Work and other life experiences build upon each

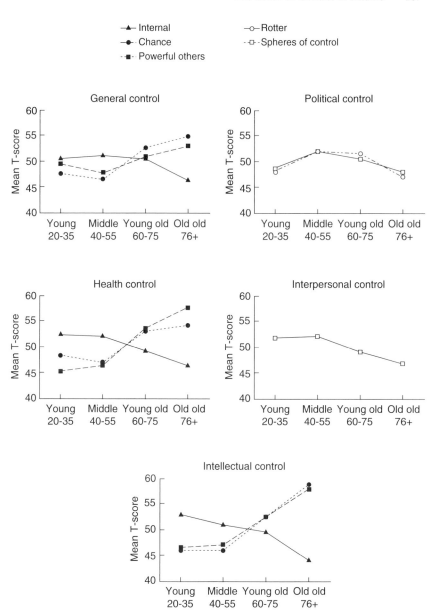

FIGURE 1   Age-group differences in general and domain-specific control beliefs. Adapted from Lachman, Ziff, & Spiro (1994).

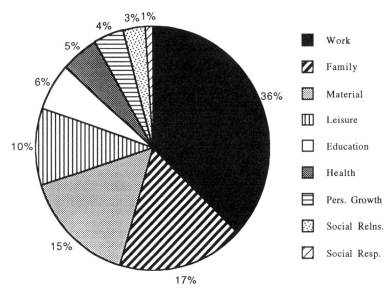

FIGURE 2   Percentages of middle-aged adults' current goals by domain. From Clark and Lachman (1994).

other during the life course, influencing and being influenced by control perceptions. If there are increased numbers of goals, roles, responsibilities, and stress during midlife, what does that mean in terms of the sense of control, particularly self-efficacy beliefs, in midlife?

Self-Efficacy

Heise (1990) asked the question, Do youths or middle-aged adults have more control over their lives? He explained that the answer is rather complex. On one hand, middle-aged adults have accumulated more roles, which allows them greater selection and opportunity to fit roles to their needs and thereby increase efficacy feelings. Also, middle-aged adults are more likely than other age groups to have powerful roles, and performing in such esteemed roles may contribute to a sense of self-efficacy. On the other hand, middle-aged adults have had more chances to have been disappointed in their roles, while young adults may just be starting out and projecting themselves into imagined, powerful future roles, thereby increasing their sense of control.

This latter idea is consistent with the work of Markus, Cross, and Wurf (1988) on possible selves. They proposed that people construct mental images of their possible selves, which, if well defined, may organize and motivate their behavior.

As reported by Ogilvie and Clark (1992), when young adults describe their best or ideal selves, they do tend to think of themselves in successful future roles. In addition, according to Levinson (1978), individuals form a Dream (usually about career success) in young adulthood, which guides them, but is then likely to be reevaluated and revised in midlife if it has not yet been fulfilled.

Consistent with this, Heise (1990) concluded:

> In short, youths may not have much control in reality, but psychologically they could feel efficacious; middle-aged folks may exercise significant control over reality, but meanwhile they may feel disappointment about failed aspirations, anxiety about vulnerable statuses, and frustration that they do not have more control in deciding which roles occupy their time. Both youths and middle-aged adults could end up with the same sense of efficacy as a result of career-related processes [career meaning an ordered sequence of roles, not necessarily work-related], but the underlying reasons are different. (p. 79)

This may partly explain the general stability of efficacy that characterizes the transition from young adulthood to middle adulthood (e.g., Brim, 1974; Lachman, 1991; Rodin, 1987).

Commenting on Heise's ideas, Foner (1990) noted that the multitude of roles that are present in midlife might also be potentially limiting to individuals' perceived freedom; that is, middle-aged adults may feel constrained by role overload. Research appears to support both views, that midlife is simultaneously a time of high stress and high control. For example, in a recent study of young, middle-aged, and older adults, Lachman, Lewkowicz, Marcus, and Peng (1994) found that midlife was perceived as "a period with many responsibilities, increased stress in several domains, and little time for leisure, but also as a peak in competence, ability to handle stress, sense of control, productivity, and social responsibility." In another recent study, Parris Stephens, Franks, and Townsend (1994) found both negative and positive effects of being in multiple roles on the mental and physical health of "women in the middle" (middle-aged women who were caregivers). Also, Burack and Lachman (1994) reported that among middle-aged adults, perceiving oneself as inefficient at planning was a significant predictor of lower levels of well-being. A sense of self-efficacy, especially in planning, is useful, if not necessary, to juggle multiple roles and responsibilities. Indeed, Jerusalem and Schwarzer (1992) found that among adults aged 21–52, those who were high in general self-efficacy had good capacities to resist stress, while those who were low in self-efficacy were especially vulnerable to difficult demand characteristics and failure experiences.

Results from various other studies also support this somewhat paradoxical view of midlife. Clark and Lachman (1994) interviewed adults aged 30–84 about their current and future goals. It was found that middle-aged adults reported having a greater number of current and future goals than did older adults, but there were no age differences in ratings of general perceived control over goals. Simon and Ogilvie (1992) interviewed young college students and middle-aged adults aged 38–47 about their personal projects (goal-related activities). Results indicated that middle-aged adults were more confident about their personal projects (especially instrumental ones) than were young college students, and there was a shift in the salience of interpersonal projects with age (interpersonal projects were rated as more stressful and time consuming, but also as more important and related to long-term goals among the middle-aged adults). Chebat (1986) also found that middle-aged adults had a higher sense of social responsibility than did younger and older adults. Such a heightened concern for others and the community is to be expected in midlife according to Erikson (1950), as individuals address the developmental issues of generativity.

Thus, in summary, concern for others and the importance of work appear to be heightened during middle adulthood. Midlife involves many roles, goals, and responsibilities. Yet there is evidence for continued, and in some cases, increased perceptions of self-efficacy, which might help individuals in dealing with increased stress. There is likewise some evidence that internal control beliefs remain stable or increase in midlife, although such apparent increases might be due to cohort differences. The very experience of successfully negotiating the demands of multiple roles may contribute to feelings of efficacy and control. Beliefs in powerful others may decrease in the decade of the 50s because it is a time when adults are likely to be in powerful positions themselves. Meanwhile, beliefs in chance appear to increase in midlife and/or later life (to be discussed further in the next section).

Later Adulthood

Old age often brings with it the increased likelihood of declines and losses (e.g., physical strength and health and certain social roles), but not necessarily an overall decrease in sense of control. According to Brandtstadter, Wentura, and Greve (1993), although adults are aware of age-related losses, they are still quite effective in maintaining a sense of control and a positive view of themselves and their development into later life. The negative effects of age-typical problems may even be buffered by a flexible, accommodating control style. In fact, Brandtstadter and Renner (1990) have found that accommodative control strategies (e.g., changing one's goals to fit a given set of circumstances) increase in importance as assimilative control strategies (e.g., changing a situation to meet one's goals) decrease in importance, beginning in midlife. In this way, they concluded that in the transition from middle adulthood to later adulthood, a sense of control is able to be preserved to a great extent.

Cross-Sectional Research

The period of later life is often characterized as a time of slow but steady decline in personal control. As with the research on perceived control in other age periods, the results in later adulthood are mixed. Some cross-sectional studies have found no differences in the internal control beliefs of middle-aged adults and older adults

(Gatz & Siegler, 1981, Study 3; Lao, 1974; Nehrke, Hulicka, & Morganti, 1980). Yet, other studies of this kind have found higher internal control beliefs in older adults than in middle-aged adults (Gatz & Siegler, 1981, Study 2; Strickland & Shaffer, 1971; Wolk & Kurtz, 1975). Also, Cicerelli (1980) found low but significant positive correlations between internality and age across 60- to 90-year-olds. Thus, it would appear that internal control beliefs either remain the same or increase in later life. However, no firm conclusions can be made about age-related stability and change from cross-sectional data.

Longitudinal Research

Lachman (1983) used cross-sequential data to examine age-related changes over a 3-year period. It was found that the oldest groups (ages 60–63 and 64–67) had the highest sense of efficacy and the middle-aged group (ages 44–59) had the lowest sense of efficacy, and these differences did not change over time. Reid and Ziegler (1981) conducted a 5-year longitudinal study of adults aged 60–100, using the Desired Control Scale. They found that 65% showed decreases, 13% showed increases, and 22% showed no differences in their personal control over time. In their 20-year longitudinal study of four generations, Gatz and Karel (1993) reported no developmental changes from midlife to later life, and the group of oldest women consistently had the most external control beliefs. They interpreted the findings as cohort effects, reflective of the older women's sociohistorical reality. Thus, these longitudinal results indicate differential patterns of changes and stability in control perceptions in later life.

Multidimensional and Domain-Specific Measures

A few studies have looked at multiple dimensions of control in later life. As already mentioned, among other results, Ryckman and Malikiosi (1975) found that internal control beliefs were stable across the middle and later decades. Saltz and Magruder-Habib (1982) found that internal and powerful others beliefs were stable among 21- to 88-year-olds, but chance beliefs were higher among older adults. Gurin and Brim (1984) found that older adults were more external in regard to environmental responsiveness, but no age differences were found for personal efficacy.

There is evidence that control beliefs vary in later life by domain as well as by source of control (e.g., findings already discussed from Bradley & Webb, 1976). A number of studies have reported finding no age differences with general measures of control, but significant age differences in specific domains (e.g., Lachman, 1986, 1991; Lachman, Baltes, Nesselroade, & Willis, 1982; Saltz & Magruder-Habib, 1982; Wallston & Wallston, 1981). Most of these studies have found that older adults had higher beliefs in external control in the domains of intelligence (particularly beliefs in chance) and health (particularly beliefs in powerful others) compared to young college students and, in a few studies, compared to middle-aged adults as well. Many of these studies that used multidimensional and domain-specific measures, however, found no age differences in internal control beliefs.

While Clark and Lachman (1994) found that age was not a significant predictor of perceptions of control over middle-aged and older adults' goals, they did find that perceived control over goals within the specific domain of leisure increased significantly with age. This is consistent with Foner's (1990) contention that as roles contract in later life, individuals may experience newfound freedoms and enjoy their unobligated time more. Evans and Lewis (1990) also noted the adaptiveness of being flexible in identifying oneself with multiple roles in later life. As put forth by Peck (1968), such flexibility may enable older adults to define themselves in meaningful ways and gain competence in domains besides work and parenting. In a study of retirement, Ogilvie (1987) found that life satisfaction was indeed a function of the amount of time spent in activities that allowed for the expression of multiple, meaningful aspects of the self. Leisure just may be the dominion in which elders have an increased sense of control and can compensate for declines in other domains.

Thus, there is not an overall steady decline of sense of control in later adulthood. Perceptions of control in certain domains, namely cognitive functioning and health, do tend to decrease. However, efficacy and internal control beliefs seem to at least remain stable in later life. As explained by Lachman (1986), older adults seem to recognize the role of external forces while still maintaining their own sense of internal control. Not only is a sense of personal control preserved, but in some areas of life, such as leisure, it may even be enhanced in old age.

INDIVIDUAL DIFFERENCES AND SENSE OF CONTROL IN MIDLIFE

Gender and Control

Sex and gender roles are linked to sense of control. In a meta-analytic review of studies using Rotter's I–E Scale, Shannon (1991) found small but statistically significant differences, with women having higher levels of external control beliefs than men. In a 1990 study of college students, DeBrabander and Boone found a similar difference, but they proposed that Rotter's scale may not adequately measure the female perception of control. Using a revised scale, they found a significant positive correlation between external locus of control and number of negative life events for men, but not for women. They concluded that women who are high in external control beliefs may be responding in culturally prescribed, socially desirable ways.

Cultural norms concerning what is socially desirable (or acceptable) for women may differ by cohort as well. For example, Bishop and Solomon (1989) found that older female Master of Business Administration (MBA) students had higher external control beliefs than did older male MBA students, but there were no sex differences among younger MBA students. Also, Simon and Ogilvie (1992) found that among middle-aged adults, women perceived greater control over interpersonal projects, while men perceived greater control over instrumental projects; no such sex differences were found among young college students. Bandura (1992) explained that stereotypes and biased cultural practices may affect women's beliefs about their occupational efficacy, but that certain changes may now be weakening these barriers; that is, there seems to be less of a discrepancy than there has been in the past between today's young men and women in their self-efficacy beliefs about successfully pursuing different kinds of careers. In addition, Burger (1992) noted that there also tend to be differences between older men and women in their general desire for control, but not among younger college students.

The sex differences in control perceptions are probably confounded by other variables in addition to cohort, such as education, income, and race. For example, Lachman (1986) reported that both sex and education contributed to the finding that elders had high external control beliefs; that is, the older sample consisted of many rural women who had low education levels. Indeed, female elders with higher education levels had lower external control beliefs than those with lower education levels, and education was negatively correlated with beliefs in powerful others within the intellectual domain. In a longitudinal study, Tashakkori and Thompson (1991) found effects of both race and sex on efficacy and control beliefs (blacks and women had higher external beliefs and lower personal efficacy beliefs than did whites and men, respectively). Crohan, Antonucci, Adelmann, and Coleman (1989) found that, among middle-aged adults, income was positively related to perceived control for black women and white men and occupational status was positively related to perceived control for both black and white women.

Socioeconomic Status and Control

Various studies have revealed that income or socioeconomic status (SES) is related to individuals' control beliefs. For instance, Schmidt, Lamm, and Trommsdorf (1978) found that among middle-aged workers, those in the middle class (rather than the lower class) believed to a greater extent that the realization of their hopes and fears depended on themselves (internal locus of control). Studies with general, unidimensional measures of control have found that low SES is related to relatively greater external control beliefs (e.g., Battle & Rotter, 1963; Franklin, 1963). Using a multidimensional scale, Levenson (1981) found that low-income students believed more in chance than did higher income students. In domain-specific studies it has been found that low-SES people also have more external beliefs about their physical health (Wallston & Wallston, 1981) and their mental health (Hill & Bale, 1981).

Some research has shown the interaction between the effects of income and race on perceived control (Battle & Rotter, 1963; Lefcourt, 1976). Battle and Rotter also found a significant, positive relationship between externality and intelligence in low-SES groups and among black individuals; that is, the individuals with higher IQ scores in these groups perceived external sources of control to a greater extent than did the group members with lower IQ scores. In this way, perhaps it is not only realistic but adaptive for some people to acknowledge external sources of control.

Cross-Cultural Influences on Control

Perceptions of control also vary as a function of the culture or country in which individuals live. In a study of nearly 12,000 adults in nine Western European countries, Jensen, Olsen, and Hughes (1990) found that there was greater variation in locus of control beliefs because of the country of residence than because of life cycle stage, sex, or social class. Levenson (1981) also reported that Japanese and German individuals were lower in internal control beliefs than were American individuals.

It has also been shown that secondary control strategies (which involve altering the self more than actively changing the environment) are more commonly used in Eastern cultures than in Western cultures, where primary control strategies (changing the environment to fit one's own needs and wishes) are more prevalent (Peng, 1994; Weisz, Rothbaum, & Blackburn, 1984). In a recent study, Peng found no age differences in primary control and increases with age in secondary control. This same pattern was found for both Americans and Chinese-Americans. However, Chinese-Americans were lower in primary control and higher in secondary control beliefs at all ages. Secondary control beliefs are indeed more consistent with Eastern thought. That is, Eastern values focus on the group and harmonious interdependence (Markus & Kitayama, 1991), which parallel the secondary control strategies of exerting control by changing the self to fit in with surrounding people and things.

In our Western culture, however, the emphasis is more on independence, achievement, and being actively in control; individuals are more likely to strive to change the environment to suit themselves. Gergen (1989) noted that personal control is at the core of our society's value system and that Max Weber (1930) equated the ideology of internal control with the Protestant Ethic, in which status is achieved through one's own independent efforts.

Cohort Effects

As previously mentioned, cohort, or generational, effects are important factors in cross-sectional research. We saw evidence of the role that cohort effects play in life-span research (e.g., Gatz & Karel, 1993) and in terms of the narrowing gender differences (e.g., Bishop & Solomon, 1989; Simon & Ogilvie, 1992). In addition, Rotter (1975) reported that college students in the mid-1970s were higher in external control beliefs than were college students in the mid-1960s, and Nigro (1987) found that from 1978 to 1983 there was a gradual shift toward greater externality among Italian college students. In this way, the relatively older individuals in cross-sectional studies may have had high internal control beliefs even when they were younger and the young adults may continue to have high external control beliefs as they get older.

Awareness of the confound of age changes and cohort differences is essential; otherwise, we may attribute control perceptions to specific age periods, which are only representative of a particular generation. Examination of cohort effects is necessary in order to fully comprehend the sense of control across the life-span, as well as to understand particular cohort groups.

Baby-Boomers in Midlife

In 1986, the generation of baby-boomers began to enter midlife, and it will be another 30 years until the youngest boomers have moved beyond this life stage. Like all middle-agers, their sense of control depends, in part, on their earlier control perceptions and experiences. What particular cohort characteristics and life experiences may have influenced baby-boomers' midlife control perceptions?

First of all, this cohort is more highly educated than its predecessors (Russell, 1987). As we know, education is positively correlated with internal control beliefs, and probably realistically so. Second, this generation grew up within a climate of hope for the future. This great hope and expectation was reflected in an address by then-President John F. Kennedy:

> Never before has man had such capacity to control his own environment, to end thirst and hunger, to conquer poverty and disease, to banish illiteracy and massive human misery. We have the power to make this the best generation in the history of the world—or to make it the last. (Kennedy, 1963, p. 696)

Thus, the baby-boomers may have perceived themselves as powerful (in sheer number, for one thing) and may have expected a lot of personal control, as they were told that their destiny (and the future of their country) was in their own hands. As Light (1988) noted, with the bright economic outlook of the 1950s, the launching of men to the moon, and the fantasy world of television, the baby-boomers grew up with great expectations about the future; they could be and do anything and everything.

But were their expectations met? They experienced the assassinations of John F. Kennedy, Robert Kennedy, and Martin Luther King, Jr., as well as race riots and the Watergate scandal. Perhaps more than anything else, this generation was greatly affected by the Vietnam War; their destinies were no longer in their own hands, but rather in those of powerful others or chance or fate.

What happens when people expect to have control and then circumstances do not allow them the opportunity to exert actual control? Several studies were reviewed by Lefcourt (1982), showing that locus of control beliefs shift with relevant environmental events, particularly with political disappointments. For example, college students in studies by Gorman (1968) and McArthur (1970) had more external control beliefs following the 1968 Democratic National Convention (when Eugene McCarthy was defeated) and the lottery for draft eligibility, respectively. In addition, Schulz and Hanusa (1978) found that older adults who experienced personal control and then had control taken away fared even worse in the long run (psychologically and physically) than did those who had started with lower personal control perceptions.

It is too soon to have a clear picture of baby-boomers' sense of control in midlife or the effects of the apparent inconsistencies between their expectations and their actual control experiences. Theoretically, however, if baby-boomers have learned that their actions do not consistently affect outcomes, they may have learned to be somewhat "helpless" (Seligman, 1975). According to the reformulated learned helplessness theory, the effects of noncontingencies depend on individuals' causal attributions (Abramson, Seligman, & Teasdale, 1978); that is, if individuals attribute negative outcomes to stable, global, and internal causes, they are more likely to be depressed.

Are middle-aged baby-boomers a particularly depressed subgroup of our population? Research has shown that depression is not necessarily tied to age, or that there is a nonlinear relationship between depression and age, with the incidence of depressive symptoms being even lower in middle adulthood than in other age periods (e.g., Kessler, Foster, Webster, & House, 1992; Mirowsky & Ross, 1992). But the baby-boomers are just entering midlife; hence their depression rates are not yet fully represented in these data. In fact, Klerman (1976) pointed out that clinical depression increased among adolescents and young adults since World War II, and may be related to the societal stresses accompanying the baby boom. Klerman raised the question of whether or not this would lead to endogenous depression in later adulthood, as these youths aged. Others have concurred, noting that the baby-boom cohort has experienced more stress than prior generations, which is reflected in high rates of delinquency, drinking and drug use, and suicides (Easterlin, 1980; Hauser, 1980; Kettle, 1981).

Easterlin (1980) also pointed to the discrepancy between expectations or aspirations and the reality faced by members of such a large cohort. There are negative effects of being part of a large generation, such as increased competition in the job market and a possible plateau in one's career during midlife. However, the popular notion that the baby-boomers will be worse off than their parents does not seem to be true (e.g., Easterlin, Macdonald, & Macunovich, 1990a, 1990b). According to a recent Gallup poll (Gallup & Newport, 1991), the overwhelming majority of baby-boomers believe that they will be, or already are, better off than their parents were at their age. In that way, perhaps baby-boomers' sense of control has not been negatively affected via disappointments in their aspirations, at least not in the economic realm.

It should be noted, though, that the baby-boom generation does span a wide range of birth years and it is a rather heterogeneous group. Not only should there be individual differences in perceived control and well-being based, for example, on attributional styles, sex, race, and SES, but in relation to age within the cohort as well. As Light (1988) observed, the younger baby-boomers have different social and political histories and economic realities than do the older baby-boomers. Politically, the youngest may not have experienced the same kinds of disillusionments; in fact, they may not have started out expecting quite as much. Socially, with higher divorce rates among their parents, the younger boomers may have learned early on that life is full of uncertainties. Economically, they grew up in a less optimistic time and Easterlin, Schaeffer, and Macunovich (1993) also pointed out that the advancements over their parental generation are not as clearly evident with the younger baby-boom group. In fact, the lower income, younger baby-boom group may indeed end up being worse off than their parental generation. Perhaps this subgroup of baby-boomers will have particularly lower levels of perceived (and actual) control when they reach middle age (although not necessarily worse mental health, given less of a discrepancy between their expectations and reality).

Thus, the pessimistic view of the baby-boomers' current and future economic welfare may be accurate in describing only a subset of that generation. In addition, according to Easterlin et al. (1993), the economic future of all baby-boomers is still somewhat under personal control through their demographic decisions; that is, many baby-boomers have chosen to postpone or avoid marriage, postpone childbearing, have fewer children, and have two working parents, thereby offsetting the negative effects of the poor economy. In this way, baby-boomers may be taking back and exerting some control over their destinies.

This is not to say, however, that such demographic decisions are entirely self-determined, nor that they necessarily entail positive consequences overall. As Easterlin et al. (1990a) pointed out, "Economic well-being is not the same as total well-being" (p. 287). They suggested that the economic success of the baby-boomers has been purchased at the expense of the noneconomic aspects of their welfare, such as family life, leisure, privacy, and independence. For instance, according to Easterlin et al. (1993), compared to previous generations, among the baby-boomers there is a noticeably smaller proportion with a spouse or adult children. This means, for one thing, there are fewer family members to whom they can turn for support or care now and in their old age. More support is, and will be, needed at the formal, societal level, such as day-care programs, flexible work schedules and leaves, universal benefits (including health care and long-term care), and various elder services. The baby-boomers, after all, are making major life adjustments in order to fare well in the current economic and social situation. They also have the expectation that society bears some responsibility to help with their economic and social needs. In this way, there is a call for a harmonious balance between individual control efforts and those of external forces. Although this cohort tends to be particularly self-reliant, like most Americans, baby-boomers also feel that there is a time and place for formal intervention (Light, 1988). Given this, plus the increased recognition of the role of external forces with age, baby-boomers would be likely to accept, perhaps even demand, such a combined effort for their future.

MENTAL WELL-BEING AND SENSE OF CONTROL

The adaptive value of a sense of control is reflected in the extensive research showing positive correlates of internal locus of control beliefs. Internality has been associated with motivation and achievement in academic situations (e.g., Lefcourt, 1982; Rotter, 1966), happiness (Brown & Granick, 1980), and physical health (Rodin, 1980). The apparent benefits of internal control beliefs may also be supported by the finding that mentally healthy individuals (as opposed to depressed individuals) tend to overestimate their degree of personal control over events that are objectively random (Langer, 1975; Langer & Roth, 1975). Such an "illusion of control" has been found to have positive effects on various types of behavior, including improvements in task performance (Monty & Perlmuter, 1975), reductions in test anxiety (Stotland & Blumenthal, 1964), adaptive coping with cancer and other diseases (Taylor, Helgeson, Reed, & Skokan, 1991), and decreases in preoperative stress (Langer, Janis, & Wolfer, 1975).

In fact, it seems that internality may be closely related to, or part of, individuals' ideal images of themselves in our society. For instance, Cowles, Darling, and Skanes (1992) had college students complete several scales (including Rotter's I–E Scale) three times each—for their real, ideal, and worst selves. It was found that the worst self was more externally oriented than was the ideal self and there was no difference between the real and ideal selves in terms of locus of control. Using a more domain-specific and multidimensional method, Clark and Ogilvie (1993) found that college students' ratings of the best and usual selves shared more in common with their mental representations of being "in control," while their ratings of the worst self shared more in common with their mental representations of being "not in control." "In control" perceptions were more highly integrated or schematized and were experienced in more areas of the young adults' lives than were the "not in control" beliefs. The more organized and pervasive the "not in control" perceptions were, the lower were the levels of self-esteem. Thus, college students in these two studies do seem to have internalized the cultural evaluation of being in control as "good" and being not in control as "bad."

Some researchers, however, have recognized that it may not always be adaptive or beneficial to have strong internal control beliefs. For example, it has been found that women who are independent and autonomous tend to delay treatment for symptoms of breast or cervical cancer (Fisher, 1967; Hammerschag, Fisher, & DeCosse, 1964). Rodin (1989) discussed the work of Glass (1977) on Type A individuals who are so driven that they continue in their control efforts even in uncontrollable situations. Rodin concluded that in some individuals, excessive efforts to be in control can have negative effects on the same physiological symptoms that have generally been shown to benefit from increased control (e.g., catecholamine levels, which have been linked to coronary disease). Various researchers have also found that high desire for, or perception of, personal control sometimes has negative effects, such as increased negative mood states (Burger, Brown, & Allen, 1983), stress, worry, and self-blame (Rodin, 1980, 1986), pressure to perform well

(Burger, 1992), feelings of inefficiency and failure (Thompson, Cheek, & Graham, 1988), and subsequent frustration in the absence of choice (Perlmuter, Monty, & Cross, 1974).

Some have proposed that giving up behavioral control or acknowledging external sources of control might be more adaptive in certain circumstances for certain people (Averill, 1974; Barrell, DeWolfe, & Cumming, 1966; Felton & Kahana, 1974; Piper & Langer, 1986; Snyder & Higgins, 1988). The fit between the individual and the environment is critical. For instance, Felton and Kahana (1974) found that external locus of control was positively correlated with adjustment within rigid environments (e.g., nursing homes) and Barrell et al. (1966) found that patients who prefer hospital staff to be authoritarian showed better emotional responses to hospitalization. Cromwell, Butterfield, Brayfield, and Curry (1977) found that heart attack patients in congruent conditions (internals in self-treatment or externals in structured treatments in which the staff made the decisions) were less likely to suffer further complications or to die than were those in incongruent conditions. Also, according to Miller and Mangan (1983), gynecologic patients' stress responses were influenced by the interaction of personal coping style and level of preparatory information provided in the situation; that is, there was less psychophysiological arousal among information seekers who were given a lot of information and information avoiders who were given little information than among individuals in either preference group who were in incongruent information situations.

Furthermore, it appears that in the extreme, neither high internal nor external control beliefs are adaptive. Rotter (1966) explained that people with beliefs at either extreme are unrealistic and "likely to be maladjusted by most definitions." Scholnick and Friedman (1993) also proposed a curvilinear relationship between control and adaptive functioning. Individuals with too high a sense of control may refrain from adaptive planning behaviors due to a false sense of security and those with too low a sense of control may not be planful because of the assumption that they cannot have any influence over the outcome. They postulated that individuals with a moderate level of perceived control would be most likely to use planning strategies. As Lachman and Burack (1993) noted, a balanced sense of control may foster adaptive planning: to be prepared for events that are highly probable, while still remaining flexible if those events do not or cannot happen. Other theorists and researchers agree that having a balance between internal and external locus of control beliefs or between assimilative and accommodative control styles is essential and adaptive in adulthood (Brandtstadter & Renner, 1990; Brandtstadter et al., 1993; Brim, 1992; Heckhausen & Schulz, 1993; Reid & Stirling, 1989; Taylor, 1983).

CONCLUDING REMARKS

Midlife is paradoxically a period in which individuals have many goals, roles, responsibilities, stress, and not enough time for leisure, and yet also experience a peak in personal control and power. Involvement in the work and social domains is heightened, along with perceived control in these areas as a result of successful experiences. In midlife, adults may begin to recognize more external sources of control and adopt more accommodative (or secondary) control strategies, while maintaining their own sense of internal control and efficacy (Brandtstadter & Renner, 1990; Peng, 1994).

If there was a prescription for "successful" control perceptions in middle age, it would most likely call for "balance." Balance, that is, between internal and external locus of control beliefs and between primary and secondary control strategies. Indeed, Jung and Erikson argued for the adaptiveness of a balanced, well-integrated self, which may not be achieved until midlife or later. In order to develop such a balanced self, individuals must accept and integrate the positive and negative aspects of themselves (see Ogilvie & Clark, 1992, for age differences in self-discrepancies). In parallel, to achieve a balanced mental state and attitude during midlife, when roles, goals, responsibilities, and stress tend to peak, individuals must believe in their own competence and effectiveness, yet also be aware of their limitations and the influences of outside factors. In fact, Krause and Stryker (1984) found that among middle-aged men, those who had *moderate* internal control beliefs coped most effectively with stress.

Clearly, there are, and will continue to be, differences in the sense of control in midlife, related to such factors as sex, race, income, education, culture, and cohort membership. In order to understand individuals' sense of control in middle adulthood, we must study their sense of control within the context of the entire lifespan, as well as within the social and historical context. Future research should include longitudinal studies of today's and tomorrow's adults, as their sense of control in midlife may differ in important ways from that of earlier cohorts of middle-agers who have been studied thus far.

ACKNOWLEDGMENTS

Preparation of this chapter was supported in part by Grant T32AG00204 from the National Institute on Aging and by the John D. and Catherine T. MacArthur Research Network on Successful Midlife Development (Orville Gilbert Brim, Director).

REFERENCES

Abeles, R. P. (1991). Sense of control, quality of life, and frail older people. In J. E. Birren, D. E. Deutchman, J. Lubben, & J. Rowe (Eds.), *The concept and measurement of quality of life in the frail elderly* (pp. 297–314). New York: Academic Press.

Abramson, L. Y., Seligman, M. P., & Teasdale, J. D. (1978). Learned helplessness in humans: Critique and reformulation. *Journal of Abnormal Psychology, 87,* 49–74.

Andrisani, P. J. (1977). Internal–external attitudes, personal initiative, and the labor-market experience of black and white men. *Journal of Human Resources, 12,* 309–328.

Andrisani, P. J., & Nestel, G. (1976). Internal–external control as contributor to and outcome of work experience. *Journal of Applied Psychology, 61*(2), 156–165.

Averill, J. R. (1974). Personal control over aversive stimuli and its relationship to stress. *Psychological Bulletin, 80,* 286–303.

Baltes, M. M., & Baltes, P. B. (Eds.). (1986). *The psychology of control and aging.* Hillsdale, NJ: Erlbaum.

Bandura, A. (1977). Self-efficacy: Toward a unified theory of behavioral change. *Psychological Review, 84,* 191–215.

Bandura, A. (1992). Exercise of personal agency through the self-efficacy mechanism. In R. Schwarzer (Ed.), *Self-efficacy: Thought control of action* (pp. 3–38). Washington, DC: Hemisphere Publishing Corporation.

Barrell, R. P., DeWolfe, A. S., & Cumming, J. W. (1966). Personnel attitudes and patients' attitudes to hospitalization for physical illness. *Journal of Psychology, 65,* 253–260.

Battle, E., & Rotter, J. (1963). Children's feelings of personal control as related to social class and ethnic group. *Journal of Personality, 31,* 482–490.

Bishop, R. C., & Solomon, E. (1989). Sex differences in career development: Locus of control and career commitment effects. *Psychological Reports, 65*(1), 107–114.

Bradley, R. E., & Webb, R. (1976). Age-related differences in locus of control orientation in three behavior domains. *Human Development, 19,* 49–55.

Brandtstadter, J., & Renner, G. (1990). Tenacious goal pursuit and flexible goal adjustment: Explication and age-related analysis of assimilative and accommodative strategies of coping. *Psychology and Aging, 5,* 58–67.

Brandtstadter, J., & Rothermund, K. (1994). Self-percepts of control in middle and later adulthood: Buffering losses by rescaling goals. *Psychology and Aging, 9*(2), 265–273.

Brandtstadter, J., Wentura, D., & Greve, W. (1993). Adaptive resources of the aging self: Outlines of an emergent perspective. Special Issue: Planning and control processes across the life span. *International Journal of Behavioral Development, 16*(2), 323–349.

Brim, O. G., Jr. (1974, September). *The sense of personal control over one's life.* Paper presented at the meeting of the American Psychological Association, New Orleans, LA.

Brim, O. G., Jr. (1992). *Ambition: How we manage success and failure throughout our lives.* New York: Basic Books.

Brown, B. R., & Granick, S. (1980, November). *Cognitive and psychosocial differences between I and E locus of control aged persons.* Paper presented at the meeting of the Gerontological Society of America, San Diego, CA.

Burack, O. R., & Lachman, M. E. (1994). *Planning and well-being across adulthood.* Unpublished manuscript, Brandeis University, Waltham, MA.

Burger, J. M. (1992). *Desire for control: Personality, social, and clinical perspectives.* New York: Plenum Press.

Burger, J. M., Brown, R., & Allen, C. K. (1983). Negative reactions to personal control. *Journal of Social and Clinical Psychology, 1,* 322–342.

Chebat, J. C. (1986). Social responsibility, locus of control, and social class. *Journal of Social Psychology, 126*(4), 559–561.

Cicerelli, V. G. (1980). Relationship of family background variable to locus of control in the elderly. *Journal of Gerontology, 35,* 108–114.

Clark, M. D., & Lachman, M. E. (1994, August). *Goals and perceived control: Age differences and domain effects.* Poster presented at the meeting of the American Psychological Association, Los Angeles, CA.

Clark, M. D., & Ogilvie, D. M. (1993, April). Multidimensional and domain specific experiences of being "in control" and "not in control" in young adult males and females. Paper presented at the meeting of the Eastern Psychological Association, Arlington, VA.

Connell, J. P. (1985). A new multidimensional measure of children's perceptions of control. *Child Development, 56,* 1018–1041.

Cornelius, S. W., & Caspi, A. (1986). Self-perceptions of intellectual control and aging. *Educational Gerontology, 12*(4), 345–357.

Cowles, M., Darling, M., & Skanes, A. (1992). Some characteristics of the simulated self. *Personality and Individual Differences, 13*(5), 501–510.

Crohan, S. E., Antonucci, T. C., Adelmann, P. K., & Coleman, L. M. (1989). Job characteristics and well-being at midlife: Ethnic and gender comparisons. *Psychology of Women Quarterly, 13*(2), 223–235.

Cromwell, R. L., Butterfield, Z. C., Brayfield, F. M., & Curry, J. J. (1977). *Acute myocardial infarction: Reaction and recovery.* St. Louis, MO: Mosby.

DeBrabander, B., & Boone, C. (1990). Sex differences in perceived locus of control. *Journal of Social Psychology, 130*(2), 271–272.

Easterlin, R. A. (1980). *Birth and fortune: The impact of numbers on personal welfare.* New York: Basic Books.

Easterlin, R. A., Macdonald, C., & Macunovich, D. J. (1990a). How have American baby boomers fared? Earnings and economic well-being of young adults, 1964–1987. *Journal of Population Economics, 3,* 277–290.

Easterlin, R. A., Macdonald, C., & Macunovich, D. J. (1990b). Retirement prospects of the Baby Boom generation: A different perspective. *The Gerontologist, 30*(6), 776–783.

Easterlin, R. A., Schaeffer, C. M., & Macunovich, D. J. (1993). Will the Baby Boomers be less well off than their parents? Income, wealth, and family circumstances over the life cycle in the United States. *Population and Development Review, 19*(3), 497–522.

Erikson, E. H. (1950). *Childhood and society.* New York: Norton.

Evans, G. W., & Lewis, M. A. (1990). The role of adaptive processes in intellectual functioning among older adults. In J. Rodin, C. Schooler, & K. W. Schaie (Eds.), *Self-directedness: Cause and effects throughout the life course* (pp. 183–197). Hillsdale, NJ: Erlbaum.

Felton, B., & Kahana, E. (1974). Adjustment and situationally-bound locus of control among institutionalized aged. *Journal of Gerontology, 29,* 295–301.

Fisher, S. (1967). Motivation for patient delay. *Archives of General Psychiatry, 16,* 676–678.

Foner, A. (1990). Social constraints on self-directedness over the life-course. In J. Rodin, C. Schooler, & K. W. Schaie (Eds.), *Self-directedness: Cause and effects throughout the life course* (pp. 95–102). Hillsdale, NJ: Erlbaum.

Franklin, R. D. (1963). Youth's expectancies about internal versus external control of reinforcement related to N variables. *Dissertation Abstracts, 24,* 1684.

Gallup, G., Jr., & Newport, F. (1991, April). Gallup mirror of America survey. *The Gallup Poll Monthly.*

Gatz, M., & Karel, M. J. (1993). Individual change in perceived control over 20 years. Special Issue: Planning and control processes across the life span. *International Journal of Behavioral Development, 16*(2), 305–322.

Gatz, M., & Siegler, I. C. (1981, August). Locus of control: A retrospective. Paper presented at the American Psychological Association Convention, Los Angeles, CA.

Gergen, M. (1989). Loss of control among the aging? A critical reconstruction. In P. S. Fry (Ed.), *Psychological perspectives of helplessness and control in the elderly* (pp. 261–290). Amsterdam: North-Holland.

Glass, D. C. (1977). Behavior patterns, stress, and coronary disease. Hillsdale, NJ: Erlbaum.

Gorman, B. S. (1968). An observation of altered locus of control following political disappointment. *Psychological Reports, 23,* 1094.

Gurin, P., & Brim, O. G., Jr. (1984). Change in self in adulthood: The example of sense of control. In P. B. Baltes & O. G. Brim, Jr. (Eds.), *Life-span development and behavior* (Vol. 6, pp. 281–322). New York: Academic Press.

Hamburg, B. A. (1980). Early adolescence as a life stress. In S. Levine & H. Ursin (Eds.), *Coping and health.* New York: Plenum Press.

Hammerschag, C. A., Fisher, S., & DeCosse, J. (1964). Breast symptoms and patient delay: Psychological variables involved. *Cancer, 17,* 1480–1485.

Hauser, P. M. (1980). Our anguished youth: Baby boom under stress. *Adolescent Psychiatry, 8,* 270–280.

Heckhausen, J. (1992). Adults' expectancies about development and its controllability: Enhancing self-efficacy by social comparison. In R. Schwarzer (Ed.), *Self-efficacy: Thought control of action* (pp. 107–145). Washington, DC: Hemisphere Publishing Corp.

Heckhausen, J., & Schulz, R. (1993). Optimisation by selection and compensation: Balancing primary and secondary control in life span development. Special Issue: Planning and control processes across the lifespan. *International Journal of Behavioral Development, 16*(2), 287–303.

Heise, D. R. (1990). Careers, career trajectories, and the self. In J. Rodin, C. Schooler, & K. W. Schaie (Eds.), *Self-directedness: Cause and effects throughout the life course* (pp. 59–84). Hillsdale, NJ: Erlbaum.

Hill, D. J., & Bale, R. M. (1981). Measuring beliefs about where psychological pain originates and who is responsible for its alleviation: Two new scales for clinical researchers. In H. M. Lefcourt (Ed.), *Research with the locus of control construct (Vol. 1): Assessment methods* (pp. 281–320). New York: Academic Press.

Howard, A., and Bray, D. W. (1988). *Managerial lives in transition: Advancing age and changing times.* New York: The Guilford Press.

Huyck, M. H. (1991). Predicates of personal control among middle-aged and young-old men and women in middle America. *International Journal of Human Development, 32*(4), 261–275.

Jensen, L., Olsen, J., & Hughes, C. (1990). Association of country, sex, social class, and life cycle to locus of control in western European countries. *Psychological Reports, 67*(1), 199–205.

Jerusalem, M., & Schwarzer, R. (1992). Self-efficacy as a resource factor in stress appraisal processes. In R. Schwarzer (Ed.), *Self-efficacy: Thought control of action* (pp. 195–213). Washington, DC: Hemisphere Publishing Corporation.

Kennedy, J. F. (1963). President John F. Kennedy, Address before the General Assembly of the United Nations, New York, September 20, 1963. *Public Papers of the Presidents of the United States: JFK, 1963,* p. 696.

Kessler, R. C., Foster, C., Webster, P. S., & House, J. S. (1992). The relationship between age and depressive symptoms in two national surveys. *Psychology and Aging, 7*(1), 119–126.

Kettle, J. (1981). The big generation: What's ahead for baby boomers? *Futurist,* p. 3.

Kivett, V. R., Watson, J. A., & Busch, J. C. (1977). The relative importance of physical psychological and social variables to locus of control orientation in middle age. *Journal of Gerontology, 32*(2), 203–210.

Klerman, G. L. (1976). Age and clinical depression: Today's youth in the twenty-first century. *Journal of Gerontology, 31*(3), 318–323.

Krause, N., & Stryker, S. (1984). Stress and well-being: The buffering role of locus of control beliefs. *Social Science and Medicine, 18*(9), 783–790.

Lachman, M. E. (1983). Perceptions of intellectual aging: Antecedent or consequence of intellectual functioning? *Developmental Psychology, 19,* 482–498.

Lachman, M. E. (1985). Personal efficacy in middle and old age: Differential and normative patterns of change. In G. H. Elder, Jr. (Ed.), *Life-course dynamics: Trajectories and transitions, 1968–1985.* Ithaca, NY: Cornell University Press.

Lachman, M. E. (1986). Personal control in later life: Stability, change, and cognitive correlates. In M. M. Baltes & P. B. Baltes (Eds.), *The psychology of control and aging* (pp. 207–236). Hillsdale, NJ: Erlbaum.

Lachman, M. E. (1991). Perceived control over memory aging: Developmental and intervention perspectives. *Journal of Social Issues, 47*(4), 159–175.

Lachman, M. E., Baltes, P. B., Nesselroade, J. R., & Willis, S. L. (1982). Examination of personality-ability relationships in the elderly: The role of the contextual (interface) assessment mode. *Journal of Research in Personality, 16,* 485–501.

Lachman, M. E., & Burack, O. R. (1993). Planning and control processes across the life span: An overview. Special Issue: Planning and control processes across the life span. *International Journal of Behavioral Development, 16*(2), 131–143.

Lachman, M. E., Lewkowicz, C., Marcus, A., & Peng, Y. (1994). Images of midlife development by young, middle-aged, and elderly adults. *Journal of Adult Development, 1,* 201–211.

Lachman, M. E., Ziff, M., and Spiro, A. (1994). Maintaining a sense of control in later life. In R. Abeles, H. Gift, & M. Ory (Eds.), *Aging and quality of life* (pp. 116–132). New York: Sage.

Langer, E. J. (1975). The illusion of control. *Journal of Personality and Social Psychology, 32,* 311–328.

Langer, E. J., Janis, I. L., & Wolfer, J. H. (1975). Reduction of psychological stress in surgical patients. *Journal of Experimental Social Psychology, 11,* 155–165.

Langer, E. J., & Roth, J. (1975). Heads I win, tails it's chance: The illusion of control as a function of the sequence of outcomes in a purely chance task. *Journal of Personality and Social Psychology, 32,* 951–955.

Lao, R. C. (1974, September). The developmental trend of the locus of control. Paper presented at the meetings of the American Psychological Association, New Orleans, LA.

Lefcourt, H. M. (1976). *Locus of control: Current trends in theory and research.* Hillsdale, NJ: Erlbaum.

Lefcourt, H. M. (1981). *Research with the locus of control construct (Vol. 1): Assessment methods.* New York: Academic Press.

Lefcourt, H. M. (1982). *Locus of control: Current trends in theory and research* (2nd ed.). Hillsdale, NJ: Erlbaum.

Levenson, H. (1974). Activism and powerful others: Distinctions within the concept of internal–external control. *Journal of Personality Assessment, 38,* 377–383.

Levenson, H. (1981). Differentiating among internality, powerful others, and chance. In H. M. Lefcourt (Ed.), *Research with the locus of control construct (Vol. 1): Assessment methods* (pp. 15–63). New York: Academic Press.

Levinson, D. J. (1978). *The seasons of a man's life.* New York: Knopf.

Light, P. C. (1988). *Baby boomers.* New York: W. W. Norton & Company.

Markus, H., Cross, S., & Wurf, E. (1988). The role of the self-system in competence. In J. Kolligan, Jr. & R. J. Sternberg (Eds.), *Competence considered: Perceptions of competence across the life span.* New Haven, CT: Yale University Press.

Markus, H., and Kitayama, S. (1991). Culture and the self: Implications for cognition, emotion, and motivation. *Psychological Review, 98*(2), 224–253.

McArthur, L. A. (1970). Luck is alive and well in New Haven. *Journal of Personality and Social Psychology, 16,* 316–318.

Miller, S. M., & Mangan, C. E. (1983). Interacting effects of information and coping style in adapting to gynecologic stress: Should the doctor tell all? *Journal of Personality and Social Psychology, 45*(1), 223–236.

Mirowsky, J., & Ross, C. E. (1992). Age and depression. *Journal of Health and Social Behavior, 33*(3), 187–205.

Monty, R., & Perlmuter, L. (1975). Persistence of the effects of choice on paired-associate learning. *Memory and Cognition, 3,* 183–187.

Nehrke, M. F., Hulicka, I. M., & Morganti, J. B. (1980). Age differences in life satisfaction, locus of control, and self-concept. *International Journal of Aging and Human Development, 11,* 25–33.

Neugarten, B. L. (1968). *Middle age and aging: A reader in social psychology.* Chicago: University of Chicago Press.

Nigro, G. (1987). Increase in external control belief in the Italian population. *Psychological Reports, 60*(1), 11–14.

Ogilvie, D. M. (1987). Life satisfaction and identity structure in late middle-aged men and women. *Psychology and Aging, 2*(3), 27–224.

Ogilvie, D. M., & Clark, M. D. (1992). The best and worst of it: Age and sex differences in self-discrepancy research. In R. P. Lipka & J. M. Brinthaupt (Eds.), *Self-perspectives across the life span* (pp. 186–222). New York: SUNY Press.

Parris Stephens, M. A., Franks, M. M., & Townsend, A. L. (1994). Stress and rewards in women's multiple roles: The case of women in the middle. *Psychology and Aging, 9*(11), 45–52.

Peck, R. C. (1968). Psychological developments in the second half of life. In B. L. Neugarten (Ed.), *Middle age and aging: A reader in social psychology* (pp. 88–92). Chicago: University of Chicago Press.

Peng, Y. (1994). *Primary and secondary control in American and Chinese-American adults: Cross-cultural and life-span developmental perspectives.* Unpublished doctoral dissertation, Brandeis University, Waltham, MA.

Perlmuter, L., Monty, R. A., & Cross, P. M. (1974). Choice as a disruptor of performance in paired-associate learning. *Journal of Experimental Psychology, 102,* 170–172.

Piper, A. I., & Langer, E. J. (1986). Aging and mindful control. In M. M. Baltes & P. B. Baltes (Eds.), *The psychology of control and aging* (pp. 71–90). Hillsdale, NJ: Erlbaum.

Reid, D. W., & Stirling, G. (1989). Cognitive social learning theory of control and aging, participatory control and the well-being of elderly persons. In P. S. Fry (Ed.), *Psychological perspectives of helplessness and control in the elderly* (pp. 217–258). Amsterdam: North-Holland.

Reid, D. W., & Ziegler, M. (1981). The desired control measure and adjustment among the elderly. In H. M. Lefcourt (Ed.), *Research with the locus of control construct (Volume 1): Assessment methods* (pp. 127–160). New York: Academic Press.

Remondet, J. H., & Hansson, R. O. (1991). Job-related threats to control among older employees. *Journal of Social Issues, 47*(4), 129–141.

Rodin, J. (1980). Managing the stress of aging: The role of control and coping. In S. Levine & H. Ursin (Eds.), *NATO Conference on coping and health.* New York: Academic Press.

Rodin, J. (1986). Health, control, and aging. In M. M. Baltes & P. B. Baltes (Eds.), *The psychology of control and aging* (pp. 139–165). Hillsdale, NJ: Erlbaum.

Rodin, J. (1987). Personal control through the life course. In R. Abeles (Ed.), *Implications of the life-span perspective for social psychology* (pp. 103–120). Hillsdale, NJ: Erlbaum.

Rodin, J. (1989). Sense of control: Potentials for intervention. *The Annals of the American Academy of Political and Social Sciences, 503,* 29–42.

Rodin, J. (1990). Control by any other name: Definitions, concepts, and processes. In J. Rodin, C. Schooler, & K. W. Schaie (Eds.), *Self-directedness: Cause and effects throughout the life course* (pp. 1–17). Hillsdale, NJ: Erlbaum.

Rotter, J. B. (1966). Generalized expectancies for internal versus external control of reinforcement. *Psychological Monographs, 80* (1, Whole No. 609).

Rotter, J. B. (1975). Some problems and misconceptions related to the construct of internal versus external control of reinforcement. *Journal of Consulting and Clinical Psychology, 43,* 56–67.

Russell, C. (1987). *One hundred predictions for the baby boom: The next 50 years.* New York: Plenum Press.

Ryckman, R. M., & Malikiosi, M. (1975). Relationship between locus of control and chronological age. *Psychological Reports, 36,* 655–658.

Ryff, C. D. (1989). In the eye of the beholder: Views of psychological well-being among middle-aged and older adults. *Psychology and Aging, 4*(2), 195–210.

Saltz, C., & Magruder-Habib, K. (1982, November). Age as an indicator of depression and locus of control among non-psychiatric inpatients. Paper presented at the meeting of the Gerontological Society of America, Boston, MA.

Schmidt, R. W., Lamm, H., & Trommsdorf, G. (1978). Social class and sex as determinants of future orientation (time perspective) in adults. *European Journal of Social Psychology, 8*(1), 71–90.

Scholnick, E. K., & Friedman, S. L. (1993). Planning in context: Developmental and situational considerations. Special Issue: Planning and control processes across the life span. *International Journal of Behavioral Development, 16*(2), 145–167.

Schulz, R., & Hanusa, B. H. (1978). Long-term effects of control and predictability-enhancing interventions: Findings and ethical issues. *Journal of Personality and Social Psychology, 36,* 1194–1201.

Seligman, M. E. P. (1975). *Helplessness: On depression, development, and death.* San Francisco, CA: Freeman.

Shannon, L. (1991). Is there a gender difference in locus of control: A meta-analysis. Poster presented at The Lives Through Time: Assessment and Theory in Personality Psychology Conference, Palm Springs, CA.

Siegler, I. C., & Gatz, M. (1985). Age patterns in locus of control. In E. Palmore, E. W. Busse, G. L. Maddox, J. B. Nowlin, & I. C. Siegler (Eds.), *Normal aging III* (pp. 259–267). Durham, NC: Duke University Press.

Simon, A. F., & Ogilvie, D. M. (1992). *Age, gender, and personal projects: A comparison of college students and middle-aged adults.* Unpublished manuscript, Rutgers University, New Brunswick, NJ.

Skinner, E., Chapman, M., & Baltes, P. B. (1982). *The causality, agency, and control interview.* Max Planck Institute for Human Development and Education, Berlin, West Germany.

Skinner, E. A., & Connell, J. P. (1986). Control understanding: Suggestions for a developmental framework. In M. M. Baltes & P. B. Baltes (Eds.), *The psychology of control and aging* (pp. 35–69). Hillsdale, NJ: Erlbaum.

Snyder, C. R., & Higgins, R. L. (1988). Excuses: Their effective role in the negotiation of reality. *Psychological Bulletin, 104*(1), 23–25.

Staats, S. (1974). Internal versus external locus of control for three age groups. *International Journal of Aging and Human Development, 5,* 7–10.

Stotland, E., & Blumenthal, A. (1964). The reduction of anxiety as a result of the expectation of making a choice. *Canadian Journal of Psychology, 18,* 139–145.

Strickland, B. R. (1989). Internal–external control expectancies: From contingency to creativity. Presidential Address in *American Psychologist, 44*(1), 1–12.

Strickland, B. R., & Shaffer, S. (1971). IE, IE & F. *Journal for The Scientific Study of Religion, 10,* 366–369.

Tashakkori, A., & Thompson, V. D. (1991). Race differences in self-perception and locus of control during adolescence and early adulthood: Methodological implications. *Genetic, Social, and General Psychology Monographs, 117*(2), 133–152.

Taylor, S. E. (1983). Adjustment to threatening events. *American Psychologist, 38,* 1161–1173.

Taylor, S. E., Helgeson, V. S., Reed, G. M., & Skokan, L. A. (1991). Self-generated feelings of control and adjustment to physical illness. *Journal of Social Issues, 47*(4), 91–109.

Thompson, S. C., Cheek, P. R., & Graham, M. A. (1988). The other side of perceived control: Disadvantages and negative effects. In S. Spacapan & S. Oskamp (Eds.), *The social psychology of health* (pp. 69–93). Newbury Park, CA: Sage.

Wallston, K. A., & Wallston, B. S. (1981). Health locus of control scales. In H. M. Lefcourt (Ed.), *Research with the locus of control construct (Volume 1): Assessment methods* (pp. 189–243). New York: Academic Press.

Weber, M. (1930). *The Protestant ethic and the spirit of captialism.* London: Unwin University Press.

Weisz, J. R., Rothbaum, F. M., & Blackburn, T. C. (1984). Standing out and standing in: The psychology of control in America and Japan. *American Psychologist, 39,* 955–969.

White, R. W. (1959). Motivation reconsidered: The concept of competence. *Psychological Review, 66,* 297–333.

Wolk, S., & Kurtz, J. (1975). Positive adjustment and involvement during age and expectancy for internal control. *Journal of Consulting and Clinical Psychology, 43,* 173–178.

CHAPTER 9

Gender Roles and Gender Identity in Midlife

Margaret Hellie Huyck

Institute of Psychology, Illinois Institute of Technology, Chicago, Illinois

In this chapter we address the question, Do men and women have different experiences during midlife? This is a complex question. This overview examines several key issues: (1) How have sex and gender been conceptualized and used as research variables in psychology and adult development? (2) What evidence is there that social and/or personal conceptualizations of gender shape the behaviors of most interest during midlife? (3) What models are useful in understanding gender differences during midlife? (4) What are the implications of our research base for research, social policy, and personal life planning?

APPROACHES TO THE STUDY OF GENDER

Some clarification in terms is necessary. *Sex* refers to the biogenetic differentiation between males and females. *Gender* refers to the social and psychological dimensions of sex. *Gender role* is used to describe the social prescriptions or stereotypes associated with each sex; it may also be used to describe the extent to which a particular individual complies with the social expectations. *Gender schema* includes all of one's beliefs about attributes of males and females and how these attributes are related.

Gender identity refers to the ways an individual defines herself or himself in terms of femininity and masculinity; this is the more personal, private sense of oneself in terms of a body self and how one relates to the gender role expectations. Readers should be aware that the use of these and related terms (e.g., sex role, sex role identity) is variable across historical time and researcher; the only reasonable stance is to note carefully the definition of these basic terms for each researcher, theorist, or advocate.

Psychologists have become sensitized to the ways in which research on gender and age often have involved biased assumptions and methods (Denmark, Russo, Frieze, & Sechzer, 1988; Schaie, 1988). Thus, any summary assessment of the kinds of gender differences evident in middle adulthood must be viewed cautiously. The patterns of differences described below are selective and suggestive; a major challenge is to enhance the research base to assess the extent and importance of age–gender interactions in the areas summarized: social stereotypes, gender identity, and behavior. In order to assess the impact of gender on behavior, we must look at data across cultures and across times; otherwise it is too easy to misattribute gender differences to features of a particular place or time. Models used to account for the observed patterns will be assessed, with emphasis on evaluating the Parental Imperative hypothesis of midlife gender shifts.

SOCIAL STEREOTYPES, GENDER IDENTITY, AND BEHAVIOR

Social Stereotypes and Gender Schema

Many psychologists argue that gender is one of the primary categories that people use to understand and think about the social world (Cross & Marcus, 1993). Gender is one of the first social categories acquired by children; by age 2½ children can differentiate boys from girls, even when they are dressed alike, and their play behaviors vary in same-sex and mixed-sex dyads (Cross & Marcus, 1993). Gender stereotypes are apparently learned very early and persist into adulthood.

Best and Williams (1993) have examined gender schemas among college students from 25 countries in North and South America, Europe, and Asia. They found substantial similarity across cultures in traits associated with each sex. In all countries the male-stereotype items were more active and stronger and the female-stereotype items were more passive and weaker. The researchers also scored the traits in terms of 15 psychological needs (as derived from Murray's theory of human behavior); 12 of the needs were clearly associated with one gender group or the other. Across countries men were described as concerned with dominance, autonomy, aggression, exhibition, achievement, and endurance; and women were described in terms of abasement, deference, succorance, nurturance, affiliation, and heterosexuality.

Although the evidence of stereotyping is very consistent, there is some variability. The stereotypes were stronger in countries that were socioeconomically less developed, where literacy was low, and the percentage of women attending the university was low. Interestingly, the male stereotype was favored in some countries (e.g., Japan, South Africa, Nigeria) and the female stereotype in others (e.g., Italy, Peru, Australia). The United States respondents viewed female stereotypes as somewhat more favorable than male ones.

Michael Kimmel (1996) argued that ideals for American manhood have shifted from an emphasis on the "self-made man" to a focus on muscles, money, or conformity. He also described a contemporary "crisis" in masculinity, wherein many men no longer feel adequately masculine.

There is also evidence that some of the social stereotypes about gender are sensitive to age. David Gutmann (1994) has documented evidence from a wide range of cultures in which older men are seen as peacemakers rather than warriors, and as more susceptible to yielding to passive comforts rather than delighting in risk taking; the middle years are seen as a period of transition and reworking the masculine style of youth. Women are also described as changing, from yielding, accommodating young women to women noted for greater assertiveness and control; stereotypes include benevolent ("grannies") and dangerous ("witches") versions of this more powerful, older woman.

Gender Identity: Feminine, Masculine, and Mixed

At the same time that one is learning social stereotypes of gender, one is also developing a sense of what it means to be male or female in a particular setting. Beliefs and expectations are embedded in each subculture, often defined by social class and ethnicity. Furthermore, each family system provides early basic images of what it means to be female or male, and how the genders relate to each other. Knowledge from all these sources is combined to form individual gender schemas (Huyck, 1994). The individual gender schemas are drawn upon to create a sense of gender self-concept, or how one's own characteristics fit into the social, subcultural, and familial gender norms.

Best and Williams (1993) examined ideal and actual self concepts of young women and men in 14 countries. They found that men felt more masculine than did women and that both men and women wished they were more masculine. The gender social stereotypes were not always reflected in strong gender differences in self-concept; that is, even when students could articulate gender stereotypes, they did not necessarily apply the stereotypes to themselves. Stereotypes become less powerful in governing behavior during the middle years. A substantial body of research has documented that midlife men and women are less likely to describe themselves in gender-stereotyped terms than are young adults; these patterns are evident when presented with self-report standardized measures of masculinity and femininity (e.g., Sinnot, 1986) and in free-response descriptions.

Gender identity has been explored among middle-aged parents and their young adult children in a study designed to assess both family similarities and possible cohort or generational differences (Huyck, 1996). The participants were drawn from caucasian American families living in midwestern "Parkville" in the early 1980s. When they were interviewed, the middle-aged women ($n = 131$) and men ($n = 107$) were aged 43–70; their children were 21 to 31. The older children will soon be entering midlife. Their concepts of themselves as masculine and feminine were explored in several ways. All the respondents responded to questions about how they defined masculinity and femininity and how they felt about themselves in terms of their own definitions of gender; and each person completed a standardized test (the PRF-Andro), which included Masculinity and Femininity Scales (Berzins, Welling, & Wetter, 1978).

The interviews reflected both changing social norms regarding gender roles and personal developmental changes. Although most could easily describe general differences between men and women, many showed some ambivalence about how consistent they thought the differences were. Responses to questions about the ways in which they were masculine (for men) or feminine (for women) were coded for the major gender-congruent style. Among the men, three major styles of masculinity were evident. The styles, along with the percent, of the middle-aged men who described themselves in terms of that style, were labeled Macho (28%), Family Man/Good Provider (47%), and Leader (26%). The women described three comparable styles of femininity: the Femme (52%), the Family Woman (23%), and the Nurturer (30%). Virtually all of the middle-aged men described themselves as masculine and virtually all the middle-aged women described themselves as feminine. A few (5% of the men and 4% of the women) said that although they were able to "pass" as appropriately masculine or feminine when the occasion demanded, they felt that they were just presenting a facade (this style was labeled Facade).

In addition, over half of the sample described ways in which they went beyond their own gender standards; the variety of these responses was even more impressive than for the gender-congruent responses. Some of these responses reflected gender expansion options. About 17% of the midlife men and 26% of the women described what we called Activity Androgyny, such as women who said they were not so feminine because they liked to paint and hang wallpaper, were better carpenters than husbands or sons, or liked sports; and men who said they were not so masculine because they didn't watch football, liked to work in the kitchen, or liked to grow flowers. About 30% of the men and 28% of the women reported Inner Androgyny themes; these included women who did not rely on men as much as they felt they were expected to, or were outspoken and critical; and men who felt they were in touch with their emotions and sensitive to the needs of others. Some of the responses were coded as gender compromised; 19% of the men reported Diminished

Masculinity ("I'm not as strong as I used to be," "I give in to my wife to keep the peace") and 15% of the women reported Diminished Femininity ("I've gotten too fat," "I no longer paint my nails"). Notably, a third (35% of men and 33% of women) denied that there was any way in which they were not masculine/ feminine.

These results lend support to models that describe acceptance of gender bimodality or androgyny in midlife, and provide many examples of the variety of ways in which an individual may move into "androgyny." Acknowledging that one has characteristics associated with the other gender is often a source of pride and pleasure; it may also be a source of embarrassment and shame. It is important to understand more about the factors that contribute to such different responses.

Several analyses with the Parkville midlife sample have been designed to explore the ways in which gender self-concept is linked to mental health. One set of analyses (Huyck, 1991a) included the 149 women and 127 men who completed self-report measures of gender-linked self-attributions (the PRF-Andro), self-esteem (Rosenberg), sense of mastery, and psychosomatic symptom distress (the SCL-90); these measures were collected prior to the personal interviews. Factor analyses revealed three major factors in the masculinity and three in the femininity scales. Factor scores were significantly related to sex and occupational status; some factor scores were associated with age. Mental health measures were related to the gender factors, with distinctive relationships for each group defined by sex, occupational status, and age. Gender-linked attributions were most predictive of mental health measures among older (55+), upper-status, "gender-sensitive" men. It was also clear that one factor was most important for men: men who admitted (on the self-report questionnaire) that they felt dependent on their wife were especially likely to have lower self-esteem, less sense of mastery, and higher psychosomatic distress scores. The older, upper-status women seemed most "gender transcendent," as none of the gender factor scores significantly predicted their mental health scores.

The second set of analyses have explored the factors that differentiate men who are "gender sensitive"—who respond with great distress to changes they perceive in themselves or in their wives in terms of gender-linked characteristics. A systematic analysis of the middle-aged men (Gutmann & Huyck, 1994) compared men who acknowledge their own femininity and are either comfortable with it or troubled by it. In part, their comfort depends on their wife: more passive men whose wives are benign or unaggressive toward them are asymptomatic; those who wives are openly assertive in the marriage are more likely to show distress symptoms. In addition, responses reflected the past, or what might be considered their early gender schemas. The men who were most troubled by their own emerging femininity and by their wives' increased assertiveness remembered their own father as weak or absent and their mother as strong; they felt tied to the strong mother, but guilty about the father and terrified that the same fate might befall them. Those who did not show symptoms of distress had internalized images of both parents as affectionate with each other (and with the son) but emotionally self-sufficient and strong in their distinctive ways. Such men were not frightened by the emergence of femininity in themselves, and they were able to tolerate more assertiveness in their wives.

A case-based analysis of the middle-aged women (Huyck, 1994) reveals similar themes. Women are responding in part to their own gender schemas, based in early family experiences as much as on cultural stereotypes, as they consider modifying their gender styles in midlife. In addition, they are responding to the realities of their contemporary situation; for midlife women, the crucial issue is whether their husband is ill. If he is ill, they feel required to continue a nurturing, accommodative mode, and to refrain from developing a more self-directed stance.

Possible differences between the generations were examined using both the PRF-Andro self-report scales and the interview ratings (Huyck, 1996). Young adults were compared with their own parents on all ten gender measures (two PRF scales and eight Gender Style ratings). Younger unmarried adult daughters differentiated themselves from their own mothers on eight of the ten gender measures; daughters who were over 26, married, and/or mothers did not differ from their own mothers on any of the gender measures. Unmarried young adult sons differentiated themselves from their own fathers by questioning their own masculinity in stereotypic terms, being more likely to define their masculinity as Macho and less likely to define it in terms of Family Man or Inner Androgyny, all of which suggest a more defensive posture of masculinity. Young men who had married were similar to their own fathers on nine of the ten gender measures, but they had higher PRF-Masculinity scores.

These analyses suggest that developmental effects (e.g., age, marriage, parenting) were more influential than generation or cohort in shaping gender styles. The results may reflect the difficulty that persons have in making substantial modifications in the gender schemas they presumably developed in the family in which they grew up. The interviews also contain many examples where both generations continue to socialize each other about gender. Middle-aged parents questioned their assumptions about gender in responses to seeing their daughters assume a professional career, or watching a son and daughter-in-law forge a more egalitarian parenting and householding arrangement. On the other hand, most of the parents felt intensely apprehensive about some of the changes, and worried either that their assertive, ambitious daughters would end up divorced or that their sons would not devote sufficient attention to career progress, and they continued to convey their concerns to their children.

Gender Impacts on Love and Intimacy in Midlife

Family and familylike relationships have always been marked both by reflections of social gender role expectations and by the opportunity to create nonstereotypic relationships based on the personal preferences of those involved. There are general patterns of gender differences in qualities prized in a marriage partner. Cross-culturally, women are less inclined toward having multiple sexual partners and more interested in older partners who have accumulated material and social resources; men are more inclined toward polygamy and promiscuity, and older men mate with women progressively more and more junior to them (Kendrick & Trost, 1993). In addition to these general patterns, behaviors may reflect the norms of a particular historical period, opportunities associated with a historical period or a particular location, or idiosyncratic desires. Behaviors may also change over the life course, with differing responsibilities and experiences or emerging desires. Here we examine gender influences in marriage and marital-like relationships, parenting, and filial care.

Heterosexual Marriage

Men are more likely than women to be married during their middle years; the gap is substantial among those aged 55–64, where 82.4% of the men and 69.3% of the women are still married. Marriage experiences differ by race. Among all adults over 18, 24.5% of white men and 17.2% of white women have never married; 36.0% of Hispanic men and 24.3% of Hispanic women have never married; and 42.1% of African-American men and 36.8% of African-American women have never married (U.S. Bureau of the Census, 1997). Black women are less likely than black men to be currently married and living with a spouse, a fact that reflects the increasingly unbalanced sex ratios after age 20; by age 40, there are approximately 120 black women for 100 black men (McAdoo, 1990).

Experience with divorce and remarriage also varies by gender and race. Most divorces still occur during young adulthood. Men are more likely to remarry, and to do so faster, than are women. During midlife, a greater proportion of divorced women have not remarried than is true for men; this is particularly true for black women.

Family systems can become very complex by midlife, particularly for "blended" families that may combine children from previous marriages with children from the current marriage. Thus, while many couples enter midlife with a marriage of 15–20 years duration and one or more adolescent children, other couples may be recovering from divorces and dealing with a small child. Men, particularly, may experience very different "ages" of themselves, as fathers of young adults from a first marriage and fathers of toddlers from a later union.

Many middle-aged couples emphasize role performance and the more instrumental aspects of the relationship, reflecting, in part, the substantial responsibilities in work, parenting, family care, and community leadership assumed by many persons during midlife. Most instrumental aspects of the relationship are gender typed, with some (but not much) evidence of lessened gender typing of household chores following retirement (Pleck, 1985). Maintaining a sex-linked division of labor within the family seems to be particularly valued by middle-aged husbands, compared to younger and older men and women, perhaps because sex-typed tasks serve to reaffirm gender identity.

Husbands and wives seem to have different perceptions of marriage (Huyck, 1995; Sheehy, 1998). Husbands typically report more marital satisfaction than do wives. Findings from qualitative studies of midlife marriage suggest that this gender difference might reflect the willingness of husbands to idealize the situation and deny existing tensions, as well as the wives' greater willingness to recognize problems and press for changes as children are launched. For example, Huyck and Gutmann (1992) conducted a study of 131 wives and 107 of their husbands, all living in Midwest "Parkville" (described earlier), who completed all phases of the study. All were in marriages of long duration (average 32 years). The families were relatively large, with an average of 4.4 children. Extensive personal interviews included questions about current perceptions of the marriage and how it had changed over time.

It was notable that the husbands and wives in the Parkville sample did not differ significantly on the self-report measure of marital satisfaction. However, there were substantial differences in the interviews. Nearly 40% of the wives were classified as Disappointed, because of the sense that their expectations of their husbands and of the marriage had not been fulfilled. The factors that contributed to their disappointment centered on: (1) inabilities of the husband to provide a standard of living that was deemed adequate to the couple; (2) a sense that the husband had been revealed as "dependent" and needing care, rather than the strong protector/provider idealized at the beginning of the marriage; (3) dismay over what was perceived as the husband's passivity and disinterest in exploring the wider world, at the point when the wives were clearly desiring release from domestic responsibilities; and (4) unwillingness to explore the possibilities of change in the relationship and in themselves. No similar themes of disappointment were evident in the husbands' interviews, though some husbands acknowledged feeling inadequate to meet their wives' expectations.

Responses to questions about the marriage were also coded in terms of Marital Politics (MP), referring to the perceptions of each partner as to whom prevails and by what rationale, particularly when potential for conflict exists in the relationship.

Five patterns of marital politics were identified for the 131 wives: (1) Patriarchal, Conceding to Husband (22.1%); (2) Passive Management of Covert Anger (22.1%); (3) Ambivalent Overt Assertiveness (30.5%); (4) Unambivalent Overt Assertiveness (14.5%); and (5) Matriarchal Nurturance (10.7%). The MP of the wives were not related to their own educational or occupational status, though husbands who had higher status positions (executives, managers, or professionals) were more likely to have wives who conceded to their authority (e.g., 1 or 2). The wife's MP style was related to marital satisfaction; satisfaction was high for both partners when the wife saw her husband as in charge (1) or when she felt she was in charge (5); marital satisfaction was lowest, not surprisingly, among couples where the wife was unambivalently assertive and challenging.

Nine different patterns were identified for the 107 husbands in the sample, each reflecting the ways in which they deal with issues of potential conflict and competing demands for resources in the marriage. The MP patterns included (1) Patriarchal (6.5%); (2) Patriarchal but under Pressure (11.2%); (3) Crisis (9.3); (4) Egalitarian (16.8%); (5) Separate Peace (4.7%); (6) Conceding Dominance Generally (19.6%); (7) Conceding Dominance because of His Ill Health (4.7%); (8) Conceding to a Domineering Wife (12.1); and (9) Nonconflictual Union (15.0%). The husband MP styles were not related to either his own or his wife's educational or occupational level, suggesting that the measures are not simply reflecting larger social status issues. Not surprisingly, satisfaction with the marital relationship varied with MP styles. The least satisfied husbands described relationships in which they were giving in to wives they perceived as domineering, or they had distanced from a troubled relationship and established a separate peace. Relatively high satisfaction was reported by men who had turned over the marital power to their wives but felt justified because of their own ill health, by men who experienced nonconflictual union, by men who resisted the pressure to change, or by men who described a differentiated but egalitarian relationship. Whether the husband is dominant, detached, or submissive, his marital satisfaction depends on the lack of conflict with his wife.

In order to assess the extent to which one might describe "their" marriage, the congruence between the MP styles of the wives and their husbands were examined. Although there was an overall moderately significant relationship ($\chi^2 = 44.4$, $p < .07$), there is also variability in their perceptions. It was clear that the persons describing the "same" marriage were conveying that relationship differently.

Same-Sex Relationships

Homosexual couples who are now middle-aged or older have been described as more likely to interact with their partners in ways that seem similar to gender-differentiated styles; such relationships seem modeled after heterosexual relationships prevalent in their age group, with a clear division of labor and one partner regarded as more dominant. In contrast, younger middle-aged partners in enduring homosexual relations tend to emphasize role flexibility, turn taking, and equity (Maracek, Finn, & Cardell, 1988). Some aspects of relationships seem linked to gender (Huyck, 1995). Many women who define themselves in middle and later life as lesbians have had prior experiences with marriage; one survey estimated that 25 to 30% of the lesbians had been married (Bell & Weinberg, 1978). Some authors suggest that middle-aged lesbians are advantaged compared to middle-aged heterosexual women because they are more likely to have a partner with whom they expect to grow old, to share the same life expectancy curve with their partner, to be less threatened by physical appearance changes, to have been employed and accumulated their own financial security, and to be involved in shared couple activities than are heterosexual couples or homosexual male couples. On the other hand, lesbian couples share experiences of growing up female and of devalued social status (Burch, 1987). Clinicians often report that heterosexual wives complain about loneliness, emotional distance, and lack of communication; lesbian partners are more likely to struggle with more intensity and sharing than is comfortable (Kirkpatrick, 1989).

Gay men who maintain long-term same-sex relationships are likely to live in proximity to other gay men who provide opportunities for contact and a supportive community. (Many men who have same-sex sexual relationships are also in heterosexual marriages; this was particularly true in the period when those who are now middle-aged were growing up.) Given a supportive homosexual community, long-term relationships can be sustained. Several studies revealed a generation gap whereby older gay men expect mentor/protege relationships marked by age and status discrepancies, and younger gay men prefer age-peers for partners (Dynes, 1990). One issue in age-discrepant relationships is making the transition from the youthful lover to the older sponsor, an issue likely to emerge in early midlife (Liebert, 1989).

Sexuality

It is clear that the most important factors affecting sexual patterns are gender and age. "Sexual scripts" involving fantasies and images of erotic arousal and gratification show gender differences early, and sexuality becomes a means of reaffirming gender identity (Marsiglio & Greer, 1994). Social images equate phallic erectness with sexual virility and powerful masculinity. Men are likely to feel demasculinized if they do not experience sexual desire and (to a somewhat lesser extent) sexual activity. In the past 30 years, there has been a shift to emphasize a man's sensitivity to the sexual needs of women; the "good man" is now expected to be a competent lover more than just a sexual animal. One consequence for middle-aged (and older) men has been increased concerns about potency and more performance anxiety (Marsiglio & Greer, 1994). Part of the concern also reflects the basic normal physiological changes in the sexual response cycle, with men showing significant changes in erectile capacity that become evident in midlife (Masters & Johnson, 1970). However, more problematic than the normal age-related changes are dysfunctions linked to health. Arthritis, prostate enlargement, and medication side effects are among the health problems that can affect sexual desire and responsivity. Such problems make midlife men very susceptible to promises of pharmacologic "renewal."

Women seem to have less difficulty with sexuality during the middle years. Women usually feel feminine even if they do not feel sexual desire and are not sexually active, though some women do link femininity with sexuality and some are very troubled by a loss of sexual partnership. Women's changes of lessened lubrication following menopause are relatively easy to compensate, and most retain the capacity to be orgasmic and multiorgasmic.

The general finding is that avowed interest in sex is quite stable throughout adulthood and old age, with men indicating stronger interest than women, on the average, and with individual differences maintained throughout life. When marital sexual relations cease, both husbands and wives agree that it is the husband who has lost interest or capability (Garza & Dressel, 1983). The minimal findings available for younger middle-aged homosexuals suggest that lesbian couples have less frequent sex than other types of couples. Gay male couples begin their relationships with the highest frequencies of sexual activity, which drops after a few years to a level lower than that of heterosexual couples in comparable-length relationships, but higher than that of lesbian couples (Blumstein & Schwartz, 1983).

Patterns of sexual activity outside the couple relationship also seem to vary. Some researchers suggest that among the younger and middle-aged gay male couples, sexual activities outside the relationship seem to be expected and tolerated (McWhirter & Mattson, 1984). Lesbian women tend to have emotionally involved outside affairs that are likely to break up the original couple (Nichols, 1987). Patterns among heterosexuals have changed over the past three decades. Younger cohorts of heterosexual men and women engage in sexual affairs in approximately equal proportions. Such affairs are likely to be kept secret and to be deeply disturbing to the relationship if disclosed. Among older middle-aged persons, men are more likely than women to have had extramarital affairs (Blumstein & Schwartz, 1983).

Mothers and Fathers

Reproductive specialization is the core reality of sexual dimorphism, and the one that underlies the socioevolutionary models of gender (Gutmann, 1994; Kendrick & Trost, 1993). The ending of reproductive potential, the menopause, is one of the hallmarks of middle age for women; in an evolutionary perspective, menopause is timed to allow the mother enough lifetime to nurture the youngest child to maturity. In fact, the ages at which women and men begin and end childbearing and childrearing, and the proportion of time and energy devoted to parenting, varies substantially across cultures, subcultures, and historical periods. Among contemporary Americans there is enough variability to make it difficult to describe gender patterns in parenting during the middle years.

By the time women are middle-aged, most have completed their childbearing. The highest birth rates remain between ages 20 and 29, though fertility rates are now almost as high between ages 30 and 34 (U.S. Bureau of the Census, 1997, Table 90, p. 75). The middle years for many women will be involved in launching children into adulthood and, perhaps, becoming grandparents. Those who have children during their teens may enter midlife as grandmothers, and enter old age as great-grandmothers; they are also more likely to be poor. Having a first child after age 30 is more common among women who have a graduate or professional degree and who have higher family incomes (U.S. Bureau of the Census, 1991, Table 103). Although there has been substantial media attention about "mature" (and even postmenopausal) motherhood, the rate is much lower after the age of 40: in 1994, from ages 20 to 24 the rate was 100.7 births/1000 women; between 40 and 44 the rate was only 9.6, and between 45 and 49 it was 0.3 (U.S. Bureau of the Census, 1997, Table 90).

Men prolong their reproductive period, but not substantially. The highest birth rate for fathers was among men aged 25–29 (116.4/1000); between age 40 and 44 the rate was 21.0, between 45 and 49 it was 7.5, between 50 and 54 it was 2.8, and after 55 it was 0.4. This indicates that men are more likely to be experiencing active fathering of small children during their middle years. Most of these are second families with a new, younger wife. The joys and terrors of such arrangements are the stuff of contemporary novels and television sitcoms.

However, to put it in perspective, cross-culturally a similar pattern is evident. Cross-culturally, polygamy is common: among 849 human cultures, 708 were polygynous, 137 were strictly monogamous, and only 4 were polyandrous (where one woman marries two or more men) (Kendrick & Trost, 1993); the contemporary pattern of serial monogamy is a compromise arrangement. The cross-cultural evidence also documents the tendency of women to be more interested in an older partner with more resources, whereas men across different cultures place more emphasis on physical attractiveness.

The experiences of mainstream parents during midlife have not been well documented, particularly compared with the research surrounding the early years of parenting. Many of the parents who are now middle-aged began their parenting with gender-differentiated responsibilities that reflected the reproductive realities (e.g., women are pregnant and can nurse), the social-structural realities (e.g., most men can earn more money and thus it seems wise to use their energy in work outside the household), and the gender schemas, which are brought into full flower with the advent of parenthood. Gutmann (1994) has described the responses of each parent to the obvious needs of a beloved, dependent child in terms of the Parental Responsibility. He argues that, cross-culturally, the standard arrangement is for mothers to be responsible for the emotional security of the child, and for fathers to be responsible for physical (and often economic) security. In order to meet these responsibilities, women must repress their own desires to be in charge, and men must repress their desires to be passive and dependent. Socialization begins early to instill these patterns in children. Gutmann also argues that as the demands of parenting phase out, as the child becomes able to care for itself, the parents can explore neglected aspects of themselves and (implicitly) evolve a new relationship. Thus, for those parents who remain together into the middle years, there is the option of reworking some of the earlier arrangements. The Parkville parents showed evidence of reworking the marital relationship. The question remains: Do fathers and mothers show persisting different approaches to parenting during midlife?

The middle-aged parents from Parkville (described earlier) were recruited into the study to describe parenting at their phase of life (Huyck, 1989). Respondents emphasized the ongoing importance of parenting, with most of the parents describing what they did in terms of providing advice and encouragement and maintaining a special interpersonal relationship with their young adult children. Compared to fathers, mothers were more involved in parenting, were more likely to provide nonfinancial assistance, and were more stressed by children who were inconsiderate or irresponsible about household chores. Whether or not children were living at home was not much related to whether the mother reported "limited" parenting, indicating that where the children live is not the primary issue in how the mothers feel about their parenting and about their children. The mothers indicated they had several bases for redefining mothering to a less-involved phase, either by the child moving out of the house or by assuming more adult responsibilities while living at home. Feelings about parenting were linked to self-esteem and sense of mastery for the younger (aged 45–53) mothers, but not for the older (aged 54–68) mothers. Responses to a self-report measure of Psychological Involvement in parenting showed that among the younger mothers, high involvement was associated with positive feelings about parenting, whereas high involvement was associated with negative feelings about parenting among the older mothers. This suggests that a shift from positive engagement to concern is measured by the same scale.

Fathers in Parkville were more likely to define their parenting in terms of providing financial assistance as needed, and providing backup help; they reported pleasures in launching children. Once children were out of the home, fathers reported less ongoing contact, advice, or encouragement; they seemed to be relieved of the burden of fathering. Their feelings about their parenting were not tied to self-esteem or sense of mastery; among older (57–70) fathers, negative feelings about their parenting were associated with more symptom distress.

Qualitative studies also suggest the ways in which parenting is redefined during the middle years. Many fathers report a mixture of pride and envy as they watch their sons grow to manhood and equal or excel them; fathers are confronted with visions of their own mortality, and their recollections of feelings experienced toward their own father when they were young adults. Themes of competitiveness are most likely to revolve around occupational achievements. Since many middle-aged men do not feel they have been as successful as they had anticipated or desired, a son represents both a "second chance" to succeed (vicariously), but also a threat that the father's inadequacy will be affirmed. Middle-aged mothers, also, confront complex feelings of pride and envy as they watch daughters become attractive, discover their sexuality (in an era that allows more information and choice), and plan their lives. Some of the women who are now in their later middle years are openly envious of the choices present for their daughters, and some feel that the daughter's options have been made possible by the mother's self-sacrifice. The happiest mothers at midlife are those who feel they have sacrificed the least—those who are married and have careers (Baruch, 1984).

These patterns suggest that the notion of a Parental Imperative is an apt one for parents like those in the Parkville sample and that mothers and fathers experience the imperative differently. Although the proportion of single middle-aged parents is rising, most midlife parenting is still done in the context of a couple.

Of course, some parents do not remain together and are not able to share parenting with a new partner; some had only a marginal relationship, or one where a stable partnership could not be established. Although some parents are working out joint parenting arrangements not reflected in household statistics, residency is one clue to parental responsibility. Women are more likely to have sustained parental responsibilities. Among households with a child under age 18 at home, 20% are headed by a mother aged 35–44, compared to 4% headed by a father. Gender differences are also evident at ages 45–54, narrowing among parents 55- to 64-years-old (U.S. Bureau of the Census, 1997, Table 80). Parental distancing is often linked to divorce, particularly when the father does not share custody and does not live close to his child.

Gender Patterns in Work: Paid and Unpaid

Employment and Economic Security

Gender differences persist in the likelihood that a man or woman will be in the paid labor force during the middle years, in the kinds of work available, and in compensation. In 1996, 92.4% of all men aged 35–44 were employed; these rates declined little by age 45–54 (89.1%), somewhat more during ages 55–64 (67.0%), and markedly after 65 (16.9%). Women were less likely to be employed than were men: 77.5% at ages 35–44, 75.4% at ages 45–54, 49.6% at ages 55–64, and only 8.6% after age 65 (U.S. Bureau of the Census, 1997, Table 620). It is important to note, however, that the labor force participation rates for women have increased substantially; for example, in 1970, only 54.4% of the women aged 45–54 were employed. The gender gap in employment rates among all those over 16-years-old is evident among Hispanic origin (79.6 vs. 53.4%), white (75.8 vs. 59.1%), and black (68.7 vs. 60.4%) groups, although the extent of the disparity varies. The gender gap has narrowed most in the black community: in 1970, 76.5% of the men and 49.5% of the women were in the labor force. The gender gap in employment rates is linked to marital status: among married persons aged 45–64, 83.2% of the men and 63.7% of the women are employed; among divorced, widowed, and separated persons that age, 73.1% of the men and 67.7% of the women are employed; and among single persons that age, 67.4% of the men and 68.5% of the women are employed.

Although many individuals are employed because they find their work fulfilling and personally satisfying, most are employed because they need to earn a living and gain access to benefits such as health care and retirement pensions. Unfortunately, the rewards for employment have been unequal for men and women. On average, middle-aged women (over 45) earn 67% of what men earn working full-time; midlife and older women employed part-time are paid 64–76% of men working part-time. The earnings gap between men and women is narrowest among the youngest workers, where women age 20 to 24 earn 95% as much as men in the same age group. The gap is higher for each successive age group of workers up to age 65 (Herz & Wootton, 1986). The gender gap in earnings is substantially greater among whites than among blacks or Hispanics, largely a reflection of the higher earnings of white men. Although more occupations are now gender neutral, persons who are now middle-aged have been operating in a labor market that has been substantially stratified by sex, race, and ethnicity.

Access to benefits associated with employment also varies by sex and family arrangement. One of the most crucial benefits is access to an employer-sponsored health care plan. Health care insurance in the United States is tied almost exclusively to full-time employment, and women are at a disadvantage because they are more likely to be employed part-time, or in service, sales, or clerical jobs where health benefits are unavailable (Older Women's League, 1992). Many women have insurance coverage as dependents of husbands whose coverage is obtained through an employer; many women lose insurance coverage when their marital status or their husband's employment status is altered. On the other hand, among never-married Americans aged 45–64, more men than women lack health insurance.

In addition to health insurance, pensions are an important benefit associated with employment. Pensions are less likely to be available to women than to men, and because they are pegged to earnings, they pay less. Currently, 46% of men and 26% of women over 65 receive a private pension; they receive a median pension benefit of $7800 and women receive a median pension income of $4200 (Older Women's League, 1998). Social Security is a mandated Federal Pension plan; benefits are based on a worker's average lifetime Social Security earnings. Women now receive lower average Social Security benefits because they have earned less money, have worked fewer hours, and have experienced more interruptions from paid work. Unless these realities change considerably, women's work patterns will continue to place them at a disadvantage in pension income (Older Women's League, 1998). By 2020, poverty among the elderly is likely to be confined primarily to women living alone. The implications for those who are now young and middle-aged are clear: plan ahead for economic resources sufficient to support the longer life expectancy of women.

Unpaid Family Work

In addition to the efforts that are recognized by the larger social system as "work" deserving of paid compensation, there is a great deal of effort expended in maintaining households and managing the affairs of daily life, caring for dependent children, and providing special care to persons who are unable to maintain themselves independently. The contributions of women and men to these two domains remains unequal, with women contributing substantially more of their time and energy to unpaid work than do men. The differences are very evident in midlife, somewhat less evident in late life, and may be changing a bit among the younger cohorts.

Housework

Women do more work at home than men do. This difference is probably most evident in what is described as "housework," which inclues all the tasks needed to maintain and manage a home as a setting for varied complex activities. There are several options for meeting the needs of home management: one partner does it all, the partners split the chores equally, they hire or assign others to do chores, or the chores and care remain undone. The focus in the past few decades has been on whether men/husbands would assume a greater proportion of householding or unpaid family care responsibilities. The evidence is that little such reallocation is evident, at least among those who are now middle-aged. The conclusion of one serious researcher into such matters is that "a person's sex continues to exert a powerful effect on the amount of family work performed" (Pleck, 1985). In fact, research indicates that, while midlife and older women theoretically would like men to participate more in the family work of household chores and caregiving, they do not really expect men to contribute as equals (Pleck, 1985).

Caregiving

The patterns for household chores are also evident in caregiving. All persons need some care, in the sense of concern, attention to our special moods and desires, and assistance to carry out special activities of daily life. In one sense, caregiving is an aspect of the everyday lives of all persons who are connected to one another by sentiment or obligation. Many people need assistance to perform tasks of daily living, but that does not make them dependent or necessarily impose a special burden on those who can provide that assistance. The special use of the term "caregiving" implies trying to meet the needs of another person who is not able to identify or articulate those needs, who needs substantial assistance in the activities of daily living, and/or who needs an advocate who can represent his or her desires with others.

Young women, as mothers, have substantial responsibility for the care of young or developmentally disabled children; such care may be extended into midlife for grandchildren or developmentally disabled adult children. Although most older persons take care of themselves (and, often others), perhaps with some assistance, with illness or very advanced age, many need additional assistance; those with dementias require protection. Women, particularly middle-aged and older women, have the major responsibility for providing assistance to frail elders. Much research has documented the provision of assistance to the frail elderly (Dwyer, 1995). Unpaid caregivers are the backbone of our nation's long-term care system because they provide between 70 and 80% of the help needed by the elderly. Most caregivers assist with instrumental activities of daily living (ADLs), which are household tasks such as housework, meal preparation, grocery shopping, and payment of bills. Many help with ADLs that are personal care tasks such as helping the older person use the toilet, bathing, grooming, oral hygiene, and feeding.

The likelihood of becoming a caregiver follows a hierarchical pattern, with spouses most likely to assume primary care; adult children take over when no spouse is available (Dwyer, 1995). Men are more likely to provide care for their wives when they are both older; son's care for frail parents is generally limited to instrumental assistance with bill payment and transportation. Women often provide both instrumental and personal care during their middle years for frail parents or parents-in-law, and for the terminal illness of a husband in his middle or later years.

Many women and men can expect to be caregivers for elders during their lifetime. Some of those will find themselves caring for children and parents at the same time, an experience that has been dubbed the "sandwich generation"; some have argued that this has become a normative experience (Brody, 1990). However, one random survey estimated that fewer than one-fourth of women fit this description, and relatively few of them felt they were "caught" or burdened (Rosenthal, Matthews, & Marshall, 1991). Unless gender patterns are changed, middle-aged women will continue to experience greater impact from family caregiving.

MODELS TO EXPLAIN GENDER DIFFERENCES

The evidence reviewed here documents many ways in which the experiences of women and men differ during midlife. We need to explain the persistent importance of gender distinctions (as reflected in stereotypes and evidence of gender discrimination), the general shift toward lessened gender distinctiveness in middle and later life, and the individual variability in the salience of gender and responses to midlife changes. There is no single model that accounts adequately for group-level sex differences and for individual variability within each sex group. There are several major models that seem most relevant to assess for understanding the phenomena reviewed. Socioevolutionary models provide some understanding of our collective heritage, both coded genetically and transmitted by learning. The cognitive models make it clear how difficult it is to overcome early learning. The cognitive-developmental models provide ways of thinking about the persistent theme of dominance in masculine development, and the more complex schemas of gender that emerge in middle adulthood. The feminist perspective challenges us to examine the roles of power and status in maintaining gender inequities.

The Socioevolutionary Perspective and the Parental Imperative Hypothesis

The socioevolutionary model assumes that the sexually dimorphic behaviors observed in any society (or species) reflect the outcome of cumulative adaptive strategies by the group as a whole. Researchers use data from many different cultures and historical periods to look for patterns of social arrangements in human communities that have managed to survive and thrive. One basic assumption is that the fact of sexual reproductive specialization has led to patterns of task specialization in order to ensure that men and women remain dependent on each other, and that both will remain essential and valued in the social system (Kendrick & Trost, 1993). Thus, while the particular tasks allocated to each sex vary somewhat across cultures, the reality (and persistence) of sex-typed tasks remains.

The most ambitious and comprehensive model of gender differentiation across the life-span has been proposed by Gutmann (1994). He suggests that the core qualities stereotypically associated with males and females have evolved in response to the demands of parenting. The observed shifts toward less sexually differentiated or more androgynous behaviors are tied to a sense of release from the "parental imperatives" associated with caring for vulnerable offspring. Elders also have gender-specific contributions to the survival of the culture, as (female) "kin tenders" and (male) "culture tenders."

Gutmann's Parental Imperative Model was tested with couples from the Parkville studies (Huyck, 1993). (Particular analyses with gender identity, marriage, and parenting are summarized earlier.) Consistent with the model, men's descriptions of themselves changed as their children matured; fathers with children living at home were more likely to describe themselves as wholly masculine, whereas fathers with no children at home were more likely to acknowledge characteristics that they did not regard as masculine. The presence of children in the home did not seem to have a direct impact on the ways men described their marriage relationship. In contrast, women who had no children under 24 living at home were more openly assertive within the marriage, but their own sense of themselves as more or less feminine did not seem affected by either the maturing of their children or their modified behavior in the marriage relationship.

In addition to parenting, several additional variables influenced the gender-linked measures. Better educated men were less likely to describe themselves as conceding in their marriage, and men with health problems were more likely to be conceding. Men with higher status occupations were more likely to describe their masculinity in terms of caring for their families. Men whose wives had more health problems were more likely to describe themselves as either Macho or having Diminished Masculinity. Postmenopausal women were less likely to describe their femininity in terms of nurturing in general, and more likely to describe it in terms of maintaining a feminine appearance and demeanor (the Femme style). Women with poorer health were more likely to describe inner androgyny and diminished femininity.

These analyses suggest a more complete, and more complex, picture of the ways in which shifts in parenting responsibilities may be linked to revisions in the sense of self and in the central marital relationship. Overall, it appears that, as their children become less vulnerable, mothers feel more confident about pressing for changes in the marital relationship; they do not, however, feel less feminine. As men phase out of paternal responsibility, they are more willing to acknowledge more "feminine" aspects of themselves.

The Cognitive Perspective

This perspective assumes that gender schemas are learned early and are maintained and reinforced by schools, work settings and the media, and by cognitive biases such as illusory correlation and belief perseverance (Geis, 1993). Gender schemas are dense with meaning, with connections to a wide variety of behaviors, feelings, and judgments. Geis argues that conscious and unconscious gender beliefs often do not match, particularly among more educated adults; conscious gender beliefs may be very egalitarian. However, most perceptions are guided by our general knowledge of the world, which includes all of the old gender stereotypes as tacit or implicit beliefs. Most processing is done automatically and subconsciously; this means that the implicit gender biases will have more influence on perception than do the conscious, rational, articulated beliefs. Furthermore, the usual cognitive consistency biases seem to operate with gender, making it difficult to "perceive" or to believe evidence that is contrary to one's schema. Geis also describes ways in which gender beliefs lead to self-fulfilling prophesies.

Cognitive Developmental Models

Early Gender Identity Development

In situations in which babies are cared for by women (which is the prevalent pattern across cultures), the earliest sense of self is feminine, or like the caregiver. Girls are able to maintain that identity, and learn the particular nuances of being feminine in that culture and family. Boys, however, must shift to a different mode; they are taught early (in words and in subtle actions) that they are not like the mother and cannot mature to be like her. Thus, many boys develop a gender schema in which the most reliable way to be masculine is to not be like females; part of resisting a feminine identification is to resist any sense of being dominated by a woman. The positive virtues and characteristics of manhood require more sophisticated learning and doing. The earliest gender schemas are acquired at a time when the child is inherently illogical and prone to overgeneralizing and making incorrect inferences. However, because they persist, subconsciously, they can exert lingering influences on later perceptions. Chodorow (1978) argued that the only way for males to develop a strong, positive sense of themselves as masculine without having to control women was to have substantial shared parenting during early years.

The power of early, internalized, parental gender schemas was evident in analyses of how men respond to midlife shifts in themselves and in their partner (Gutmann & Huyck, 1994). Among the Parkville men who acknowledge their own femininity, some are troubled (as evidenced by psychosomatic symptom distress) and some are comfortable. In part, their comfort depends on their wife: more passive men whose wives are benign or unaggressive toward them are asymptomatic; those whose wives are openly assertive in the marriage are more likely to show distress symptoms. In addition, responses reflected the past, what might be considered their early gender schemas. The men who were most troubled by their own emerging femininity and by their wives' increased assertiveness remembered their own fathers as weak or absent and their mothers as strong and tied to the son; those who did not show symptoms of distress had internalized images of both parents as affectionate with each other (and with the son) but emotionally self-sufficient. Such men were not frightened by the emergence of femininity in themselves, and they were able to tolerate more assertiveness in their wives.

Adult Cognitive Development

Some of the models of cognitive development document the ways in which adults, by early midlife, develop more complex modes of thinking and problem solving (Labouvie-Vief & Hakim-Larson, 1989). They are particularly able to rethink old dualities. Masculine–feminine is such a duality, and this perspective may help explain why some individuals are able to reappraise their earlier, more abstract, gender schemas.

The Feminist Perspective

Beall (1993) advises against taking a socioevolutionary view too seriously. A social constructionist view of gender argues that conceptualizations of the world may be popular or persistent because (1) it mirrors "reality" empirically, or (2) it rationalizes differential treatment of groups or the current social order. The data reviewed above can be interpreted as reflecting power and status systems more than differences tied intrinsically to reproductive specialization: because men are larger and stronger, they have been able to establish social systems that institutionalize their greater access to scarce resources, and to make women's access to resources contingent on their compliance with male preferences. In this model, self-interest alone could account for the reluctance of men to share more equally in family work, and the greater empathy attributed to women can be seen as a reflection of lower status, as lower status persons (regardless of sex) are more apt to be deferential and expend more energy learning how to decode the behavior of higher status persons. In this perspective, we are challenged to examine closely how social structures may restrict the options for desired changes.

IMPLICATIONS FOR RESEARCH, SOCIAL POLICY, AND PERSONAL LIFE PLANNING

Research

One obvious implication for research on midlife is that gender must be a central variable. Research carried out using only one sex and generalizing results to the other cannot be tolerated. Furthermore, we must have more research that focuses on what aspects of gender contribute to observed differences; this implies a full investigation of gender.

It is, of course, important to avoid errors of overstating gender differences, as well as underestimating differences by not taking into account the full context.

Social Policy

Social policies are established to create collective responses to what are often experienced as individual problems. During midlife, there are evidences that men and women confront different levels and kinds of challenges. Social policies should be constructed that reduce the inequities linked to age, gender, race and ethnicity, and sexual orientation; here we are concerned primarily with those linked to gender, but we have seen that gender inequities are often compounded by other inequities.

"Caregiving is an act of love—with consequences" (Sommers & Shields, 1987, p. 18). Some of the consequences have been identified above: the unpaid family work performed by women leaves them vulnerable to health problems, inadequate access to health care, lower incomes when employed, and a high risk of poverty in later life. One of the major social challenges is to forge social policies that will support the work of caregivers; this means creating partnerships. Within families, this means a partnership in which men and boys learn to provide hands-on care for older relatives. In the private sector, it means developing programs such as long-term health care insurance, leaves of absence with no loss of pension credits for employees who take time off for caregiving (and making these leaves available to both male and female employees), part-time employment for people combining work with care, and funding for programs such as adult day-care centers. In the public sector, this partnership means a comprehensive program for long-term health care for the chronically ill, including a support program for caregivers providing economic assistance, when necessary, to make it all possible. For caregivers, it means building a movement with all available allies to make these changes possible (Sommers & Shields, 1987).

Personal Life Planning

Perhaps the most crucial issue is to remember that, although the groundwork for the middle years is laid earlier, the middle years offer new opportunities for personal growth and more egalitarian partnerships. Women and men come to the middle years with more life experience, cognitive maturity, and both knowledge about what is likely to work effectively and the confidence to challenge the status quo from an informed standpoint. Most are not yet confronting the serious illnesses of later life. The questioning of social stereotypes and norms attached to age, sex, and other categories (e.g., sexual orientation, race, ethnicity, disability) has made it more possible to explore new options.

It is also crucial to think ahead, and to make decisions that will be good for old age. Men generally find it much to their advantage to be in a stable, relatively stress-free marriage. However, given the realities of fate and a sense of equity, midlife men should be preparing themselves to be good personal caregivers, for a wife or other family member who needs their assistance. Women need to plan for a long life. Economic security has to be a top priority, and becoming informed about financial issues and financial planning during midlife is a good start. Women who enjoy the company of other women will have a great variety of companions in later life; women who feel validated only by a man are likely to be more lonely. Women need to think about who will care for them if they survive the usual caregivers, or if they have chosen not to marry or rear children; this requires working actively for humane, available nonfamily care.

ACKNOWLEDGMENTS

The intergenerational research project, "Aging Parents, Young Adult Children and Mental Health," was funded by a U.S. Public Health Services grant from the Center on Aging, National Institute of Mental Health, Grant Number ROI MH36264, to the Illinois Institute of Technology from 1982–1986, M. Huyck and S. Frank, Co-Principal Investigators. We especially appreciate the guidance of Dr. Nancy Miller and Dr. Barry Lebowitz from NIMH for their guidance in establishing the project. I thank all the respondents who participated and shared their lives with us; Susan Frank for her contributions in establishing the data set; Amy Shapiro for her work as Project Coordinator; and the students who have helped collect the data and prepare it for analysis. Interviewers included Cathy Butler Avery, Scott Andrews, Jeffrey Angevine, Larry Antoz, Mike Bloomquist, Yael Buchsbaum, Paul Carney, Lidia Cardone, Rita Decker, Jim Duchon, Helen Dredze, Susan Frank, Gail Grossman, Dee Heinrich, Jeri Hosick, Margaret Huyck, Mark Laman, Hunter Leggitt, Bill Pace, Kate Philben, Timothy Pedigo, Martha Scott, and Mary Jane Thiel.

REFERENCES

Baruch, G. (1984). The psychological well-being of women in the middle years. In G. Baruch & J. Brooks-Gunn (Eds.), *Women in midlife.* New York: Plenum.

Bell, A. P., & Weinberg, M. S. (1978). *Homosexualities: A study of diversity among men and women.* New York: Simon & Schuster.

Berzins, J., Welling, M., & Wetter, R. (1978). A new measure of psychological androgyny based on the Personality Research form. *Journal of Consulting & Clinical Psychology, 46(1).*

Best, D. L., & Williams, J. E. (1993). A cross-cultural viewpoint. In A. E. Beall & R. J. Sternberg (Eds.), *The psychology of gender* (pp. 215–250). New York: Guilford.

Blumstein, P., & Schwartz, P. (1983. *American couples: Money, work, sex*. New York: Morrow.

Brody, E. M. (1990). *Women in the middle: Their parent-care years*. New York: Springer.

Burch, B. (1987). *Barriers to intimacy: conflicts over power, dependency and nurturing in lesbian relationships*. In Boston Lesbian Psychological Collective, *Lesbian psychologies* (pp. 126–141). Chicago: University of Illinois Press.

Chodorow, N. (1978). *The reproduction of mothering: Psychoanalysis and the sociology of gender*. Berkeley: University of California Press.

Cross, S. E., & Marcus, H. R. (1993). Gender in thought, belief, and action: A cognitive approach. In A. E. Beall & R. J. Sternberg (Eds.), *The psychology of gender* (pp. 55–98). New York: Guilford.

Denmark, F., Russo, N., Frieze, I., & Sechzer, I. (1988). Guidelines for avoiding sexism in psychological research. *American Psychologist, 43,* 582–585.

Dynes, W. R. (Ed.). (1990). *Encyclopedia of homosexuality*. New York: Garland.

Dywer, J. W. (1995). The effects of illness on the family. In R. Bleiszner & V. H. Bedford (Eds.), *Handbook of aging and the family* (pp. 401–421). Westport, CN: Greenwood.

Garza, J., & Dressel, P. (1983). Sexuality and later life marriages. In T. Brubaker (Ed.), *Family relationships in later life* (pp. 91–108). Thousand Oaks, CA: Sage.

Geis, Fl. L. (1993). Self-fulfilling prophecies: A social psychological view of gender. In A. E. Beall & R. J. Sternberg (Eds.), *The psychology of gender* (pp. 9–54). New York: Guilford.

Gutmann, D. L. (1994). *Reclaimed powers: Toward a new psychology of men and women in later life*. Evanston, IL: Northwestern University Press.

Gutmann, D. L., & Huyck, M. H. (1994). Development and pathology in postparental men: A community study. In E. H. Thompson, Jr. (Ed.), *Older men's lives* (pp. 65–84). Thousand Oaks, CA: Sage.

Herz, D., & Wootton, B. H. (1996). Women in the workforce: An overview. In C. Costello & B. Krimgold (Eds.), *The American woman 1996–97: Women and work* (pp. 44–78). New York: Norton.

Huyck, M. H. (1989). Midlife parental imperatives. In R. Kalish (Ed.), *Midlife loss: Coping strategies* (pp. 10–34). Newbury Park, CA: Sage.

Huyck, M. H. (1991a). Gender-linked self-attributions and mental health among middle-aged parents. *Journal of Aging Studies, 5(1),* 111–123.

Huyck, M. H. (1991b). Parents and children: "Post-parental" imperatives. In B. B. Hess & E. W. Markson (Eds.), *Growing old in America* (4th ed., pp. 415–426). New Brunswick, NJ: Transaction.

Huyck, M. H. (1993). *Evaluating the parental imperative model of gender-linked midlife changes: Couples in Parkville, U.S.A.* Unpublished manuscript.

Huyck, M. H. (1994). The relevance of psychodynamic theories for understanding gender among older women. In B. F. Turner & L. E. Troll (Eds.), *Women growing older: Psychological perspectives* (pp. 202–238). Thousand Oaks, CA: Sage.

Huyck, M. H. (1995). Marriage and close relationships of the marital kind. In R. Bleiszner & V. Bedford (Eds.), *Handbook on aging and the family* (pp. 181–200). Westport, CT: Greenwood. (Reissued in paperback, 1996)

Huyck, M. H., & Gutmann, D. L. (1992). Thirtysomething years of marriage; Understanding experiences of women and men in enduring family relationships. *Family Perspectives, 26,* 249–265.

Huyck, M. H. (1996). Continuities and discontinuities in gender roles and gender identity. In V. Bengston (Ed.), *Continuities and discontinuities in the adult life course and aging*. New York: Springer.

Kendrick, D. T., & Trost, M. R. (1993). The evolutionary perspective. In A. E. Beall & R. J. Sternberg (Eds.). *The psychology of gender* (pp. 148–172). New York: Guilford.

Kimmel, M. (1996). *Manhood in America: A cultural history*. New York: Free Press.

Kirkpatrick, M. (1989). Lesbians: A different middle age? In J. M. Oldham & R. S. Liebert (Eds.), *The middle years: New psychoanalytic perspectives* (pp. 135–148). New Haven: Yale University Press.

Labouvie-Vief, G., & Hakim-Larson, J. (1989). Developmental shifts in adult thought. In S. Hunter & M. Sundel (Eds.), *Midlife myths: Issues, findings, and practice implications* (pp. 69–96). Newbury Park, CA: Sage.

Leonard, F. (1994). *Money and the mature woman: How to hold on to your income, keep your home, plan your estate* (rev. ed.). New York: Addison-Wesley.

Liebert, R. S. (1989). Middle aged homosexual men: Issues in treatment. In J. M. Oldham & R. S. Liebert (Eds.), *The middle years: new psychoanalytic perspectives* (pp. 149–159). New Haven: Yale University Press.

Lott, B., & Maluso, D. (1993). The social learning of gender. In A. E. Beall & R. J. Sternberg (Eds.), *The psychology of gender* (pp. 99–126). New York: Guilford.

Maracek, J., Finn, S., & Cardell, M. (1988). Gender roles in the relationships of lesbians and gay men. In J. DeCecco (Ed.), *Gay relationships* (pp. 169–175). Kirkwood, NY: Hawthorn.

Marsiglio, W., & Greer, R. (1994). A gender analysis of older men's sexuality. In E. Thompson, Jr. (Ed.), *Older men's lives* (pp. 122–140). Thousand Oaks, CA: Sage.

Masters, W. H., & Johnson, V. E. (1970). *Human sexual inadequacy.* Boston: Little, Brown.

McAdoo, H. P. (1990). A portrait of African American families in the United States. In S. Rix (Ed.), *The American woman 1990–91: A status report* (pp. 71–93). New York: Norton.

McWhirter, D., & Mattison, A. (1984). *The male couple: How relationships develop.* Englewood Cliffs, NJ: Prentice Hall.

Morgan, L. A. (1991). Economic security of older women: Issues and trends for the future. In B. B. Hess & E. W. Markson (Eds.), *Growing old in American* (4th ed., pp. 427–440). New Brunswick, NJ: Transaction.

National Committee to Preserve Social Security and Medicare. (1994). *Facts at your fingertips.* Washington, DC: Author.

Nichols, M. (1987). *Lesbian sexuality.* In Boston Lesbian Psychologists Collective, *Lesbian psychologies* (pp. 97–125). Chicago: University of Illinois Press.

Older Women's League. (1992). *Critical condition: Midlife and older women in America's health care system.* Washington, DC: Author.

Older Women's League. (1998). *Women, work, and pensions: Improving the odds for a secure retirement.* Washington, DC: Author.

Pleck, J. H. (1985). *Working wives/working husbands.* Thousand Oaks, CA: Sage.

Rhode, D. L. (1990). Gender equality and employment policy. In S. Rix (Ed.), *The American woman 1990–91: A status report* (pp. 170–202). New York: Norton.

Rosenthal, C. J., Matthews, S. H., & Marshall, V. W. (1991). Is parent care normative? The experiences of a sample of middle-aged women. In B. B. Hess & E. W., Markson (Eds.), *Growing old in America* (4th ed., pp. 427–440). New Brunswick, NJ: Transaction.

Schaie, K. W. (1988). Ageism in psychological research. *American Psychologist, 43(3),* 179–183.

Sheehy, G. (1998). *Understanding Men's Passages.* New York: Random House.

Sinnott, J. D. (1986). Sex roles and aging: Theory and research from a systems perspective. *Contributions to Human Development (15).* New York: Karger.

Sommers, T., & Shields, L. (1987). *Women take care: The consequences of caregiving in today's society.* Gainesville, FL: Triad.

U.S. Bureau of the Census. (1997). *Statistical abstract of the United States: 1997* (117th ed.). Washington, DC: Government Printing Office.

CHAPTER 10

Intellectual Functioning in Midlife

Sherry L. Willis and K. Warner Schaie

The Pennsylvania State University, University Park, Pennsylvania

One of the paradoxes of middle age is that it is viewed both as the "best of times" and as the beginning of the "worst of times." Middle age is often described as the "prime of life," when individuals are at the zenith of their careers, are at the highest levels of income and are most likely to be in leadership positions (Neugarten, 1968). Indeed, the founding fathers deemed that the United States presidency should be occupied by a person no younger than middle age; given the lower life expectancy in colonial times, 35 years would have been considered well into middle age. On the other hand, the approach of age 50 in our culture is characterized as "being over the hill."

These opposing views of middle age represent concerns not only with the physical aging process, but also with fears of possible downward shifts in competency and mental ability in midlife. Those beyond young adulthood are targeted for food supplements and herbal remedies said to increase mental alertness, to aid memory, and to maximize mental performance. Decreases in estrogen because of menopause are said to result in memory loss and possible dementia; women entering menopause are advised to adopt hormonal replacement therapy as an antidote for incipient mental decline (Kampen & Sherwin, 1994).

Does the research literature on cognition in middle age support either or both of these opposing views of changes in competency in midlife? Are middle-aged adults at their "prime" in mental ability, or are they "over the hill"? Do longitudinal studies report loss of cognitive functioning in women at the time of menopause? Do women exhibit earlier and more dramatic rates of decline in abilities than do men?

In this chapter we summarize selectively an extensive body of longitudinal research on cognitive functioning spanning the adult life course from young adulthood to old age. The Seattle Longitudinal Study will serve as the primary database for our discussion. Particular focus will be given to the middle years. It is critical, however, to examine cognitive functioning within a life-span context in order to address the questions of whether performance in midlife is at the "prime" or "over the hill."

Five major questions regarding cognitive functioning in middle age will be addressed. First, we examine the life-span trajectories of several basic mental abilities across adulthood and address the question of at what age is peak level of performance reached for each ability. Second, we consider changes in mental abilities from young adulthood to middle age. Third, we discuss in some detail the nature of change in mental abilities within middle age. Gender differences in trajectories, in peak performance, and in change are considered. Fourth, we shift from basic mental abilities to cognitively demanding tasks of daily living and consider changes in competency in midlife for these higher order, more complex life skills. Finally, we examine generational differences in basic mental abilities. Specifically, we address the question of whether the baby boom cohorts now in middle life are functioning at higher levels than their parents' generation when at the same age—thus testing the perpetuation of the American dream of each generation doing better than the last.

THE SEATTLE LONGITUDINAL STUDY

Research findings from the Seattle Longitudinal Study (SLS; Schaie, 1996) serve as the primary database for this chapter. The SLS is a longitudinal, cohort sequential study of adult cognitive functioning, examining changes in performance on a number of basic mental abilities from young adulthood (early 20s) to very old age (90s). Changes in participants' cognitive performance are followed at 7-year intervals, representing seven major testing cycles (1956, 1963, 1970, 1977, 1984, 1991, 1998). The study began in 1956 with 500 individuals being assessed, with mean ages of 22 to 67. Individuals are recruited at random from a large health maintenance organization in Seattle. At each testing cycle the parent population is stratified by age and sex and 25 men and 25 women are randomly selected at each cohort interval from young adulthood to old age. At each testing cycle all participants from prior cycles are retested and a new sample is drawn. Across the course of the study, individuals have been studied for 35-, 28-, 21-, 14-, and 7-year intervals.

Basic Mental Abilities

The focus of the SLS has been on individual change and generational differences in functioning on a set of basic mental abilities. These abilities have been studied primarily within a psychometric approach to cognition (Thurstone, 1938); however, several of the abilities are also recognized and studied within other approaches to cognition (Cattell, 1963; Horn, 1982). The findings summarized in this chapter focus on six of these basic mental abilities: Vocabulary, Verbal Memory, Number, Spatial Orientation, Inductive Reasoning, and Perceptual Speed.

Brief descriptions of each of the ability domains are given below.

Vocabulary

This ability represents the competence to understand ideas expressed in words. The range of a person's passive vocabulary used in activities such as reading and listening is represented. Vocabulary is assessed by the individual identifying a synonym for the stimulus word. Vocabulary is an ability that is not only salient in a psychometric approach to cognition, but is also central in text processing research (Dixon, Hultsch, Simon, & von Eye, 1984; Hultsch & Dixon, 1990; Meyer, Marsiske, & Willis, 1993) and in neuropsychology (Folstein, Folstein, & McHugh, 1975).

Verbal Memory

This domain represents ability to encode and recall meaningful language units, such as lists of words. The ability to recall lists of words under immediate and delayed conditions is assessed. Verbal memory is a domain of study also in an information processing approach to cognition (Craik & Salthouse, 1992). Moreover, deficits in verbal memory are one of the hallmarks of early dementia within a neuropsychology approach (American Psychiatric Association, 1994; McKhann et al., 1984).

Number

The ability to perform simple mathematical computations including addition, subtraction, and multiplication. The focus of the assessment is on computations being done quickly and accurately.

Spatial Orientation

This is the ability to visualize and mentally manipulate (rotate) stimuli in two- and three-dimensional space. It involves the ability to maintain orientation with respect to spatial objects and to perceive relationship among objects in space. Spatial orientation has also been studied with an information processing approach to cognition

(Craik & Salthouse, 1992) and is of concern in clinical studies of neuropathology (McKhann et al., 1984). This ability is central to applied skills such as map reading, way finding, and occupational skills such as navigation and dentistry.

Inductive Reasoning

This is the ability to recognize and understand patterns and relationships within a problem and to utilize these relationships to solve other instances of the problem. It involves the ability to foresee, to analyze, and plan, and to solve logical problems. Within the study of expertise, inductive reasoning represents a form of procedural knowledge. Within neuropsychology, it is represented as an executive function, and is believed to exhibit early decline in dementia (Marson, Ingram, Cody, & Harrell, 1995; McKhann et al., 1984). Reasoning as manifested in executive function is of critical importance in the study of decision making.

Perceptual Speed

This ability involves competence in quickly and accurately making simple discriminations in visual stimuli. This ability is also represented in information processing (Craik & Salthouse, 1992) and neuropsychological approaches to cognition.

It should be noted that each of these ability domains is represented at the latent construct level with respect to the findings presented in this chapter. That is, the data reported are for factor scores representing these abilities, rather than for single tests of the ability (Schaie, 1996).

AGE-RELATED CHANGE IN BASIC MENTAL ABILITIES

A Life-Span View of Cognitive Functioning: Peak Performance in Midlife

Overview

We begin by examining the life-span trajectory for cognitive functioning from young adulthood to old age. Figure 1 shows that the highest level of functioning for four of the six mental abilities considered occurs in midlife. For both men and women, peak performance on inductive reasoning, spatial orientation, vocabulary, and verbal memory is reached in middle age. It is only for two of the six abilities examined—perceptual speed and numerical ability—that the stereotypical trajectory of life-span change occurs. Perceptual speed is the ability showing the earliest, most linear pattern of decline, beginning in young adulthood.

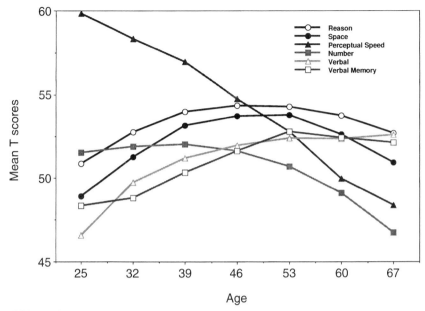

FIGURE 1   Longitudinal change in six abilities: Ages 25 to 67. From Schaie, K. W. (1994). The course of adult intellectual development. *American Psychologist, 49,* 304–313. Copyright © 1994 by the American Psychological Association. Reprinted with permission.

A life-span perspective of cognitive development suggests that midlife, the age interval of the 40s through the early 60s, is a period of maximum performance on some of the more complex, higher order mental abilities, such as inductive reasoning, spatial orientation, and vocabulary. Interestingly, peak performance levels occur in midlife for abilities traditionally characterized as representing both fluid intelligence (inductive reasoning, spatial orientation) and crystallized intelligence (vocabulary; Cattell, 1963). While both fluid and crystallized abilities reach a peak in midlife, the fact remains that across the life-span fluid abilities show an earlier trajectory of decline than crystallized; that is, fluid abilities begin to show reliable decline in the mid-60s, while crystallized abilities do not show reliable decline until the 70s (Schaie, 1996).

Gender Differences

Peak performance is reached somewhat earlier on average for men than for women for the four abilities reaching maximum levels in midlife. For men, peak performance on spatial orientation, vocabulary, and verbal memory is reached in the 50s. For women, peak performance on spatial orientation, vocabulary, and verbal memory is reached in the early 60s.

It is notable that women on average exhibit decline in perceptual speed some-what earlier than men, with women reaching peak performance in the 20s with steady linear decline occurring thereafter through middle and old age. Decline for men on perceptual speed does not begin until the 30s.

There are gender differences not only in timing of peak performance but also in level (i.e., mean score) of functioning. Across much of young and middle adulthood the mean score of women is higher than that of men for vocabulary, verbal memory, perceptual speed, and induction (Schaie, 1996; Willis & Schaie, 1988). The largest gender differences in favor of women are on vocabulary and verbal memory. In contrast, men consistently have higher average scores on spatial orientation.

Given the focus of this chapter on middle age, it is important to consider age-related change trajectories at two intervals: (1) from young adulthood to middle age, and (2) short-term change within the middle-age period. Consideration of short-term change (i.e., change over 7 years) versus long-term change (i.e., change over 14 to 21 years from young to middle adulthood) may provide insight into the differing perspectives on cognition in middle age that have appeared in the literature.

Longitudinal Change from Young Adulthood to Midlife: Gain and Loss

Gain from Young Adulthood

Contrary to stereotypical views of intelligence and the naive theories of many educated laypersons, young adulthood is not the developmental period of peak cognitive functioning for many of the higher order cognitive abilities (Schaie, 1996). Figure 2 shows the cumulative change in T-score points between performance at age 25 (represented as 0 on the y-axis) and performance at six subsequent ages: 32, 39, 46, 53, 60, and 67 years.

The figure shows that for four (vocabulary, spatial orientation, verbal memory, and inductive reasoning) of the six abilities studied, middle-aged individuals are functioning at a higher level than they did at age 25. Improvement from young adulthood to peak performance in middle age is on the order of .30 to .60 standard deviation units. Gain from young adulthood to peak for inductive reasoning is approximately .35 standard deviation units, gain for verbal memory and spatial orientation is approximately .40 standard deviation units; and gain for vocabulary is .60 standard deviation units.

The increase in performance from young adulthood to middle age is particularly noteworthy for women. Women in midlife are performing on average one-half a standard deviation above their scores at age 25 on spatial orientation, vocabulary, and verbal memory. For vocabulary, women continue to exhibit at least one-half a standard deviation of increase from their performance in young adulthood into the 60s and early 70s. Men also are performing at peak levels in midlife, but the increase

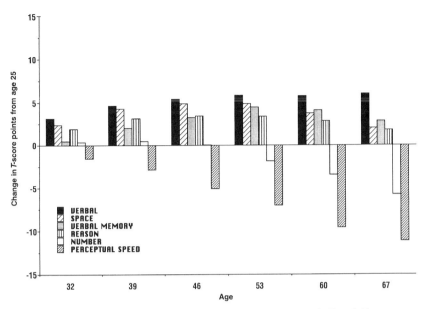

FIGURE 2   Cumulative change from age 25 to ages 32, 39, 46, 53, 60, and 67.

from performance in young adulthood is not quite so dramatic; the increase for spatial orientation and verbal memory is on the order of .20 to .30 standard deviation units.

Loss from Young Adulthood

In contrast, perceptual speed ability shows a steady and increasing decline from age 25 to middle age. By the late 50s to early 60s, individuals on average are functioning one standard deviation below their performance level at age 25. Women in particular show a decline in perceptual speed from young adulthood. Women show a decline of approximately 1.00 standard deviation unit, compared to a loss of .70 for men. Numerical ability that was measured by speeded arithmetic tasks also shows age-related decline, although the magnitude of the decline is much smaller than for perceptual speed. A decline of approximately .40 to .50 standard deviation units is shown by the mid-60s for both men and women.

Change across 7-Year Intervals during Middle Age

While there is significant cumulative positive change from young adulthood through much of midlife for many important abilities, the middle-aged adult may

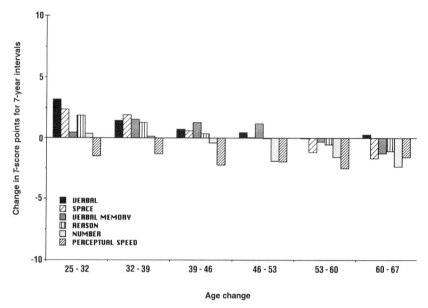

FIGURE 3   Ability change in 7-year intervals.

be more aware of short-term changes occurring *during* the 40s and 50s. Examination of short-term (i.e., 7-year) changes in the middle years suggest a different pattern of trajectories (Schaie, 1996).

Figure 3 presents the magnitude of changes occurring at each of six 7-year intervals in adulthood (i.e., 25–32, 32–39, 39–46, 46–53, 53–60, and 60–67 years). For each of the first three 7-year intervals (25–32, 32–39, and 39–46 years), there is positive change across the 7-year interval, with the exception of perceptual speed, and of numerical ability in the third interval. By the interval of 53–60 years of age, however, all abilities are exhibiting stability (i.e., vocabulary) or modest decline over the 7 years, while at the same time being at the peak level of performance compared to young adulthood! Men and women in their 50s are on average at their highest level of performance (compared to their scores in young adulthood), yet they are beginning to experience very modest short-term decline.

The middle-aged individual may have very different perceptions of his or her cognitive functioning, whether a long-term or short-term view of current status is taken (Schaie, Willis, & O'Hanlon, 1997). In a similar vein, findings from longitudinal data that covers the full adult life-span present a different picture of developmental trajectories in middle age than may short-term studies of change in midlife. The middle-aged individual's perception of his or her intellectual functioning may be more pessimistic than the longitudinal data would suggest for several reasons. Comparisons of change in functioning may be more likely to be made over shorter intervals. One may have a more vivid or accurate perception of oneself 7 years ago than 20 years ago. Moreover, comparison events (e.g., work and family responsibilities) may be more similar and more comparable over shorter time intervals.

COHORT DIFFERENCES IN ABILITIES: PARENT VERSUS BABY BOOM COHORTS

Study of developmental changes in cognitive functioning in midlife must include not only consideration of age-related (intraindividual) change, which has been described in the preceding sections, but also discussion of generational or cohort differences in level of cognitive functioning (Schaie, 1990, 1996). Prior cohort research has found that the nature of cohort effects varies across different mental abilities. Abilities such as inductive reasoning and verbal ability have shown strong positive cohort trends, with successive cohorts in the first quarter of the 1900s performing on average at a higher level when at the same chronological age as prior cohorts. In contrast, a negative cohort trend has been found for number ability, with earlier birth cohorts performing at a higher level than succeeding cohorts. Continuing changes in advances in health care, technology, educational experience, and cultural events suggest that cohort trends will continue to change with successive cohorts.

Given that those currently in middle age represent the large baby boom cohorts (Easterlin, 1987; Easterlin, Schaeffer, & Macunovich, 1993), it is of interest to compare their level of functioning in midlife to prior cohorts at the same chronological ages. Of particular interest are comparisons of level of cognitive functioning in the parent cohorts (median birth cohort 1924) of the baby-boomers versus the baby-boomers, when at the same chronological age. The baby boom cohorts have been defined as spanning the period from 1946 to 1960 and hence data on three baby boom cohorts (1945, 1952, 1959) are available in the SLS (Easterlin, 1987).

Figure 4 presents mean *differences* in *T*-score points between parent (birth cohort 1924) and baby boom cohorts (birth cohorts 1945, 1952, 1959) for the six basic mental abilities discussed previously. The parent cohort is set to 0. The figure addresses two types of issues: (1) trends between parent and baby-boomer cohorts, and (2) trends among the three boomer cohorts.

Parent versus Baby Boom Cohorts

Strong positive cohort trends are shown for two of the abilities, Verbal Memory and Inductive Reasoning, with baby boom cohorts scoring one-half a standard deviation or more above the performance of the parent generation. A positive cohort trend but of a lesser magnitude (approximately .25 standard deviation units) is shown for Spatial Orientation. Fairly flat cohort differences are shown for Vocabulary and

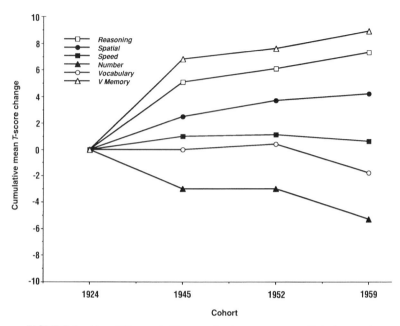

FIGURE 4   Mean differences in *T*-score points between parent and baby boom cohorts.

Perceptual Speed. Particularly notable is the negative cohort trend for Number (approximately one-third standard deviation).

The strong positive cohort trend for Inductive Reasoning has been found in cohort research with earlier cohorts, as has the negative cohort trend for Number (Schaie, 1996). The relatively flat cohort trend for Vocabulary is particularly notable since cohort research with earlier cohorts has shown a stronger positive trend. Prior research on cohort trends for Verbal Memory and Perceptual Speed are limited.

Trends within Baby Boom Cohorts

The differences among baby boom cohorts, spanning a 15-year interval, appear particularly modest, compared to the magnitude of cohort differences between parent and baby boom cohorts. Very slight positive trends (.10 standard deviation unit) are noted for three of the abilities, Inductive Reasoning, Spatial Orientation, and Verbal Memory. A negative cohort trend, particularly in what is known as the "tail" of the boomer cohorts (1959 cohort; Easterlin, 1987) was found for Vocabulary and Number. The negative cohort trend for Number continues a negative trend first observed in the late 1930s cohorts—a trend now extending over 25 years.

LONGITUDINAL CHANGE IN EVERYDAY SKILLS AND COMPETENCIES

Basic Mental Abilities and Everyday Activities

The mental abilities discussed above rarely manifest themselves in the daily lives of adults in the form in which they are studied in the psychological laboratory. Cognitive functioning in everyday life takes the form of tasks, such as comprehending medication labels, balancing a checkbook, remembering a shopping list, or figuring out an airline schedule (Barberger-Gateau et al., 1992; Fillenbaum, 1985). In the study of cognitive aging, these daily tasks have been studied as a form of everyday problem solving (Willis, 1991). Although these basic abilities and everyday problem solving appear, at first glance, to be distinctly different phenomena, research has shown that everyday problem solving often involves constellations of these basic abilities (Willis, Jay, Diehl, & Marsiske, 1992). For example, comprehending a medication label has been shown to involve inductive reasoning, verbal ability, and sometimes numerical skill. In some instances, perception speed is also involved.

Age-Related Change in Tasks of Daily Living

Are there age-related changes in the middle-aged adult's ability to carry out cognitively demanding tasks of daily living? Research on everyday problem solving is more recent and longitudinal data are more limited. The existing data within the SLS suggest that reliable age-related change does not occur until the mid-60s for everyday problem solving on tasks such as those described above (Schaie, 1996). A steeper pattern of decline becomes evident in the 70s and 80s.

The previous findings on decline in perceptual speed are of importance in relation to everyday problem solving (Willis et al., in press). Recent research indicates that those with slower perceptual speed show greater decline in everyday problem solving. Specifically, individuals who are slower when at baseline assessment or who exhibit a greater magnitude of decline on speed also show a greater decline on everyday problem solving. Decline in perceptual speed in relation to everyday problem solving has been found to be particularly salient for adults over the age of 70.

SUMMARY

When the trajectory of the six mental abilities is examined over the entire adult life course from young adulthood to old age, middle age is a life stage in which peak performance is found for several important basic mental abilities. In midlife both men and women score the highest on measures of four mental abilities—vocabulary, verbal memory, inductive reasoning, and spatial orientation. Of particular note is that these four abilities represent the more complex, higher order domains of cognitive functioning. Inductive reasoning and, in some circumstances, spatial orientation represent the executive functions that are viewed within clinical and neuropsychology as the essential components for independent living and a productive lifestyle. These ability domains have been found to be significantly associated with success in professional occupations such as computer programming, dentistry, and piloting.

The peaking of verbal memory in midlife is of particular interest because memory deficit is one of the most common cognitive concerns among adults of all ages (Hertzog, Dixon, & Hultsch, 1990). Young adults, as well as middle-aged and older adults report similar types of memory problems, with the frequency of the problems reported increasing with age. Age at peak verbal memory performance is particularly noteworthy for women, as the highest scores occur in the early 60s, toward the later end of middle age. Although memory *complaints* in midlife do not appear to be well founded in most cases (with the exception of depression), *objective* memory loss in middle age is a major concern, given the norm of peak performance during this age period (Folstein et al., 1975). Hence, objective memory deficits prior to the 60s are one of the earliest and most salient factors associated with onset of dementia. It is perhaps because the "average" middle-aged adult is doing so well with memory performance that difficulties with verbal memory measures are so striking and often indicative of onset of pathologies.

Those familiar with the fluid–crystallized intelligence distinction may question the finding of peak performance for both abilities represented as fluid (e.g., inductive reasoning, spatial orientation), and crystallized (vocabulary). While both fluid and crystallized abilities reach a peak in midlife, the fact remains that across the lifespan fluid ability shows an earlier trajectory of decline than crystallized. Fluid ability begins to show reliable decline in the mid-60s, whereas crystallized abilities do not show reliable decline until the 70s or 80s.

The peaking of abilities in midlife suggests that, in some cases, substantial improvement in functioning has occurred since young adulthood, the stereotypical age for peak performance. The question arises of how much improvement, on average, occurs from young adulthood to middle age? Women in midlife are performing on average one-half a standard deviation above their scores at age 25 on spatial orientation, vocabulary, and verbal memory. The gain for men is on the order of one-fifth to one-third of a standard deviation. This gain appears to be most prominent from the 20s into the 30s. The significant increase in level of functioning in early middle age suggests that experiences associated with early career development and the assumption of adult responsibilities (e.g., managing finances) may contribute significantly to cognitive functioning. This gain in functioning appears to occur after the end of postsecondary education for most adults. The larger gain for women may reflect the increasing numbers of women entering the professions and maintaining careers during the childbearing years.

Equally noteworthy to the positive trajectories is the decline trajectory for perceptual speed, beginning in the 20s, particularly for women. Speed of responding has been characterized as closely related to central processing resources (Craik & Salthouse, 1992) and to basic neuropsychological functioning. Speed has shown to be associated with the rate of processing involved in more complex, higher order skills. For example, some form of speed of processing is involved in mental rotation and in working memory, associated with inductive reasoning. Decline in perceptual speed from age 25 to age 53 is on the order of one standard deviation for women and one-third of a standard deviation for men. Statistically, the magnitude of decline is impressive. The question arises of the extent to which statistically significant decline represents clinically meaningful changes. Some have suggested that considerable decline representing statistically significant changes can occur with relatively limited practical implications in some situations (Schaie, 1989a, 1989b); further inquiry is merited.

The opposing developmental trajectories for speed and for some higher order mental abilities suggest that cognitive functioning in the middle years may reflect that compensatory mechanisms are at work. Middle-aged adults peaking in abilities such as inductive reasoning and verbal memory may be employing higher order skills to compensate for loss in speed of responding. Salthouse has reported that older typists compensated for slower responding with the viewing of longer spans of information. These compensatory strategies may be possible due to high levels of functioning on abilities such as verbal memory and inductive reasoning.

The early decline in speed may also suggest the need to explore behavioral cognitive interventions in middle age. Most cognitive interventions may been focused on older adults, given that most complex abilities do not show reliable decline until the mid-60s (Willis, 1990). However, the earlier trajectory of decline for speed may argue that interventions in speed in midlife are warranted. The modifiability of processing speed, particularly in old age, has been demonstrated in the work of Ball and Owsley (1991), and enhancement of speed of responding has been demonstrated by Hoyer, Labouvie, and Galtes (1973).

A paradox occurs in middle age in that most adults are functioning significantly above their performance in young adulthood, yet by the late 50s some very modest instances of decline are occurring. These very early and modest instances of decline must be interpreted with considerable caution. First, the level of decline does not become statistically reliable until the 60s for spatial orientation and reasoning and until the 70s for verbal memory and vocabulary (Schaie, 1996). Thus, the decline, although detectable, is within the error of measurement. Nevertheless, it is possible that these early hints of decline are perceived by the middle-aged adult and serve as the basis for some of the anxiety regarding "being over the hill" expressed in midlife. These short-term changes may also be represented in recent reports of declines in the control group in the study of the effects of hormone replacement therapy (HRT) on cognition. It will become increasingly important in interpreting these

HRT studies that changes in performance be considered within the context of longitudinal research, noting the trajectory of functioning over longer intervals than is possible within short-term experimental studies.

Finally, we considered generational differences in cognitive functioning for the baby boom cohorts and their parents. Positive cohort trends for the baby-boomers were noted for inductive reasoning, spatial orientation, and verbal memory. These findings continue the positive generational trends that have been noted in comparisons of prior birth cohorts. Of particular concern, however, are the slowing of cohort differences for vocabulary and the negative cohort trend for number. The implication of the slowing of positive cohort trends is that fewer age differences (in comparison with younger cohorts) will be evident for the baby-boomers should they need to remain in the work force or in other forms of productive endeavors. The stereotypes of negative age decline will not be as readily reinforced if there is less difference concurrently between younger and older generations.

REFERENCES

American Psychiatric Association. (1994). *Diagnostic and statistical manual of mental disorders* (4th ed.) (DSM-IV). Washington, DC: Author.

Ball, K., & Owsley, C. (1991). Identifying correlates of accident involvement for the older driver. *Human Factors, 33*, 583–595.

Barberger-Gateau, P., Commenges, D., Gagnon, M., Letenneur, L., Sauvel, C., & Dartigues, J. (1992). Instrumental activities of daily life as a screening tool for cognitive impairment and dementia in elderly community dwellers. *Journal of the American Geriatrics Society, 40*, 1129–1134.

Cattell, R. B. (1963). Theory of fluid and crystallized intelligence: A critical experiment. *Journal of Educational Psychology, 54*, 1–22.

Craik, G., & Salthouse, T. A. (Eds.). (1992). *The handbook of aging and cognition.* New York: Erlbaum.

Diehl, M., Willis, S. L., & Schaie, K. W. (1995). Everyday problem solving in older adults: Observational assessment and cognitive correlates. *Psychology and Aging, 10*, 478–491.

Dixon, R. A., Hultsch, D. F., Simon, E. W., & von Eye, A. (1984). Verbal ability and text structure effects on adult age differences in text recall. *Journal of Verbal Learning and Verbal Behavior, 23*, 569–578.

Easterlin, R. A. (1987). *Birth and fortune: The impact of numbers on personal welfare* (2nd ed.). Chicago: University of Chicago Press.

Easterlin, R. A., Schaeffer, C. M., & Macunovich, D. J. (1993). Will the baby boomers be less well off than their parents? Income, wealth, and family circumstances over the life cycle in the United States. *Population and Development Review, 19*(3), 497–523.

Fillenbaum, G. (1985). Screening the elderly: A brief instrumental activities of daily living measure. *Journal of the American Geriatric Society, 33*, 698–706.

Folstein, M. F., Folstein, S. E., & McHugh, P. R. (1975). Mini-Mental State: A practical method for grading the cognitive state of patients for the clinician. *Journal of Psychiatric Research, 12*, 189–198.

Hertzog, C., Dixon, R. A., & Hultsch, D. (1990). Metamemory in adulthood: Differentiating knowledge, belief, and behavior. In T. M. Hess (Ed.), *Aging and cognition: Knowledge, organization and utilization.* Amsterdam: Elsevier.

Horn, J. L. (1982). The theory of fluid and crystallized intelligence in relation to concepts of cognitive psychology and aging in adulthood. In F. I. M. Craik & S. Trehub (Eds.), *Aging and cognitive processes* (pp. 237–278). New York: Plenum.

Hoyer, W., Labouvie, G., & Baltes, P. B. (1973). Modification of response speed and intellectual performance in the elderly. *Human Development, 16,* 233–24.

Hultsch, D. F., & Dixon, R. A. (1990). Learning and memory in aging. In J. E. Birren & K. W. Schaie (Eds.), *Handbook of the psychology of aging* (3rd ed., pp. 258–274). San Diego, CA: Academic Press.

Kampen, D. L., & Sherwin, B. B. (1994). Estrogen use and verbal memory in healthy postmenopausal women. *Obstetrics and Gynecology, 83,* 979–983.

Marson, D. C., Ingram, K. K., Cody, H. A., & Harrell, L. E. (1995). Assessing the competency of patients with Alzheimer's disease under different legal standards: A prototype instrument. *Archives of Neurology, 52,* 949–954.

McKhann, G., Drachman, D., Folstein, M., Katzman, R., Price, D., & Stadlan, E. M. (1984). Clinical diagnosis of Alzheimer's disease: Report of the NINCDS-ADRDA Work Group under the auspices of the DHHS Task Force on Alzheimer's disease. *Neurology, 34,* 939–944.

Meyer, B. J. F., Marsiske, M., & Willis, S. L. (1993). Text processing variables predict the readability of everyday documents read by older adults. *Reading Research Quarterly, 28*(3), 235–248.

Neugarten, B. L. (Ed.). (1968). *Middle age and aging.* Chicago: University of Chicago Press.

Schaie, K. W. (1989a). Perceptual speed in adulthood: Cross-sectional and longitudinal studies. *Psychology and Aging, 4,* 443–453.

Schaie, K. W. (1989b). The hazards of cognitive aging. *Gerontologist, 29,* 484–493.

Schaie, K. W. (1990). Intellectual development in adulthood. In J. E. Birren & K. W. Schaie (Eds.)., *Handbook of the psychology of aging* (3rd ed., pp. 291–319). San Diego, CA: Academic Press.

Schaie, K. W. (1996). *Intellectual development in adulthood: The Seattle longitudinal study.* Cambridge: University of Cambridge Press.

Schaie, K. W., Willis, S. L., & O'Hanlon, A. (1994). Perceived intellectual performance change over seven years. *Journal of Gerontology: Psychological Sciences, 49,* 108–118.

Thurstone, L. L. (1938). *The primary mental abilities.* Chicago: University of Chicago Press.

Willis, S. L. (1990). Current issues in cognitive training research. In E. A. Lovelace (Ed.), *Aging and cognition: Mental processes, self awareness and interventions* (pp. 263–280). Amsterdam: Elsevier.

Willis, S. L. (1991). Cognition and everyday competence. In K. W. Schaie & M. P. Lawton (Eds.), *Annual Review of Gerontology and Geriatrics, 11* (pp. 80–109). New York: Springer.

Willis, S. L. (1996). Assessing everyday competence in the cognitively challenged elderly. In M. A. Smyer, K. W. Schaie, M. Kapp (Eds.), *Older adults' decision-making and the law* (pp. 87–126). New York: Springer.

Willis, S. L., Jay, G. M., Diehl, M., & Marsiske, M. (1992). Longitudinal change and prediction of everyday task competence in the elderly. *Research on Aging, 14*(1), 68–91.

Willis, S. L., & Schaie, K. W. (1988). Gender differences in spatial ability in old age: Longitudinal and intervention findings. *Sex Roles, 8,* 189–203.

Willis, S. L., Schaie, K. W., Yanling, Z., Kennett, J., Intrieri, B. & Persaud, A. (1998). *Longitudinal studies of practical intelligence.* University Park: The Pennsylvania State University.

CHAPTER 11

A Life-Span Framework for Assessing the Impact of Work on White-Collar Workers

Bruce J. Avolio

Center for Leadership Studies and School of Management, State University of New York at Binghamton, Binghamton, New York

John J. Sosik

School of Management, Penn State Great Valley

The focus of this chapter is on examining the interaction of individuals and the life/ work context that they accrue over the course of their respective careers. Both present and past experiences are used in this chapter to discuss the future impact of life and work contexts on individual worker behavior. Predictions are offered to link changes that are evolving in the life and work context for middle-aged white-collar employees throughout the remainder of this decade, and on into the next millennium, addressing anticipated changes in ability, behavior, and work performance in this target group.

For the purposes of this chapter, our focus will be on examining workers who are between 40 and 65 years of age. Age 65 is used as the upper cutoff for middle age, although as the age of retirement increases, middle age may extend past the traditional cutoff of age 65.

The multilevel framework used in this chapter to examine the middle-aged worker includes the individual and his or her work/life context as representing two distinct levels of analysis, a third level representing the accrual of work context/life experiences over time, a fourth level representing cohort membership, and a fifth level that extends the multilevel framework into future work settings. At this fifth and final level, we are taking a prospective view of aging and work behavior, where we will extrapolate from current changes in the nature of work to the expected impact of those changes on future middle-aged workers in the next millennium.

The term level is used in this chapter to represent qualitatively different entities hierarchically arranged at distinctly different points in time (Miller, 1978). For instance, age norms can be operationalized at an *individual level,* or what an individual believes is "age appropriate" behavior. They can also be operationalized at the *work group, organization,* and/or even *societal* level. Each *level* requires that we conceptualize and measure the concept of age norms differently, depending on the most appropriate level of analysis chosen.

By incorporating a levels-of-analysis perspective with respect to studying aging and work issues, we can avoid what Robinson (1950) called an "ecological fallacy" or the "fallacy of the wrong-level" (see Rousseau, 1985). It seems reasonable to interpret the relationship between the type of work an individual does in a certain job and level of turnover as being causally linked, when in fact the broader context in which individuals are embedded may drive the turnover rates observed in an organization, for example, poorer supervision at higher levels of the organization, or inequities in the pay system.

The inclusion of time and a levels-of-analysis framework provides a basis for hypothesizing the impact of *accrued* work experiences from early phases in an individual's career, on up to and including his or her current work environment on subsequent levels of ability, motivation, and performance. This framework should enable us to explain with greater precision the evolution of work behavior patterns over time for white-collar professional employees, who are currently embedded in jobs that are rapidly changing in terms of the processes being used and the challenges for those workers. Examining the context in which behavior has been and is currently embedded will also allow us to generalize from assessing the impact of accrued experiences on observed work behavior and performance to predicting patterns of work behavior and performance at the upper stages of an individual's career on into the next millennium.

In addition to examining current and prior life/work experiences, we also focus this chapter on the evolving and changing characteristics of white-collar positions. The ongoing and anticipated changes over the next 20–30 years have significant short-term and long-term implications for studying the development and employment patterns of the current generation of young to middle-aged white-collar employees.

We begin this chapter by taking a prospective view of the evolving work context, with respect to white-collar semiprofessional and professional positions. Next, we discuss previous findings reported in the aging and work literature concerning this target group, focusing on trends in work behavior, motivation, performance, and ability. Then, we emphasize the necessity for examining the accrued work context within a levels-of-analysis perspective to explain the pattern of relationships reported in previous literature for this target group.

For the purposes of this chapter, we define white-collar workers as semi- to professional workers, including in this group higher level clerical occupations on up to professional positions, such as management and supervision.

THE CHANGING NATURE
OF WHITE-COLLAR WORK

Forecasting the future is always risky. Yet, in order to fully understand the potential age and work behavior patterns expected for white-collar workers in the next millennium, we need to put forth some predictions regarding the characteristics of careers and work contexts individuals will be expected to accrue, on up to the point in time where we examine future work behavior.

Taking a prospective view of aging and work behavior seems essential given the type of findings reported by Schaie (1994) and his colleagues, which point to positive shifts in cognitive abilities at higher ages, in more recent cohorts, particularly those including the "baby-boom" generation. Schaie's results indicated that more recent cohorts of workers are showing a positive trend in terms of the maintenance of cognitive abilities at more advanced ages in the life-span. Similarly, significant increases in average educational levels, as well as a rise in continuing education at later points in the life-span for more recent cohorts, may also affect future age and cognitive ability relationships to the extent that education impacts on maintaining those abilities (Avolio & Waldman, 1990). Specifically, if current trends continue, we would expect that younger cohorts of white-collar professionals now entering the work force will exhibit a more positive relationship between age and cognitive ability as they reach the middle to upper end of their respective life-span.

As noted by Schaie (1990), "For those abilities showing a curvilinear pattern, shifts in educational strategies and intensity of exposure to relevant materials may be the most important antecedent to cohort differences" (p. 309). Of course, what we don't know at present is the long-term impact of continuous education coupled with an intellectually stimulating job/home environment on individual differences in cognitive ability observed at different points across the working life-span. However, we do know that some environmental contexts are more conducive to successful aging than are others (Baltes & Baltes, 1990). The key issue is to identify what aspects of the work and life context promote the most successful patterns of aging; then, we can enhance those aspects of the context with the goal of positively impacting how individuals develop and age over time.

Kohn and Schooler (1983) reported a positive relationship between job complexity and levels of intellectual flexibility found at older ages. Similarly, Avolio and Waldman (1987) reported differences in age–test correlations for semiprofessional *skilled* versus *unskilled* blue-collar workers. Avolio and Waldman (1990) demonstrated that occupational type moderated differences in the relationship between age and cognitive test performance with a large representative sample comprised of *unskilled* to *skilled employees*. Their sample included workers from all states within the United States, who ranged in age from 16 to 74. Supporting these trends, Schaie (1990) predicted that up to one-third of the variance in changes in cognitive ability over the life-span may be due to external factors such as education, occupation, and socioeconomic status, as opposed to biological or "natural" correlates of aging. Taken together, there is mounting evidence that the work and life context we accumulate over the life-span can impact on the level of ability, motivation, and performance we observe in individuals at the upper reaches of the life-span.

In sum, one could argue that jobs should be redesigned to promote challenge, intellectual stimulation, and room for development, as each of these factors has been linked to the maintenance of higher levels of both cognitive and physical functioning at later points in the life-span. In fact, this type of job redesign is already under way in many organizations. The trends toward empowering the white-collar work force, and the redesign of jobs to provide more meaning in the work that is completed, could contribute to a future work context that could promote such challenges across the working life-span.

Today, the overriding focus in many organizations is to develop a flexible, adaptable, learning organization, a multifunctional team-based structure, multiskill training and cross-training across careers, and rapid transfer of information and communications across all organizational levels (Avolio, 1997; Bass, 1994). A 1994 article in *Fortune* magazine by William Bridges offered a glimpse at the magnitude of change occurring in the job market. Bridges states,

> Many organizations are today well along the path toward being dejobbed. . . . To an extent that few people have recognized, our world is no longer a pattern of jobs, the way a honeycomb is a pattern of those little hexagonal pockets of honey . . . jobs are no longer socially adaptive. That is why they are going the way of the dinosaur." (p. 64)

Employees are being prepared to take on more than one function to provide the basis for a more flexible and adaptive organization. They will also be measured in terms of the intellectual capital they bring to the organization and develop over time (Senge, 1990).

There is a significant shift occurring in most organizations from being designed around narrow specialties within functional areas to developing workers to take on greater responsibility for the entire product service. Division of labor is now being conceived in terms of broader assignments, with much greater responsibility for the coordination and completion of tasks being assigned to individual employees at lower levels of the organization. The idea that there is only one best way to produce a product or service has given way to an integration of the social and rational approaches to work design. Today, employees and work teams are being empowered to plan, direct, and control their own work processes. The new approaches to job/organization redesign and reengineering involve the development of self-directed/self-managed teams. As noted by Bass (1994), "responsibilities of the team may include everything (including the paperwork) required to obtain an order from a customer, design, assemble, inspect and ship the product, as well as finding out how satisfied the customer is with it" (p. 22). These new employees are more highly trained, involved, and committed to their work than what would be typically found in traditional structures that characterized organizations within the United States throughout most of the industrial revolution.

Evolution and Changing Patterns in the White-Collar Workplace

There are several distinct patterns that have emerged over the last decade that have had a profound impact on the nature of white-collar work. These trends include, but are not limited to, the downsizing of organizations, particularly with decreases in white-collar positions, and the develeling of management layers in organizations from 8 to 10, down to 3 or 4, which in combination have dramatically increased the *span of control* and responsibility of white-collar workers who remain employed. Corresponding with the trend toward deleveling, there has also been a shift in the philosophy of management toward empowerment, continuous improvement, an acceleration in career transitions, and promoting diversification of the work force (e.g., only 15 percent of new entrants into the work force will be white males by the year 2000). Collectively, these trends have led to a focus on the individual career needs of workers, and greater emphasis on developmental strategies extended over the working life-span (Daft, 1992; Schermerhorn, Hunt, & Osborn, 1994).

The current as well as future middle-aged white-collar worker faces several major challenges in the new workplace of the next millennium. These challenges include but are not limited to an increased focus on continuously improving work processes and the quality of products/services, globalization of work, rapid developments in information technologies, new ways of organizing, and increased attention to individual rights in the workplace (Schermerhorn et al., 1994). Each of these major trends is taken up below.

Changes in the Nature of Work

Productivity involves a comparison of the quality and quantity of output produced with the utilization of inputs required to achieve a certain level of output. Total quality management (TQM) scholars, such as W. Edwards Deming and Joseph Juran, have emphasized that the performance of organizational systems depends on the effectiveness of training employees to streamline organizational processes to only those activities that add value to the ultimate product and/or service (Sosik & Wilson-Dionne, 1994). Their recommendations focus on developing work systems that allow for greater flexibility to respond to rapidly changing needs in the market, as well as a focus on continually updating the knowledge and capabilities of the work force. Organizations are currently undergoing a dramatic shift in the way they structure work that is not only having a significant impact on what is expected of employees, but how they are evaluated and developed. For example, the move toward designing organizations with less hierarchical levels and more cross-functionality in terms of the composition of teams, is having a significant impact on what is expected of these workers. For example, employees often need to learn two or three different jobs that span several functional areas, while being rewarded for what they have learned in "pay for skills" reward programs, as well as pay for performance.

Globalization involves the expansion of the business and economic market to all geographic regions of the world. Globalization has prompted organizations to develop global thinking skills, while developing a broader understanding of multicultural perspectives. Globalization has replaced the traditional white male work force with people of different races, ethnic and national backgrounds, lifestyles, physical abilities, and ages (Bruxelles & Torres, 1992).

Today, it is not uncommon for even relatively small businesses in the United States to consider overseas markets as their primary place of business. The shift to a more global work force has the potential to break down many cultural barriers that previously existed between different countries. This trend is leading to a whole new range of interactions between different cultural groups that had never before existed. The interaction of these diverse cultures will certainly have an impact on the various preconceptions and stereotypes of individuals in different cultures—particularly age stereotypes. In some cultures, middle-aged to older workers may be viewed more positively and allowed opportunities to take on more challenging assignments at later stages in their careers. To the extent that they are successful in these assignments, the impact of negative age stereotypes on selection and evaluation decisions may be altered. In this vein, societies that have more negative stereotypes regarding older workers may be confronted with information and data that would necessitate a revisiting and substantial revision in those stereotypes.

Information Technology

Other factors driving the make-over in organizational structures include recent developments in information and computer technologies that are changing the way organizations process work. The advent of computer networking has broken down the flow of information in hierarchies into widely dispersed and loosely coupled systems of "information highways." Computer networks have facilitated an astounding explosion of information that empowers employees at lower levels, who previously were denied access to critical information flows. Consequently, decisions are now being made at lower organizational levels and closer to the point of contact with the customer. Thus, workers at increasingly lower levels of the organization have a much broader view of product development and how to address the needs of their customers (Avolio, 1997; Kiechel, 1993).

Computer networks can eliminate some psychological barriers that previously existed between functional departments by providing communication channels that result in a greater sharing of information across entire organizations. For example, new networks of employees from accounting, marketing, and production may be forged by computer technology that facilitates the operation of cross-functional teams (Sims & Lorenzi, 1992). Moreover, the proliferation of computer technology compels employees to develop higher levels of computer literacy in order to adapt to this changing aspect of their work. Indeed, perhaps the biggest change under way is the one in which the future white-collar worker will find him- or herself more well informed.

Diversification of Work Force Characteristics and Values

Changing demographics and work force diversity will also characterize the future nature of work and organizations. Changes such as the decrease in the size of the population and work force, and increases in the number of women, minorities, immigrants, and temporary workers in the work force impact the job mix and career opportunities in industry and society-at-large (Denton, 1992; Khojasteh, 1994). Management of a multicultural workplace will present challenges to managers and employees alike. The specific challenge facing managers is how to transform a slower, growing labor force composed of more female, immigrant, minority, and older workers into a skilled, efficient, and flexible resource (Elmati, 1993). Employees will need to develop sensitivity to working closely with individuals from different cultures and national origin. Moreover, managers will have to: (1) be more inclusive in recruiting workers; (2) invest in training employees to work with a much broader range of individuals; and (3) tap into the latent abilities of a much broader and diversified range of individual workers across the life-span. With less employees, who have greater cross-functional responsibilities, there will be more emphasis on tapping into the knowledge skills and abilities of the entire work force (Keen, 1992).

Focusing on Individual Rights

Organizations are now paying an increasing amount of attention to human rights issues in the workplace. Both union and nonunion work forces are pressing for increases in self-determination, employee rights, and equal employment opportunity (Schermerhorn et al., 1994). Self-determination involves active employee participation in both organization decision making and career planning and orientation. For example, some public accounting firms are now allowing their employees to determine job-related aspects such as clients they prefer to handle, hours they wish to work, and periods of time-off during the slow season (Mingle, 1994).

In sum, if current trends continue, we can expect to have middle-aged workers who: (1) have a broader array of skills because of cross-training across functional areas; (2) are more amenable to continuous training and development; (3) are used to working with individuals from a diverse range of cultures; (4) are comfortable using the newest technologies and information-processing equipment; and (5) are likely to be individuals who have a more proactive view on how to develop and maintain the knowledge, skills, and abilities required for competing in the "new" organizational systems of tomorrow.

Move toward Self-Managed Teams

Sims and Lorenzi (1992) have predicted that by the early part of the next millennium, *50%* of all organizations in the United States will be designed around the concept of self-directed/managed teams. The move toward self-directed teams requires that management share greater responsibility for decision making with employees of all ages, that there be a greater emphasis on continuous education, training, and development, and that rewards be designed to provide incentives for developing skills and knowledge across one's career, rather than just rewarding performance outcomes. In this regard, companies such as Corning, Inc. are dedicating 5% of the working year to educating its work force, thus continually developing its work force's capabilities and motivation to tackle problems across their careers (Daft, 1992).

Based on these current trends, the "new generation" of older white-collar workers that will appear in the next millennium will have been provided with rewards to not only maintain their capabilities but also to improve them over time. This represents a radical shift from earlier reward practices in organizations that have traditionally focused on "pay for performance" versus "pay for development."

As described by Senge (1990), the *learning organization* is one that facilitates the personal development of all employees, while continuously transforming and upgrading itself over time. The ideal organizational learning system is one in which development is designed to facilitate an individual's progression through various life stages/passages, thus maximizing the development and performance of individuals embedded in the system, as well as the overall organization's performance. Along these lines, Ray Stata, president and chairman of Analog Devices suggested "that the rate at which individuals and organizations learn may be the only sustainable, competitive advantage especially in knowledge intensive industries" (p. 74).

Based on current trends, one can easily imagine future organizations that are "learning enterprises," composed of a collection of interdependent self-sustaining employees who have the ability to apply their accumulated experience to handling novel situations (Morris, 1993). To the extent that training and education focuses on developing worker capabilities across the life-span to handle novel situations, we can expect to see a shift in patterns that have been typically observed at higher ages for problem-solving capabilities associated with those situations.

To the degree the work context has been shown to have a *direct* and *indirect* impact on worker motivation, ability, performance, and potential, one can only speculate what these dramatic shifts in the nature of work will have on the current and, more important, future middle-aged/older white-collar worker of the next millennium. However, prior research already noted earlier has shown linkages between the work/life context and current older worker ability, behavior, and performance, suggesting that changes accruing in the work environment may have a profound impact on the characteristics of the middle-aged worker of the next millennium.

Toffler (1990) talks of the shift occurring today in organizations from the "low brow" to the "high brow" firm. Toffler's prediction is consistent with trends noted earlier, in that he describes a work environment in which job knowledge is rapidly turning over, resulting in a significant need for continuous education and greater worker involvement in decision making at lower and lower levels in organizational hierarchies.

It is hard to imagine one achieving the type of total quality organization discussed by Edward Deming (1986), the learning organization discussed by Senge (1990), or the empowered work team discussed by Sims and Lorenzi (1992) without a continuous investment in the development of an organization's human resource potential. Indeed, we can represent the changes under way as a large-scale experiment that parallels those that have been conducted numerous times in the life-span literature. In those experiments, investigators typically have examined the impact of training and task modification on differences in intellectual ability for older versus younger adults (Schaie, 1990), except that in the current experimental setting, the training and task modifications are happening *in vivo*, with some organizations like Motorola committing to invest over 4% of its revenues into the continuous development of its work force. In contrast, in our hypothetical experiment, the other condition is represented by the many organizations that have yet to downsize, delevel, and empower their work force.

It is by no means an exaggeration that some organizations are at least 15 years ahead of others on this emerging development curve within the United States, and even further out if you compare those leading organizations to ones in comparable industries that operate in less developed nations. Given what we already know about the relationship between training interventions, task characteristics, and the maintenance of intellectual capacity across the life-span, it is interesting to speculate what one might observe in our middle-aged white-collar worker of the next millennium, who grew up in an empowered and intellectually rich organizational environment. The key question is: how will the focus on work force development and continuous improvement impact the motivation to learn and the cognitive abilities of future middle-aged to older workers, as compared to the current cohort of white-collar workers?

All other things being equal, and given the magnitude of the ongoing "experimental manipulation," we would predict that the patterns of intellectual aging may be significantly altered at later points in the life-span for white-collar workers who accrue a portfolio of enriched experiences across their careers. Supporting this prediction, there already is preliminary data summarized by Schaie (1990), which shows such positive trends for aging and cognitive abilities in more recent cohorts. Thus, to the extent that one's occupational environment impacts on cognitive aging patterns, we would expect the emergence of a more positive trend with aging white-collar workers in the next millennium.

Tieger (1989) suggests that our focus must now shift toward differentiating "natural aging" at work, that one might consider "context free," versus aging that is induced by the nature of work context. The distinction we make between natural aging and contextually based aging is to emphasize a belief of ours, that the context and its changes over time have not received adequate attention in the aging and work literature. Moreover, there has been no adequate longitudinal research examining the impact of the evolving context on worker ability, motivation, and performance. Given the dramatic shifts in the nature of work that are under way and predicted to occur, greater attention to the impact of the work context on white-collar ability, motivation, and performance seems well worth the effort. Future research must link individual and organizational learning patterns in a more explicit and structured way to fully understand the impact of the ongoing changes in the nature of work on middle-aged to older white-collar employees (Lowenthal, 1994; Morris, 1993).

We have summarized in Figure 1 the global structural changes occurring in organizations today and those anticipated in the next millennium. A more specific summary of events involved in those changes is presented in Figure 2.

A Shift in Generational Focus

Deutschman (1992), in his article entitled, "The Upbeat Generation," describes the current cohort of younger workers in college and/or their first full-time jobs, as placing greater importance on receiving development and continuing education opportunities. Dubbed "Generation X," this group repeatedly places greater value on careers as well as on lifestyles that provide for more intellectual enrichment and meaning (Woodruff, 1992).

In a 1990 American Management Association survey of 7200 business managers, 50% of this sample indicated that they measured success in terms of having more meaningful work to accomplish. These "new age" workers described having an interesting and meaningful job as being more important to them than advancing up organizational hierarchies (Goddard, 1991). According to Goddard, the new population of employees entering the work force today are more interested in solving worthwhile problems that get at root cause, and have their sights on continuous

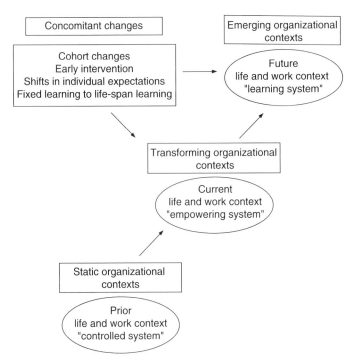

FIGURE 1   Macrochanges in organizational contexts.

change and improvement, compared to earlier cohorts. Finally, the current cohort of younger workers are more prone to question authority, similar to the emerging trends observed within the late 1970s' cohort of AT&T managers reported by Howard and Bray (1988).

The patterns noted for the upcoming generation are in fact not all that different from ones that are already emerging with the current generation of middle-aged workers (Paul & Townsend, 1993). For example, Paul and Townsend reported that 75% of middle-aged workers want to continue working in meaningful roles, and 50% desire to continually upgrade their skills throughout their careers.

SUMMARY

What are some basic patterns that are occurring in organizations today that will likely affect the nature of white-collar work and the worker into the next millennium? First, and foremost, the characteristics of the work force will change dramatically by the year 2005: white male professional and managerial workers will go from comprising 55% of the work force to 44%; white women professionals will go

- Expansion of each individual's zone of discretion

- Shift toward thinking versus doing (Corning, Inc. dedicates 5% of the work year to education)

- Rewards for development, learning, and performance

- Revenue shift from capitol improvements to continuous people improvement

- Recipients of information to creators and seekers

- Demands for higher perspective-taking capacity

- Requirements to learn job families versus tasks within jobs

- The nature of superior and follower interactions is changing and will change by cohort

FIGURE 2   Overview of impact at the individual level of analysis.

from comprising 37% to 42%; Hispanics will go from 6% to 11%, with a similar increase for blacks. Unfortunately, in the current literature, there is very little data on aging and work patterns for these minority groups to guide decision making and/or organizational policies (Avolio & Waldman, 1994; Warr, 1994). Other trends discussed in this section include the changing nature of white-collar jobs with increase in decision-making responsibility being pushed to lower organizational levels for higher level problems; at the same time there is greater attention placed on developing employees' knowledge, skills, and capabilities to continuously address new and emerging problems.

Organizational contexts are changing, with more emphasis being placed on learning and rewarding individuals for expanding their skill, knowledge, and competency base, as opposed to strictly rewarding performance outcomes (see Figure 2). We can only speculate at the present time what impact continuous development of future middle-aged and older workers will have on age stereotypes and age grading associated with both individuals and occupations.

CURRENT AGING AND WORK BEHAVIOR/ PERFORMANCE PATTERNS

We now turn our focus toward providing a general overview of age and work behavior patterns that have been reported in previous research. Specific reference is made in this section to the aging and work literature rather than the broader life-span literature on topics such as age and cognitive ability. Our purpose here is to summarize what we know about the relationship between age and work behavior so that we may have a basis for examining the gap between what we know and will need to know given the changing nature of work discussed earlier.

At present, much of the data on age and work behavior patterns indicates that there is greater variability within age groups than that observed between age groups, particularly at the upper reaches of the life-span. The pattern of findings observed in this literature supports taking a closer look at the context in which such patterns have emerged.

In most reviews of this literature, correlations reported between age and ability, motivation, and work performance are rather low, and are often better explained by taking into consideration job-relevant factors; for example, Fossum, Arvey, Paradise, and Robbins (1986) argued that declines in ability and/or performance for jobs whose content knowledge changes rapidly are more likely due to older technicians getting less exposure to training, education, and the most intellectually and challenging job assignments, than to "natural" aging processes. Thus, it is the "unexercised potential" that Denney (1982) referred to that may account for a portion of both the between- and within-age-group differences noted in this literature.

AGE GRADING/NORMS AND THEIR IMPACT ON WORK BEHAVIOR

The current cohort of older workers may not only be "selected out" by others from opportunities to learn new skills and competencies in their respective organizations, but they may also "self-select out," further accelerating the aging patterns noted in this literature. The self-selection that occurs may be partially attributed to the general notion among the current older white-collar professionals that they see themselves as being less suited for new learning experiences. Based on current age norms/grading of occupations, older white-collar workers may believe the stereotypes about intellectual aging leads them to make job choices that accelerate declines in ability, motivation, and ultimately work performance (Waldman & Avolio, 1993).

Age grading may affect not only the individual's confidence to take on various tasks of varying difficulty, but also those individuals who evaluate older workers in terms of their performance capabilities (Ferris, Judge, Chachere, & Liden, 1991). Such age norms may work against individuals in terms of performance evaluations, promotion, and/or initial selection decisions (Shore & Bleicken, 1991).

For instance, Saks and Waldman (1994) examined whether age norms worked against individuals entering entry-level white-collar professional positions, which have historically been filled with very young professionals, for example, public accounting. In their study of age-performance relationships involving a sample of public accountants, Saks and Waldman examined performance ratings for individuals ranging in age from 20 to 41, reporting a negative relationship between age and overall ratings of performance. This negative relationship was eliminated when they controlled for individual grade point averages and number of previous jobs held by these accountants.

Preliminary findings reported by Saks and Waldman (1994) indicate that certain age norms may exist for professional positions, which can bias the evaluations of "older" workers when there is a preponderance of younger workers occupying those positions. These results support earlier arguments presented by Lawrence (1988), concerning the impact of age norms on performance evaluations. Such age norms may bias not only initial selection decisions, but also promotion and training opportunities, and decisions made by individuals to select themselves in and out of such occupations.

With the rapid changes occurring in organizational structures today that are affecting white-collar occupations, some age norms may change more or less in favor of older professional white-collar workers, depending on the particular context in which these workers are embedded. For example, the rapid changeover in knowledge-intensive occupations may result in less older white-collar workers being selected into those positions. The "young" age norm that becomes established may work against the older employee, as was shown in the study reported by Saks and Waldman (1994) with public accountants. Consequently, the issue of whether previous age norms will apply to current and future white-collar occupations is still very much open to further debate and analysis.

Age and Job Satisfaction

Kacmar and Ferris (1989) have reported that satisfaction with work increased with age after controlling for job and organizational tenure. Similarly, Warr (1994) reported that there was a positive relationship between age and job contentment/occupational well-being, after controlling for tenure, job level, and work demands.

Sterns, Marsh, and McDaniel (1994) summarized the results of a meta-analysis, which is a quantitative method for aggregating previous research findings (see Hunter & Schmidt, 1990), of the age/job satisfaction literature with a sample totaling 30,069 individuals. Sterns, Marsh, and McDaniel (1994) reported a low positive correlation between age and job satisfaction ($r = .07$). Sterns et al. (1994) recommended that some of the variation observed across samples in the relationship between age and job satisfaction was probably due to occupational type. Specifically, for white-collar professionals the age and satisfaction correlation was *.16,* while for blue-collar positions the correlation was reduced to *.02.*

Age and Work Values

Engle, Miguel, Steelman, and McDaniel (1994) reported results of a meta-analysis of previous literature, which examined the relationships between age and work values. Engle et al. (1994) reported a positive relationship ($r = .23$) between age and Protestant Work Ethic, and a negative relationship ($r = -.07$) between age and growth need strength. These results suggest that the accrued context as well as stage of one's career development may contribute to the pattern of relationships observed at later points in an individual's life-span. For instance, the type of job and/or extent of family responsibilities at different career stages may moderate the relationship between age and growth need strength, satisfaction, and commitment to one's job, career, and organization (Engle et al., 1994).

Age and Turnover

In a similar vein, Healey, Lehman, and McDaniel (1994) reported results of a meta-analysis of the age and turnover literature with a sample that included 42,625 individuals. Healey et al. (1994) reported that age was negatively correlated with turnover ($r = -.08$), and that this relationship did not vary substantially for jobs coded at high ($r = -.07$), medium ($r = -.11$), and low complexity levels ($r = -.09$). Age provided relatively little added value in determining when individuals voluntarily chose to leave an organization. These results supported earlier findings reported by Cotton and Tuttle (1986) and Rhodes (1983).

Age and Work Performance

Meta-analyses of the age and work performance literature have also produced a similar pattern of results to those described previously. Two previous meta-analyses of this literature have reported relatively low correlations between age and work performance (McEvoy & Cascio, 1989; Waldman & Avolio, 1986).

Waldman and Avolio (1986) reported evidence to support (1) occupational type as a moderator of the age and work performance relationship, and that (2) the relationship between age and work performance varies depending on whether the job was a professional versus a nonprofessional occupation. Similarly, Sparrow and Davies (1988) indicated that the strength of the relationship between age and the quality of job performance varied depending on level of job complexity. Specifically, peak performance occurred later on in jobs requiring (1) greater levels of task complexity, and (2) levels of complexity that are typically associated with knowledge-based white-collar occupations.

Avolio, Waldman, and McDaniel (1990) showed that length of job-relevant experience across a broad range of 111 nonprofessional to semiprofessional occupations was a significant, if not better, predictor of performance than age over the working life-span. Avolio et al. (1990) reported that there was a small moderating effect for different occupational types on age–performance relationships, whereby both age and experience were shown to be better predictors for jobs requiring higher levels of cognitive ability and mastery of skills. Some drop-off in performance with age was noted for lower level clerical occupations, although, in general, work performance plateaued over the working life-span.

Results from each of these meta-analyses point to the importance of examining the work context/experiences an individual accrues over time on individual attitudes, behavior, and performance. Specifically, when we find that the work context moderates the relationship between age and work behavior/performance, we are suggesting that the context is relevant to understanding, if not explaining, the pattern of this relationship. Unfortunately, in most prior research, job and contextual experiences have typically been measured in number of years an employee has been in a job/occupation, not in terms of the nature of the work context, thus limiting its explanatory value (Avolio et al., 1990; Waldman & Avolio, 1993). Future research will need to examine both the quantity and the quality of experiences accumulated over time, at one level of analysis, to determine the impact of occupational and job type characteristics on subsequent age and work behavior/performance relationships.

AGE DIFFERENCES IN COGNITIVE ABILITY

One of the most widely researched areas in life-span psychology has involved the examination of differences and declines in cognitive and intellectual abilities at older ages. As noted at the outset of this chapter, some of the recent research in this area has demonstrated that the most significant declines in cognitive ability occur very late in the life-span, and may therefore have relatively little impact on actual work performance competencies (Avolio & Waldman, 1994; Schaie & Willis, 1993).

Schaie and Willis (1993) summarized the literature in the area of age and cognitive abilities, indicating that ability levels peaked, on average, around midlife, and then plateaued for the next 25–30 years, after which they demonstrated some acceleration in decline. Schaie and Willis suggested that future research should focus on determining the extent of interindividual differences, rather than attempting to confirm and/or disconfirm decremental patterns of aging in various cognitive abilities.

For nearly half a century, the literature on age and cognitive abilities has examined alternative explanations for age–test differences. For example, Lorge (1945) suggested that differences observed between older and younger cohorts, educational levels, and years since being involved in formal educational programs would account for age–test differences in intellectual performance at various points across the life-span. Most prior research, however, has confounded age and average educational levels when analyzing age–test differences in cognitive ability. Specifically, prior research has not separated out how recently workers attended educational programs, nor examined the quality of those programs. Moreover, there has been relatively little emphasis on systematically examining the impact of an individual's work and broader life context on age–cognitive ability relationships (Avolio & Waldman,

1990, 1994). The lack of data on these issues is magnified when dealing with underrepresented minorities.

In line with arguments to refocus future research on the accrued context and its impact on age–test differences in cognitive ability, Bronfenbrenner (1979) suggests that, "the assumption is that the nature of the attribute does not change, irrespective of the context in which one finds oneself" (p. 207). Similarly, Salthouse (1991) suggests that "the role of experience as a causal factor responsible for age differences in cognition is therefore still very much an open question" (p. 153). Yet, Salthouse goes on to say that it is unlikely that age differences in cognitive ability measures at various points across the life-span will be appreciably altered and/or eliminated by controlling for differences in individual experience. We agree with Salthouse's major premise, that at some point in the life cycle some decline in functional capacity will occur no matter what the experiences an individual has accrued. However, our interest is in examining those factors that can enhance the maintenance of ability and performance among white-collar workers, by taking a closer look at the impact of the evolving context on patterns of aging from the earliest stages of one's career to retirement, with respect to ability, motivation, and performance. The data does not yet exist to examine these factors.

Several studies have demonstrated a connection between specific experiences with certain job characteristics and differences observed in ability across the life-span (e.g., Denney, 1982, 1984, 1989; Salthouse, Babcock, Mitchell, Skrovronek, & Palmon, 1990; Schaie, 1984; Schooler, 1984). For example, Schooler (1984) reported that individuals who worked in job environments represented by higher levels of task complexity maintained higher levels of cognitive functioning over the life-span. Similarly, Schaie (1984) concluded that both the degree of engagement with one's environment and level of environment complexity accounted for some of the interindividual differences in cognitive functioning observed at later points in the life-span. Similarly, Salthouse et al. (1990) reported that architects preserved higher levels of spatial ability at later points in the life-span, when compared with a group of nonarchitects of similar ages. However, consistent with our earlier comments, even architects who accrued continuous experience in working with their spatial abilities showed declines in those abilities at older ages.

In line with the impact of the environment on age–test performance, Schooler (1990) suggested that occupations supporting greater self-direction can have a significant impact on the level of intellectual flexibility observed at later points in the life-span. Schooler summarized this position, stating that, "the findings of cross-cultural, social and cognitive research indicate that the nature and effectiveness of adult cognitive processes are affected by socially structured and culturally determined experiences" (p. 353).

To date, the role of the experiences one accrues on and off the job, in explaining age–test differences, is still poorly understood. Moreover, the evolving and ongoing changes in white-collar positions and the impact of those changes on the future middle-aged work force is not, and almost by definition cannot be, fully understood in terms of its impact on aging processes until we have been able to track patterns with this target group over time.

At the present time, we need much better documentation of the types of experiences individuals accrue both in and out of the job setting, and the relationship of those experiences to the maintenance of ability across the life-span. Of equal importance is the linking of those experiences to the white-collar worker's knowledge base that has accrued over time, and its *direct* and *indirect* impact on the maintenance and/or decline of certain key abilities. For example, through continuous training, we expect that the knowledge base an individual accrues should result in their maintaining higher levels of cognitive functioning at later points in the life-span (Charness, 1988).

Schmidt, Hunter, and Outerbridge (1986) suggest that specific experiences result in the creation of knowledge, which can in turn impact on levels of cognitive ability observed at later points in the life-span. Miller, Slomczynski, and Kohn (1985) reported that people who did more intellectually stimulating work learned from the job and developed knowledge sets that they could generalize to non-job-related activities. In a similar vein, Miller, Schooler, Kohn, and Miller (1979) examined the closeness of supervision an employee had received over time, concluding that the level of occupational self-direction positively affected future levels of intellectual performance for both males and females in their sample.

Lee (1991) has also shown a positive relationship between the level of task complexity associated with occupations and cognitive ability level. Similarly, Avolio and Waldman (1990) reported that occupational type moderated age–test differences for a nationally representative sample of American male and female workers aged 18–65. Specifically, they reported a low negative relationship between age and General Aptitude Test Battery (a widely used standard measure of individual cognitive ability) performance for employees from white-collar clerical occupations, while for individuals in health care occupations, there was a much greater drop-off in cognitive test performance at older ages. Avolio and Waldman (1990) hypothesized that the accumulation of high levels of stress over one's career and burnout may have had a negative impact on the maintenance of cognitive abilities observed in their sample at the upper end of the life-span. Avolio and Waldman (1990) recommended that future research "examine the connection between specific life and occupational experiences and how such experiences may influence an individual's cognitive abilities over time" (p. 49).

Collectively, previous studies indicate that future research should take an "interactionist" view toward studying aging and work patterns, whereby the job context and life experiences are examined in terms of their impact on ability, motivation, and performance over the life-span. At the same time, we must view the individual as an active agent in shaping his or her own life and work context. Specifically, some individuals may choose to stay in jobs in which there is little if any intellectual stimulation, while others may continually upgrade jobs, having a more positive impact on the maintenance of their intellectual/cognitive abilities at later points in the career/life-span. A main point in this chapter has been that irrespective of what the individual chooses to do, the context is changing so dramatically in white-collar occupations that future research will need to take into consideration these evolving trends to fully explain patterns in aging and work behavior, ability, and performance observed into the next millennium.

Some Extensions to Earlier Results

To expand on the comparisons reported by Avolio and Waldman (1990) with their sample of white-collar and blue-collar workers employed in 111 different jobs, and to build on earlier findings that have shown differences in ability and performance for these target groups, we have reanalyzed the data reported in Avolio and Waldman by comparing white-collar ($n = 2363$) to blue-collar ($n = 18,391$) employees on both cognitive ability and job performance measures (see Avolio and Waldman, 1990, for a more detailed description of their original study).

Test patterns for workers presented in terms of young standard deviation units (less than or equal to 19) are provided in Figures 3 and 4. Using this standard for comparison, we can examine how each successive age group compares to the youngest age group. Figure 3 summarizes findings for white-collar/semiprofessional occupations, demonstrating differences in ratings of overall work performance between the six age groupings (Figure 3a), and differences in cognitive ability as measured by the General Aptitude Test Battery (GATB) (Figure 3b).

Figure 3a shows relatively little variation in age–test performance patterns up to and including age 65. For General, Verbal, and Numerical abilities (Figure 3b), differences across the working life-span on all three measures of cognitive ability were less than 1 standard deviation unit.

The data presented in Figure 4 demonstrate a similar pattern of results, in that performance remained relatively stable over the typical working life-span, while cognitive ability showed relatively small drop-offs up to and including age 65. Consequently, patterns of work performance and cognitive ability for nonprofessional blue-collar positions indicated that the drop-offs in both ability and performance were relatively small when comparing each of five older age groups to the youngest workers in the sample.

Building on our earlier comments, the extent to which occupations in this sample become more self-directed and require continuous learning, the more likely the context accrued by the current group of young to middle-aged workers will have a positive impact on age–test patterns observed at older ages. Changing our focus from intraindividual change to interindividual change will require that we take a closer look at interindividual differences and the "common causes" that have an impact on age changes in cognitive ability across the working life-span (Salthouse, 1992). Some of the "common causes" already discussed in this article with respect to changes in the nature of white-collar jobs will be particularly interesting

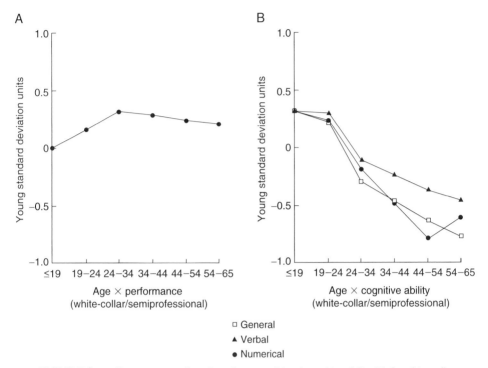

FIGURE 3   Differences in overall work performance (A) and cognitive ability (B) for white-collar semiprofessional workers in six age groupings.

to track over time in terms of their impact on ability, motivation, and performance. For example, it will be interesting to examine shifts in age–test differences in cognitive ability that have been demonstrated for earlier cohorts that grew up in an environment in which empowerment, continuous learning, and self-directed work teams were not part of management practices, versus the current cohort of workers who are involved in empowering organizational cultures.

SUMMARY

In this section, we reviewed a number of studies on aging and work behavior/performance that indicated that a much closer look at the context in which white-collar employees are embedded was required. To a large extent, chronological age accounted for relatively little variance in ability and performance differences across the typical working life-span.

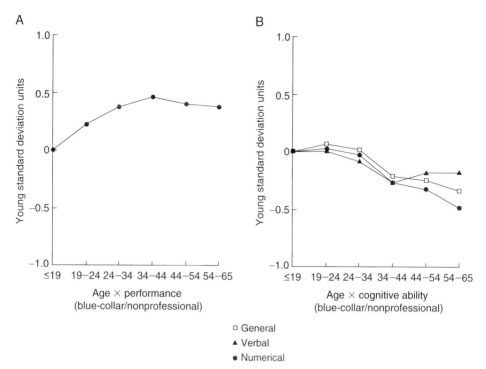

FIGURE 4   Differences in overall work performance (A) and cognitive ability (B) for blue-collar nonprofessional workers in six age groupings.

USING "LIFE STRUCTURES" TO EXAMINE CONNECTIONS BETWEEN INDIVIDUALITY AND CAREER DEVELOPMENT

Recent discussions in the career development literature have begun to take a much closer look at how we might separate life and career stages of individuals to explain distinctly different patterns of development (Cytrynbaum & Crites, 1989). For example, a female white-collar employee reentering the work force at age 50 may be going through a *maintenance stage* of her career when she is in her late 50s, rather than her early 40s, as implied by most career development models. In this way, career development processes can be viewed as being relative, based on one's accrued life and work context. Furthermore, we can then extend this view of career development to constructing clusters of individuals, who display similar and/or prototypical career development patterns.

   One useful approach is to consider the "life structure" of individuals, to determine the basis for their individuality. Similar to our earlier discussion on the impact of one's accrued life and work context on individual development, Levinson and Gooden (1985, p. 5) have discussed the concept of life structure as representing the "underlying pattern or design of a person's life at a given point in time." Such life structures are in flux and malleable, based on the contextual experiences an individual is exposed to over the course of his or her life-span.

Most career life-span models represent what Vrondracek, Lerner, and Schulenberg (1986) referred to as "developmental contextualism." Specifically, the focus is on examining where internal "natural aging" effects end and social forces begin, with respect to life-span development. Thus, we can examine the "life structure" of individuals who have accrued certain experiences that would set them apart from other subgroups. This sort of framework has been discussed in more general terms in Schein's (1978) career anchor model, in the sense that Schein focused on individual differences and similarities within certain career points and anchors, discussing adult socialization with respect to careers as a moving synthesis across different occupational and career stages.

Schein's model has its roots in the work of authors such as Dill, Hilton, and Reitman (1962), who developed a career model based on the premise that development could be explained only by carefully examining the interaction over time between the individual and his or her environment. In line with the main thesis of the current chapter, development is significantly affected by the opportunities organizations provide and will provide into the future with respect to opportunities to learn and build knowledge and skills. Dill et al. (1962) also viewed the environment as a complex shifting reality over time, in which individuals learn (more or less) to interact effectively with the changing demands and challenges of their respective contexts.

Going back to some of the emerging trends in organizations predicted for the next millennium, we can speculate how de-leveling might positively impact the exploration stage associated with younger employees, while negatively impacting an individual's need for advancement. Consequently, the changes in organization structure alone may create a very different life structure than has been observed in the current or previous cohorts of white-collar workers (Arthur & Kram, 1989). In a very real sense, the past may no longer be an adequate indicator of future age and work/career patterns.

SOME IMPLICATIONS AND CONCLUSIONS

There have been two major themes articulated in the current chapter. The first focused on the changing nature of white-collar occupations and the impact those changes may have on the development of individuals occupying those positions. The second major theme focused on taking a multilevel view of individual development with much greater attention being paid to the context and its impact on individual development over time. Suggestions for further analysis and construction of subgroups based on different life structures provide at least one practical alternative to existing life-span models of human development that are currently available in the literature. Such models of development will go a long way toward helping to classify situations and contexts that have long been shown to have both a *direct* and an *indirect* impact on worker ability, motivation, and performance across the life-span.

REFERENCES

Arthur, M. B., & Kram, K. E. (1989). Reciprocating at work: The separate, yet inseparable possibilities for individual and organizational develop. In M. B. Arthur, D. T. Hall, & B. S. Lawrence (Eds.), *Handbook of career theory* (pp. 66–89). Cambridge: Cambridge University Press.

Avolio, B. J. (1997). *The great leadership migration to a full-range leadership development system.* Kellogg Leadership Studies Project, University of Maryland, College Park, MD.

Avolio, B. J., & Waldman, D. A. (1987). Personnel aptitude test scores as a function of age, education and a job type. *Experimental Aging Research, 13,* 109–113.

Avolio, B. J., & Waldman, D. A. (1990). An examination of age and cognitive test performance across job complexity and occupational types. *Journal of Applied Psychology, 75,* 43–50.

Avolio, B. J., & Waldman, D. A. (1994). Variations in cognitive abilities across the working lifespan: Examining the effects of race, experience, education and occupational type. *Psychology and Aging, 9,* 430–432.

Avolio, B. J., Waldman, D. A., & McDaniel, M. A. (1990). Age and work performance in nonmanagerial jobs: The effects of experience and occupational type. *Academy of Management Journal, 33,* 407–422.

Baltes, P. B., & Baltes, M. M. (1990). *Successful aging.* Cambridge, UK: Cambridge University Press.

Bass, B. M. (1994). Continuity and change in the evolution of work and human resource management. *Human Resource Management, 33*(1), 3–31.

Bridges, W. (1994). The end of the job. *Fortune, 130*(6), 62–74.

Bronfenbrenner, U. (1979). *The ecology of human development: Experiments by nature and design.* Cambridge, MA: Harvard University Press.

Bruxelles, M. & Torres, C. (1992). Capitalizing on global diversity. *HR Magazine, 37*(12), 30–33.

Charness, W. (1988). The role of theories of cognitive aging: Comment on Salthouse. *Psychology and Aging, 3,* 17–21.

Cotton, J. L., & Tuttle, J. M. (1986). Employee turnover: A meta-analysis and review with implications for research. *Academy of Management Review, 11,* 55–70.

Cytrynbaum, S., & Crites, J. O. (1989). The utility of adults development theory in understanding career adjustment process. In M. B. Arthur, D. T. Hall, & B. S. Lawrence (Eds.), *Handbook of career theory* (pp. 66–89). Cambridge: Cambridge University Press.

Daft, R. L. (1992). *Organization theory and design.* St. Paul, MN: West Publishing Company.

Deming, W. E. (1986). *Out of the crisis.* Cambridge: MIT Institute for Advanced Engineering Study.

Denney, N. W. (1982). Aging and cognitive changes. In B. B. Wolman (Ed.), *Handbook of developmental psychology* (pp. 807–827). Englewood Cliffs, NJ: Prentice-Hall.

Denney, N. W. (1984). A model of cognitive development across the life span. *Developmental Review, 4,* 171–191.

Denney, N. W. (1989). Everyday problem solving: Methodological issues: Research findings and a model. In L. W. Poon, D. C. Rubin, & B. A. Wilson (Eds.), *Everyday cognition in adulthood and later life* (pp. 330–351). Cambridge, UK: Cambridge University Press.

Denton, W. (1992). Workforce 2000. *Credit World, 81*(1), 14–18.

Deutschman, A. (1992). The upbeat generation. *Fortune, 26*(1), 42–54.

Dill, W. R., Hilton, T. L., & Reitman, W. R. (1962). *The new managers.* Englewood Cliffs, NJ: Prentice-Hall.

Elmati, D. (1993). Managing diversity in the workplace: An immense challenge for both managers and workers. *Industrial Management, 35*(4), 19–22.

Engle, E., Miguel, R., Steelman, L., & McDaniel, M. A. (1994, April). *The relationship between age and work needs: A comprehensive research integration.* Paper presented at the National Meetings of the Society for Industrial and Organizational Psychology, Nashville, TN.

Ferris, G. R., Judge, T. A., Chachere, J. G., & Liden, R. D. (1991). Work unit age composition, supervision, age and subordinate outcomes. *Psychology and Aging, 6,* 616–622.

Fossum, J. A., Arvey, R. D., Paradise, C. A., & Robbins, N. E. (1986). Modeling the skills obsolescence process: A psychological/economic integration. *Academy of Management Review, 11,* 362–374.

Goddard, R. W. (1991). A new view of work. *Supervision, April,* 14–26.

Healey, M., Lehman, M., & McDaniel, M. A. (1994, April). *Age and job-relevant training performance.* Paper presented at the National Meetings of the Society for Industrial and Organizational Psychology, Nashville, TN.

Howard, A., & Bray, D. W. (1988). *Managerial lives in transition: Advancing age and changing times.* New York: Guilford Press.

Hunter, J. E., & Schmidt, F. L. (1990). *Methods of meta-analysis: Correcting errors and bias in research findings.* Newbury Park, CA: Sage.

Kacmar, K. M., & Ferris, G. R. (1989). Theoretical and methodological considerations in the age-job satisfaction relationship. *Journal of Applied Psychology, 74,* 102–207.

Keen, C. (1992). The changing nature of work. *Financial World, 16*(13), 66–75.

Khojasteh, M. (1994). Workforce 2000: Demographic change and then impact. *Industrial Journal of Public Administration, 17*(3), 465–505.

Kiechel, W. (1993). How will we work in the year 2000? *Fortune, 127*(10), 38–52.

Kohn, M. L., & Schooler, C. (1983). The cross-national universality of the interpretive model. In M. L. Kohn & C. Schooler (Eds.), *Work and personality: An inquiry into the impact of social stratification* (pp. 281–295). NJ: Ablex.

Lawrence, B. S. (1988). New wrinkles in the theory of age: Demography, norms, and performance ratings. *Academy of Management Journal, 31,* 309–337.

Lee, J. S. (1991). *Abstraction and aging.* New York: Springer-Verlag.

Levinson, D. J., & Gooden, W. E. (1985). The life cycle. In H. I. Kaplan & B. J. Sadocle (Eds.), *Comprehensive textbook of psychology* (4th ed.). Baltimore, MD: Williams and Williams.

Lorge, L. L. (1945). Schooling makes a difference. *Teachers College Record, 46,* 483–492.

Lowenthal, J. (1994). *Reengineering the organization.* Milwaukee, WI: ASQC Quality Press.

McEvoy, G. M., & Cascio, W. F. (1989). Cumulative evidence of the relationship between age and job performance. *Journal of Applied Psychology, 74,* 11–17.

Miller, J. G. (1978). *Living systems.* New York: McGraw-Hill.

Miller, J., Schooler, C., Kohn, M. L., & Miller, K. A. (1979). Women and work: The psychological effects of occupational conditions. *American Journal of Sociology, 85,* 66–94.

Miller, J., Slomczynski, K. M., & Kohn, M. L. (1985). Continuity of learning-generalization throughout the life span: The impact of job on intellectual processes in the United States. *American Journal of Sociology, 91,* 593–615.

Mingle, J. (1994). The shape of firms to come. *Journal of Accountancy, July,* 39–46.

Morris, L. (1993). Learning organizations: Settings for developing adults. In J. Denide & P. Miller (Eds.), *Development in the workplace* (pp. 179–197). Hillsdale, NJ: Erlbaum.

Paul, R. J., & Townsend, J. B. (1993). Managing the older worker: Don't just rinse away the gray. *Academy of Management Executive, 1,* 67–74.

Rhodes, S. R. (1983). Age-related differences in work attitudes and behavior: A review and conceptual analysis. *Psychological Bulletin, 93,* 328–367.

Robinson, W. S. (1950). Ecological correlations and the behavior of individuals. *American Sociological Review, 15,* 351–357.

Rousseau, D. M. (1985). Issues of level in organizational research: Multi-level and cross-level perspectives. In B. Staw & L. Cummings (Eds.), *Research in organizational behavior* (Vol. 7, pp. 1–37). Greenwich, CT: JAI Press.

Saks, A. M., & Waldman, D. A. (1994, April). *The relationship between age and job performance for entry-level professionals.* Paper presented at the National Meetings of the Society for Industrial and Organizational Psychology, Nashville, TN.

Salthouse, T. A. (1991). *Theoretical perspectives in cognitive aging.* Hillsdale, NJ: Erlbaum.

Salthouse, T. A. (1992). *Mechanisms of age-cognition relations in adulthood.* Hillsdale, NJ: Erlbaum.

Salthouse, T. A., Babcock, R., Mitchell, D. R., Skrovronek, E., & Palmon, R. (1990). Age and experience effects in spatial visualization. *Developmental Psychology, 26,* 128–136.

Schaie, K. W. (1984). Midlife influences upon intellectual functioning in old age. *International Journal of Behavioral Development, 7,* 463–478.

Schaie, K. W. (1990). Intellectual development in adulthood. In J. E. Birren & K. W. Schaie (Eds.), *Handbook of the psychology of aging* (pp. 291–310). San Diego: Academic Press.

Schaie, K. W. (1994). The course of adult intellectual development, *American Psychologist* (Vol. 49, pp. 304–314).

Schaie, K. W., & Willis, S. L. (1993). Age difference patterns of psychometric intelligence in adulthood: Generalizability within and across ability domains. *Psychology and Aging, 8,* 44–55.

Schein, E. H. (1978). *Career dynamics: Matching individual and organizational needs.* Reading, MA: Addison-Wesley.

Schermerhorn, J., Hunt, J. G., & Osborn, R. (1994). *Managing organizational behavior.* New York: John Wiley.

Schmidt, F. L., Hunter, J. E., & Outerbridge, A. N. (1986). Impact of job experience and ability on job knowledge, work sample performance, and supervisory ratings of performance. *Journal of Applied Psychology, 71,* 432–439.

Schooler, C. (1984). Psychological effects of complex environments during the life-span: A review and theory. *Intelligence, 8,* 259–281.

Schooler, C. (1990). Psycho-social factors and effective cognitive functioning in adulthood. In J. E. Birren & K. W. Schaie (Eds.), *The handbook of aging* (pp. 347–358). San Diego: Academic Press.

Senge, P. (1990). *The fifth discipline.* New York: Doubleday.

Shore, L. M., & Bleicken, L. M. (1991). Effect of supervisor age and subordinate age on rating congruence. *Human Relations, 44,* 1093–1105.

Sims, H. P., Jr., & Lorenzi, P. (1992). *The new leadership paradigm: Social learning and cognition in organizations.* Newbury Park, CA: Sage.

Sosik, J. J., & Wilson-Dionne, S. D. (1994, April). *Deming's total quality leadership: Assessing the appropriateness of a single leadership style.* Paper presented at the National Meeting of the Academy of Management, Dallas, TX.

Sparrow, P. R., & Davies, D. R. (1988). Effects of age, tenure, training, and job complexity on technical performance. *Psychology and Aging, 3,* 307–314.

Sterns, A. A., Marsh, B. A., & McDaniel, M. A. (1994, April). *Age and job satisfaction: A comprehensive review and meta-analysis.* Paper presented at the National Meeting of the Society for Industrial and Organizational Psychology, Nashville, TN.

Tieger, C. (1989). Le vieillissement différentiel dans et par le travail. *Le Travail Humain, 52,* 21–56.

Toffler, A. (1990). *Powers shift.* New York: Bantam Books.

Vrondracek, F. W., Lerner, R. M., & Schulenberg, J. E. (1986). *Career development: A lifespan development approach.* Hillsdale, NJ: Erlbaum.

Waldman, D. A., & Avolio, B. J. (1986). A meta-analysis of age differences in job performance. *Journal of Applied Psychology, 71,* 33–38.

Waldman, D. A., & Avolio, B. J. (1993). Age and work performance in perspective: A cross-sequential model. In K. N. Rowland & G. Ferris (Eds.), *Research in personnel and human resource management* (pp. 133–162). Greenwich, CT: JAI Press.

Warr, P. (1994). Age and employment. In H. C. Triandis, M. D. Dunnette, and L. M. Hough (Eds.), *Handbook of industrial and organizational psychology* (Vol. 4, pp. 485–558). Palo Alto, CA: Consulting Psychologists Press.

Woodruff, M. (1992). Understanding and supervising the 20 something. *Supervision, April,* 10–12.

CHAPTER 12

Middle Age: New Thoughts, New Directions

James D. Reid

Department of Psychology, Washington University, St. Louis, Missouri

Sherry L. Willis

The Pennsylvania State University, University Park, Pennsylvania

As the millennium approaches, a greater understanding of human growth and development during middle age is of crucial importance. With the passage of the baby-boom generation from adulthood into midlife and late life, the need for an expanded knowledge base about midlife development becomes even more important. In this volume, we have attempted to present a picture of the dynamic nature of biological, psychological, and social functioning in midlife. A model of holistic functioning in adult development has guided our progress through the various chapters. The human organism, not unlike a flower or field of grain, undergoes seasons of growth and development. Not unlike the lovely flower, the midlife individual remains full of life but becomes increasingly aware of the reality of frost. It is in this season of life that the individual finds himself or herself poised in the middle: somewhere between the dynamic energy of youth on one hand and the inevitability of eventual decline and death on the other. It is this middle ground, stable yet always dynamically changing, that now presents new challenges for the individual to face during middle age.

As we look back across the chapters of *Life in the Middle,* some major themes emerge. We now turn our attention to these themes as well as new thoughts about middle age, and new directions for scholarly inquiry into this increasingly important era of the life-span.

DEVELOPMENT IN MIDLIFE IS UNDERSTOOD WITHIN A HISTORICAL AND SOCIOCULTURAL CONTEXT

As noted throughout this book, contributors have emphasized the importance of the contextual milieu of the developing individual. At middle age, the individual finds herself or himself within an environment molded and shaped by cultural, social, economic, political, and historical forces. The developmental setting including the local community—churches, educational institutions, neighborhoods, cities, states, and countries—influences the individual's experience. In addition, the interpersonal environment—families, peers, and relationships with co-workers— are contextual influences that profoundly shape the lives of individuals.

The baby-boom generation has witnessed and experienced dramatic historical changes that have influenced the developmental process. In addition to the unprecedented size of the current cohorts, changes in life expectancy and longevity have resulted in remarkable opportunities and challenges. Political and social change, as well as changes in technology, and the shifting demographic or ethnic profiles of American citizens have shaped and molded the experience of the developing individual in ways that are very different from those of previous generations.

For the first time in history, adults finds themselves living in a global village in which cultural and political dynamics in various parts of the world become influential informational sources for making sense of one's own life. Our understanding of midlife will increase as we expand our openness to consideration of these important multicultural issues. Further research on midlife will be enriched by focusing greater attention on variability due to race, ethnicity, gender, and sexual orientation. By better understanding cultural and ethnic variability, aspects of midlife development that are universal can be teased apart from those developmental experiences that are constrained by culture-specific influences.

MIDLIFE DEVELOPMENT IS INFLUENCED BY AN INTERACTION OF HEREDITY AND ENVIRONMENT

Particularly in the area of biological development, but also in other areas of inquiry such as personality traits, variability attributed to genetic influences has been the subject of increasing interest. Just as cultural and environmental factors influence development in midlife, so do genetic factors. The interactive effects of genetic and environmental influences are areas of continued, as well as future, research.

Perhaps the literature on midlife development will be spared the nature/nurture debate to the extent that it has traditionally been present in thinking about childhood and adolescence. The quality of the conversation is elevated by the important contribution of behavior geneticists who carefully study heredity—environment interactions as they relate to midlife development.

MIDLIFE DEVELOPMENT INVOLVES BOTH CONTINUITY AND DISCONTINUITY

Developmental theory presents contradictory accounts of the process of development. Some theorists suggest that the nature of development across the life-span involves gradual change that is cumulative or incremental. Other theorists characterize the course of development as progressing through qualitatively distinct stages.

Similarly, the literature on midlife presents contradictory descriptions of change. Whereas some theorists suggest that change is progressive, other theorists hold the view that development is characterized by periods of stability followed by abrupt shifts. Future research will improve our understanding by focusing attention to those specific domains of biopsychosocial functioning best characterized by continuity or discontinuity.

THE "MIDLIFE CRISIS" HAS BEEN OVERDRAMATIZED

As has been noted, learning to grow is often a struggle. However, the popular notion of a "midlife crisis" as a normative developmental experience is not strongly supported by current literature. Perhaps a more accurate description would suggest that midlife is a time of reevaluation, introspection, and prioritization. Some individuals, it is true, find the reality of faded youth and lost opportunities to be distressing. In addition, the growing realization of the inevitability of one's own mortality may lead to a sense of hopelessness and despair. However, for many individuals, the beauty of development during midlife involves an emerging sense of perspective regarding one's own place within the life cycle.

The cultural and historical period in which the notion of a "midlife crisis" first emerged was a time of rapid and immense social change. The United States of the 1960s and 1970s witnessed dramatic social and personal introspection as well as the desire, by many, to take a look within and make personal changes in order to live more fully. In addition, this was a historical period that directed attention to mental health as well as psychological and personal growth.

In contrast, the relative stability and affluence of the 1980s and 1990s have witnessed a reemergence of unbridled capitalism that tends to view humans as machines to be used up and replaced with newer and cheaper parts when they wear down. Survival of the economically fittest is the rule of the current game. Unfortunately, corporate and government entities now place little emphasis on emotional well-being and fostering of optimal mental health. If midlife is a time of reevaluation, introspection, and prioritization, it will be interesting to observe how future cohorts of midlife individuals react to their own aging and assess their own lives.

MIDLIFE DEVELOPMENT IS DETERMINED BY BOTH EARLY AND LATER EXPERIENCES

The individual at middle age is shaped by both early developmental experiences and ongoing life events. Some theorists place heavy emphasis on the importance of early childhood experiences as critical determinants of development in adulthood. As such, relationship quality and deficiencies in parental relationships are believed to create needs in the child that reemerge across developmental eras. Other theorists seem to reject the notion that previous experience shapes development in adulthood in significant ways. These theorists point to events and experiences in adulthood as the major determinants of development during midlife. This debate is ongoing.

THE FAMILY PLAYS A LARGE ROLE IN MIDLIFE DEVELOPMENT

A large part of being in the middle during midlife, refers to the position of the individual within the family. What has been referred to as the "sandwich generation" places emphasis on the unique challenges and stresses of the midlife individual who is faced with pressures from younger and older generations. The individual at midlife may have children who place demands on their middle-aged parents for time, energy, and financial support. On another front, aging parents may place pressures and demands that are different but equally taxing.

Relationship issues, both good and bad, influence development during midlife. Romantic and marital relationships may be sources of rich fulfillment, as well as considerable psychological pain. Divorce and separation, conflicts with children and step-children, sibling rivalry and difficulties with step-siblings, interactions with parents and grandparents, as well as relationships with extended family members all make important contributions to ongoing experiences in middle age.

Despite the stresses and strains of family life, the family is an important source of identity, self-esteem, and well-being. Research designed to describe more fully and explain in greater detail the influence of family relationships on midlife development will contribute greatly to understanding of the individual at midlife.

GENDER DIFFERENCES AND GENDER
EQUALITY ARE IMPORTANT ISSUES

Issues of gender and gender equality are important areas of understanding that have not received enough attention within the literature on midlife. Many of the studies of normative development during middle age have used samples of only men. In addition, attention to women's development and the influence of the ubiquitous tyranny of a rigid gender dichotomy will greatly expand our understanding of development during this era of the life-span. Similarly, greater study of issues of gender can ultimately lead to liberation from rigid gender roles that constrain behavior and influence mental health in negative ways.

In addition, attention to gender and gender issues can direct attention not only to the role that gender and sex roles play in shaping identity, but to greater attention to sexuality in general. The reality of variability in sexual interests, sexual identities, and sexual orientation cannot be ignored in future research on midlife. The relative invisibility of core issues of sexuality in discussions of midlife cannot be sustained in the mainstream arena of academic inquiry.

MIDLIFE DEVELOPMENT IS DETERMINED
BY AN INTERACTION OF BIOLOGICAL,
PSYCHOLOGICAL, AND SOCIAL PROCESSES

Biological processes involve changes in external appearance and internal organ system functioning. The influences of genetic processes, which may have been set in motion at earlier times or emergent only latter in life, are dynamic and ongoing sources of developmental change during middle age. Diet and lifestyle factors, which are often begun at earlier developmental eras, result in changes in physical health during midlife. In addition, hormonal changes impact physical functioning, health, appearance, and identity.

Personality changes as well as emotional and subjective well-being are important issues that relate to psychological functioning during middle age. Continued inquiry into the nature of the developing self, identity, and self-esteem is of critical importance for future research. Continuity and change in cognitive processes, including changes in mental abilities and thought processes of individuals during midlife, will remain an important area of inquiry. Strategies and techniques for the maintenance of optimal cognitive functioning, as well as reversal of decrements in intelligence and problem-solving skills are important areas of applied interest. Emerging data on individual difference variability point to exciting intervention strategies to prevent or reverse unwanted decrement in abilities. Social changes involve changes in relationships with romantic partners, family, co-workers, and friends. As noted previously, the interpersonal context is an important component of psychological well-being, and an important area of future inquiry.

Biological, psychological, and social functioning can best be understood as processes of dynamic interaction. These interactions are complex and constantly changing. The challenge of future research is to characterize the complex patterns of change and stability in biopsychosocial functioning during middle age.

MIDLIFE INDIVIDUALS DESERVE BETTER HEALTH CARE

As in almost all areas of the life-span, adequate and appropriate health care is of critical importance. Unfortunately, for many individuals during midlife, their health care is sadly inadequate. With the exception of wealthy individuals, most Americans are unhappy with the quality and quantity of current health care systems. At midlife, changes in physical functioning raise the issue of continued optimum functioning. Particularly for women, contradictory and confusing recommendations for maintenance of optimal physical health is currently the norm. In addition, the current system of "managed care" is perceived by many to be a system designed to deny care. Finally, in this era of "reform" of government programs, many individuals have no access to health care at all. Midlife individuals deserve better health care.

In summary, development during midlife represents a potential period of rich interpersonal functioning, personal productivity, and psychological growth. Some individuals, however, experience developmental trajectories that are less than optimal. The goal for the future is to stimulate greater interest in all areas of biological, psychological, and social functioning during middle age. Both basic and applied research will increase our understanding of life in the middle.

Author Index

Subject Index